Neurodegenerative Processes: The Role of Sex Hormones

Neurodegenerative Processes: The Role of Sex Hormones

Editor: Luke Moore

MURPHY & MOORE
www.murphy-moorepublishing.com

www.murphy-moorepublishing.com

MURPHY & MOORE

Cataloging-in-Publication Data

Neurodegenerative processes : the role of sex hormones / edited by Luke Moore.
p. cm.
Includes bibliographical references and index.
ISBN 978-1-63987-383-8
1. Nervous system--Degeneration. 2. Hormones, Sex. 3. Neurohormones. 4. Neurosciences. 5. Neurology. I. Moore, Luke.
RC365 .N48 2021
616.804 7--dc23

Murphy & Moore Publishing,
1 Rockefeller Plaza,
New York City, NY 10020, USA

ISBN 978-1-63987-383-8 (Hardback)

Contents

Preface

Over the recent decade, advancements and applications have progressed exponentially. This has led to the increased interest in this field and projects are being conducted to enhance knowledge. The main objective of this book is to present some of the critical challenges and provide insights into possible solutions. This book will answer the varied questions that arise in the field and also provide an increased scope for furthering studies.

Neurodegenerative diseases are a class of diseases in which the neurons of the brain are affected. They are generally incurable since the neurons in the brain do not reproduce in most cases. Therefore, damaged neurons cannot be replaced by the body. A few of the common neurodegenerative diseases are Parkinson's, Huntington's and Alzheimer's disease. Studies have shown that there is a connection between the progression of a few particular types of neurodegeneration and sex steroids. The effect of estrogens, through their action on cognate nuclear and membrane receptors, was shown to be neuroprotective in nature. The effect of male hormones on neuronal cells has been negative in some cases, whereas in other cases it exhibited neuroprotective behavior. This book contains some path-breaking studies in the research related to neurodegenerative processes. Also included herein is a detailed explanation of the role of sex hormones in neurodegenerative processes. Scientists and students actively engaged in this field will find this book full of crucial and unexplored concepts.

I hope that this book, with its visionary approach, will be a valuable addition and will promote interest among readers. Each of the authors has provided their extraordinary competence in their specific fields by providing different perspectives as they come from diverse nations and regions. I thank them for their contributions.

Editor

1

Cellular and Molecular Mechanisms of the Effects of Sex Hormones on the Nervous System

Slavi Delchev and Katerina Georgieva

Abstract

The mechanisms of the action of sex steroid hormones on the nervous system are related to both classical, intracellularly mediated effects and non-classical membrane effects due to binding to membrane receptors. Some steroids are capable of inducing rapid neu rotransmitter-like effects, similar to those of dopamine or glutamate that alter the activity of neuronal systems via different types of receptors. The neuroactive steroids are endogenous neuromodulators synthesized in the brain and rapidly affecting neuronal excitability. Sex steroids exert many pleiotropic effects in the nervous system: they modulate main neurotransmitter systems, promote the viability of neurons, play an important role in myelination, and influence cognitive processes. Estradiol protects neurons from excitotoxic damage and increases neuronal survival. Progesterone stimulates neurological and functional recovery. Androgens also exhibit a wide array of neuroprotective effects in motoneurons, including supporting cell survival, axonal regeneration, and dendritic maintenance. Despite the considerable increase of sex hormones and neurosteroids research in recent years and the ongoing discovery of biochemical mechanisms of action, their role in neurodegenerative processes remains not well determined.

Keywords: sex hormones, neurosteroids, genomic effects, non-genomic effects, neuroprotection, neurodegenerative diseases

1. Introduction

Sex hormones are synthesized from cholesterol mainly in the gonads and adrenal cortex. In the brain, different sex steroids can also be further metabolized to different neurosteroids or be produced anew in neurons and glial cells, with an even more potent effect on the nervous system. The mechanisms of action of the sex steroid hormones on the brain are related to both classical, intracellularly mediated effects and non-classical (non-genomic) membrane effects due to their binding to membrane receptors. Some steroids are capable of inducing rapid neurotransmitter-like effects. Sex steroids exert diverse pleiotropic effects on the nervous system: they modulate major neurotransmitter systems, promote the viability of neurons, play an important role in myelination, and influence cognitive processes. Estradiol increases neuronal survival and recovery. It protects neurons from excitotoxic damage, amyloid β (Aβ) toxicity, oxidative stress, and glucose deprivation. The defense induced by estrogens is mediated by complex mechanisms. Progestins have also been found to exert neuroprotective effects similar to those of estrogens. Androgens exhibit a wide range of neuroprotective effects in motoneurons, including supporting cell survival, axonal regeneration, and dendritic maintenance. The relationship between sex steroids and the brain-derived neurotrophic factor (BDNF) has garnered a growing interest due to the role BDNF plays in the pathogenesis of neurodegenerative diseases.

2. Steroidogenesis

Sex hormones are steroid compounds synthesized from cholesterol mainly in the testes, ovaries, and adrenal cortex. The male sex hormones (androgens) and female sex hormones (estrogens and gestagens) have a common biosynthetic pathway (**Figure 1**).

The final product of the steroidogenesis of sex hormones depends on whether or not specific metabolizing enzymes are available in the respective cell [1]. The sex steroids in human blood include androgens (testosterone, dehydroepiandrosterone (DHEA), dehydroepiandrosterone sulfate (DHEAS), androstenedione, and dihydrotestosterone), estrogens (estradiol, estriol, and estrone), and gestagens (progesterone and 17α-hydroxyprogesterone). The major male hormone, testosterone, is produced by the Leydig cells in the testes. Dihydrotestosterone (DHT) is a potent androgen, derived from testosterone by the enzyme 5α-reductase (type 1 and type 2) in some peripheral tissues, mediating some testosterone-induced effects. This enzyme is expressed in the skin, scalp, prostate, epididymis, liver, and nervous system (neocortex, subcortical white matter, and hippocampal tissues) [2]. DHEA, DHEAS, and androstenedione are secreted mainly by the adrenal cortex in the same amounts in both sexes. DHEA and androstenedione are steroids involved in the sex hormones' biosynthesis pathway; both are primary endogenous precursors of testosterone and estrogens. Although they are weak androgens, they are circulating steroids that can be converted into active androgens and estrogens in the peripheral tissues [1, 3].

Estrogens are produced by aromatization of androgens, including those derived from adrenal steroidogenesis. Although the ovaries produce large amounts of androgens, they secrete little of these into the blood, while the rest are aromatized to estradiol, which is the major estrogen. The theca cells in the ovaries synthesize testosterone and androstenedione, which then diffuse into the granulosa cells of the follicles. There androstenedione is converted into testosterone, which in turn is aromatized to estradiol that enters the blood stream. A portion of the androstenedione is aromatized to estrone, which in turn is converted into estradiol. Androgen aromatization is realized under the influence of the enzyme aromatase, which is

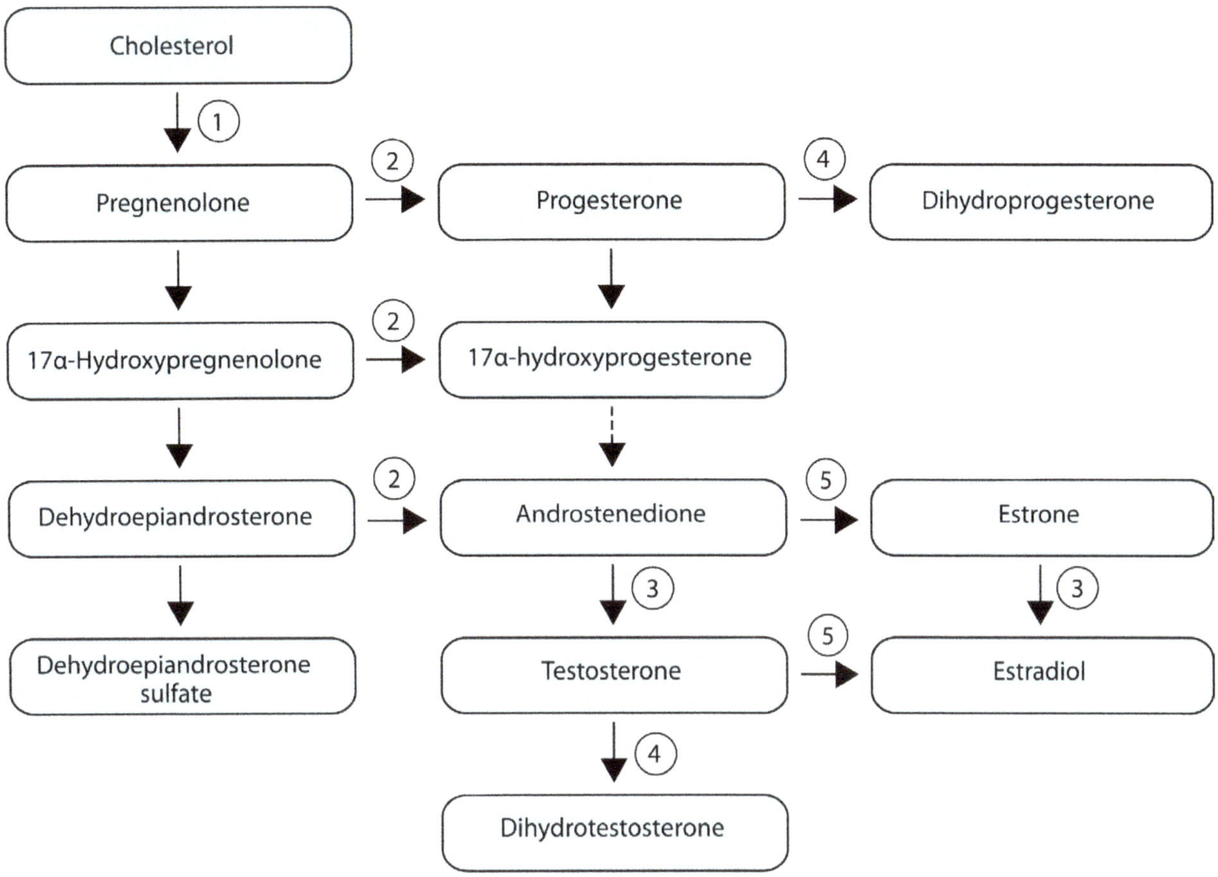

Figure 1. Sex steroid biosynthesis pathway. Enzymes are shown as follows: (1) P450 side-chain cleavage enzyme; (2) 3β-hydroxysteroid dehydrogenase; (3) 17β-hydroxysteroid dehydrogenase; (4) 5α-reductase; (5) aromatase. The dashed arrow indicates poor flux. Not all intermediate steroids, pathways, and enzymes are included (modified from Refs. [1, 55]).

expressed in steroidogenic tissues, the brain, and nonsteroidogenic tissues, especially fat and bone. Progesterone is the major progestogen and is produced in both theca and granulosa cells, the adrenal gland, and testes [1, 3].

The neuroactive steroids are brain-synthesized endogenous neuromodulators that rapidly alter neuronal excitability. Some of them reach the brain from adrenals and gonads and are further metabolized locally just like the aromatization of testosterone into estradiol [4]. They have been referred to as neurosteroids as they can be derived anew from cholesterol in neurons and the glial cells [5]. The synthesis of neuroactive steroids requires the translocation of cholesterol across the mitochondrial membrane [6]. This process occurs through a molecular complex formed by the translocator protein 18 kDa (TSPO), the steroidogenic acute regulatory protein (StAR), the voltage-dependent anion channel protein (VDAC), and the adenine nucleotide transporter protein (ANT).

In the mitochondria, cholesterol is converted into pregnenolone by the P450 side-chain cleavage enzyme (P450scc). Soluble pregnenolone diffuses into the cytosol (the endoplasmic reticulum) where it is further metabolized into various neuroactive steroids such as progesterone,

5α-dihydroprogesterone, DHEA, androstenedione, etc. The enzyme 3β-hydroxysteroid dehydrogenase, required for further conversion of pregnenolone into progesterone, has been found in the brain [7]. The enzyme 17β-hydroxysteroid dehydrogenase type 10 catalyzes the oxidation of neuroactive steroids in mitochondria with NAD^+ as the coenzyme. This enzyme catalyzes most effectively the oxidation of allopregnanolone and allotetrahydrodeoxycorticosterone, which is essential for the homeostasis of these neuroactive steroids [8].

Although TSPO is highly expressed in microglia and astrocytes and is less abundant in neurons, neurosteroidogenesis occurs primarily in principal neurons of several brain areas that have the necessary set of enzymes to convert cholesterol into neuroactive steroids [9].

3. Mechanisms of action

The first thing a hormone does is to bind to specific receptors on the target cell. Cells without receptors for the hormone do not respond to the action. The receptors for certain hormones are localized on the cell membrane, while others are located in the cytoplasm or nucleus. After binding to the specific receptor, the hormone triggers a cascade of cellular responses that become increasingly potent with each successive stage. Thus even small concentrations of the hormone can produce a significant effect [3].

3.1. Genomic action via steroid receptors

According to the classic genomic theory of action, sex hormones as steroid hormones bind preferentially to specific protein receptors within the cell rather than to receptors located on the cell membrane. These hormones are fat-soluble and can easily pass through the cell membrane and bind to specific receptors in the cytoplasm. Depending on the steroid and tissue, however, unbound steroid receptors may be located in the nucleus as well. The particular distribution of the receptor between the cytoplasm and nucleus varies. When the cytoplasmic receptors bind to their specific steroid hormone ligands, they translocate to the nucleus. Depending on their mechanism of action and subcellular distribution, nuclear receptors may be classified into at least two groups [10]. Nuclear receptors that bind to steroid hormones are all classified as type I receptors. Only type I receptors have a heat shock protein (HSP) associated with the inactive receptor that will be released when the receptor interacts with the ligand. Type II nuclear receptors have no HSP and in contrast to the classical type I receptor are located in the cell nucleus. The activated hormone-receptor protein complexes then bind to a specific regulatory section of DNA, called hormone response element, by activating or inhibiting the transcription of specific genes and the formation of messenger RNA. Later on, after an extended period of time (usually from a few hours to a few days) counted from the entry of the hormone into the cell, new proteins develop in the cell and alter the cell functions.

The complexity of the steroid action can be accounted for by the abundance of identified steroid receptors and their affinity for the hormone. The excess/deficiency of the respective sex steroid regulates the number of the active receptors (downregulation/upregulation) in the target cells. Testosterone and DHT exert their functions via binding to the androgen receptor

(AR), resulting in conformational change of the receptor and translocation of the androgen/AR complex from the cytosol to the nucleus. Various AR coregulators can further modulate the transcriptional regulation of target genes [11]. AR receptors are expressed in neurons and glial cells and their expression can be regulated by injury and by circulating testosterone concentration [12–14]. AR mRNA is downregulated post-orchidectomy and after axotomy [12]. AR levels also decrease with aging, especially in the nucleus basalis of Meynert (which degenerates in Alzheimer's disease (AD)) and the diagonal band of Broca [15].

The estrogen receptor-α (ERα) was characterized as an intracellular, ligand-regulated transcription factor located primarily in the nucleus [16]. Once bound to estradiol, ERα dimers were shown to regulate gene expression via interaction with estrogen response elements. Following a series of discoveries, a structurally related estrogen receptor-β (ERβ) was identified [17]. Sites of estrogen receptor expression identified in the brain comprised the hypothalamus, pituitary, and preoptic area, among others, which, based on a series of lesion and stimulation studies, were known to affect physiology and behavior related to endocrine function [18]. Apart from the great number of various isoforms, the classic intracellular receptors have also many splice variants that have been studied and characterized. For example, for estrogens besides the ERα and ERβ isoforms, multiple splice variants (e.g., ER$\alpha\Delta4$) can initiate signaling from the membrane [19]. Experiments demonstrated that the same protein is capable of mediating both intracellular and membrane actions of estradiol. For progesterone, a whole new class of progesterone receptors (PRs) has been identified—the membrane PRs localized on the membrane and involved in the reproductive actions of progesterone [20].

3.2. Non-genomic action

The classic genomic mechanism of the action of steroid hormones alone cannot account for all subsequent changes in the target cells; hence, it has been updated to include an additional (non-classic) explanation of the rapid, non-genomic, membrane-initiated action. For decades, steroid hormones have been known to induce acute changes (within minutes) in the physiological functions [21], neuronal activity [22], and behavior [23].

Recent research demonstrated that steroids can function in a "neurotransmitter-like" way, being synthesized at precise spatial locations within neural circuits in the brain and acting within minutes as local neuromodulators that rapidly regulate cognitive functions and behavior [24–27].

Some steroids, such as progesterone, are capable of inducing rapid neurotransmitter-like effects, similar to those of dopamine or glutamate, which alter the activity of neuronal systems via multiple types of receptors [19, 25, 28]. Some of these steroid receptors have been classified as extranuclear or membrane receptors, which signal through G-proteins or other second messenger systems [29, 30]. There is recent evidence of these classical steroid receptors binding to response elements on DNA to regulate gene expression, showing that they contain palmitoylation sequences allowing them to be trafficked to the plasma membrane to quickly alter cellular activity [19, 31]. After being trafficked, these nuclear transcription factors interact with other proteins to initiate their signaling at the level of the plasma membrane. From here, intracellular signaling cascades involving effectors (e.g., the mitogen-activated protein kinase (MAPK) and cAMP response element binding protein (CREB)) are initiated via the transactivation of cell surface–bound receptors, most notably the metabotropic glutamate receptors (mGluRs). Subsequently, estrogen membrane–initiated signaling can in turn activate the regulatory section of DNA and trigger transcription processes.

The modern understanding of a cell response to a steroid action is that it occurs within the same time frame as that of the G protein–coupled receptors influencing a variety of cellular functions such as gating membrane channels, increasing the intracellular calcium release, activating tyrosine-protein kinase (Src), MAPK, and others [27]. Many studies support a model of integrated signaling that couples signal transduction cascades to transcription in the nucleus, providing an integrated view of hormone signaling in the brain [32].

Recently, extensive research focused on the rapid, non-genomic action of estrogens has raised the question of how rapidly the increase of these steroids can occur in the brain. Of course, estrogens, just like any other steroids, cannot be stored in synaptic vesicles prior to their rapid release, due to their lipophilic nature [4]. It has been suggested, therefore, that the rapid effects of estrogens require a corresponding rapid change of local steroid concentration via rapid changes in their rate of synthesis by androgen conversion [24, 33], which implies changes in aromatase activity. Changes of aromatase activity reflect changes in aromatase protein concentrations. For instance, sex steroids control the hypothalamic aromatase expression in most vertebrates: weak aromatase expression is detected in castrated male animals, while testosterone replacement increases significantly aromatase protein and enzyme activity [34, 35]. There is strong evidence suggesting that aromatase activity can be rapidly modulated via translational modifications, most notably via phosphorylation. The rapid modulation of aromatase activity by phosphorylation is a widespread mechanism present in certain tissues of various species, including humans [4]. The enzymatic changes lead to a rapid local modulation of estrogen availability and consequently to a modification of cellular estrogen-dependent processes that are not mediated by the genomic actions of these steroids. The phosphorylation/dephosphorylation processes provide a new widespread mechanism by which estrogen concentration could be rapidly altered in the brain and other tissues.

Although most of the research on neurotransmitter-like actions of steroid hormones is focused on sex hormones and reproduction, other steroids also induce effects through non-classic mechanisms. As with estrogens and progestins, glucocorticoids can act on the membrane to alter physiology, functioning more like neurotransmitters than classical steroid hormones.

Neurosteroids are also capable of interacting with cell surface neurotransmitter receptors to modulate neural cell physiology. Two of the endogenous neurosteroids, pregnenolone sulfate and pregnanolone sulfate, can potentiate or inhibit N-methyl-D-aspartate (NMDA) receptor responses [36]. $GABA_A$ receptors represent one of the most elaborate neurotransmitter receptor structures, harboring multiple binding sites for allosteric modulators, neuroactive compounds, and neuroactive steroids [37]. Allopregnanolone has been shown to promote neurogenesis in both rodent and human neuroprogenitor cells, most likely through binding to the $GABA_A$ receptor [38]. The modulation of the activity of receptors by neurochemicals such as allopregnanolone has been extensively studied in the context of neurodegenerative disorders [39].

Another mechanism of steroid action takes effect at the level of the microtubules via a proposed receptor microtubule-associated protein of type 2 (MAP2) [40]. Neuronal microtubules play an important role in the growth and maintenance of neurites during neuronal differentiation. They are composed of tubulin and microtubule-associated proteins (MAPs). MAPs determine neuronal shape and control the balance between rigidity and plasticity in neuronal processes. Neurosteroids may be involved in the formation and stabilization of microtubules and thus neuronal plasticity and function [40]. Experimental data demonstrate that progesterone treatment attenuated the injury-induced loss of MAP2 [41].

4. Biological effects of sex hormones on the nervous system

Testosterone and its metabolite estradiol induce numerous effects during critical periods of pre- and perinatal brain developments (organizational effects) that are necessary for brain sexual differentiation. Testosterone exposure is an essential requirement for masculinization of the brain. Nuclear volume, neuronal morphology, and astrocyte complexity are examples of the wide range of effects by which testosterone and estradiol can induce permanent changes in the function of neurons [42]. In the developing male rat, testosterone secreted from the testes is not bound by α-fetoprotein and freely enters the brain where it is locally converted into estradiol in specific nuclei. Consequently, neonatal males have more than double the levels of estradiol than females in brain regions subject to sexual differentiation [43]. High levels of the ER are concentrated in the same brain regions and ER is essential for transducing the steroid signal [44]. The gain or loss of function upon developmental estradiol exposure corresponds to the specific cellular morphological changes observed during the critical period, and the dendritic spines and astrocytes seen in each brain region retain that "memory" of early steroid exposure [42].

4.1. Effects of female sex steroids

It is generally accepted that estrogen acts as a conditional neuroprotectant with a complex pattern of biological actions, which are modulated by several interacting factors [45]. It has been found that administration of estradiol increases neuronal survival and recovery in adult animals and different lesion models [46, 47]. Estradiol protects neurons from excitotoxic damage due to seizures and stroke, as well as in AD [48]. One of the suggested mechanisms of this effect is the ability of estrogens to enhance neuropeptide Y (NPY) expression and release, as NPY has antiexcitatory effects [49]. In vitro estradiol was found to protect neurons from glutamate toxicity and Aβ peptide toxicity, oxidative stress, and glucose deprivation [50–53]. The defense state induced by estrogen is mediated by complex mechanisms that converge upon regulation of mitochondrial function. Estrogen preserves ATP levels via increased oxidative phosphorylation and reduced ATPase activity, thereby increasing mitochondrial respiration efficiency. Estrogen increases antiapoptotic proteins, Bcl-2 and Bcl-xL, which prevent formation of the permeability transition pores protecting against estrogen-induced increase in mitochondrial Ca^{2+} sequestration and triggering of apoptotic processes [54]. Therefore, the decreased levels of estrogen could most likely contribute to the increased risk of developing neurodegenerative diseases, especially in postmenopausal women [52, 55].

It is suggested that in addition to having a direct effect on neurons, estrogens may affect the astrocytes by stimulating them to release protective growth factors and regulate the astrocytes genes and proteins associated with the glutamate level control. Other mechanisms implicated here may include the anti-inflammatory effect associated with suppression of microglia, inflammatory cytokines, and free radicals production, which cause inflammatory damage to the neurons, effects on endothelial cells realized by increasing the mitochondrial efficiency and stimulating angiogenesis, genomic influence on anti-apoptotic protein genes of Bcl family and reduction of apoptotic trends and effect of free radical scavenging. These are the hypothetical models of estrogen neuroprotection in cerebral ischemia and in other neurodegenerative disorders such as Parkinson's disease (PD) and AD [52, 56].

There is growing evidence that estrogen may have a neuroprotective role in PD. Experimental studies have demonstrated that estrogen is neuroprotective in 1-methyl-4-phenyl-1,2,3,6-tetrahydropyridine (MPTP)-induced nigrostriatal lesions, an animal model of idiopathic PD [57, 58]. In these and other studies, 17β-estradiol was used and its effect was shown to be stereospecific. An isomer with weak estrogenic activity, 17α-estradiol, was ineffective with regard to the prevention of MPTP-induced dopamine loss [52]. What is worthy of note is that the receptors ERα and ERβ are sparsely localized in the striatum and substantia nigra of mice, and treatment with MPTP or estrogen does not change the distribution and density of the estrogen receptor. Despite the low availability of ER in these parts of the brain, estrogen has managed to induce a protective effect on the striatum against MPTP-induced loss of dopaminergic neurons [59].

Studies in humans showed that short-term estrogen treatment in postmenopausal women increased dopamine transporter availability in the caudate putamen [60] and that women who had taken postmenopausal estrogen replacement therapy were less likely to develop PD than those who had not [61].

There is evidence of inducing differentiation of human neural stem cells, which develop in the tyrosine hydroxylase (dopaminergic) neurons, and the effect was blocked by application of an estrogen receptor antagonist [62, 63].

As it is supposed that oxidative stress plays an important role in the processes of neuronal degeneration in the PD, it is interesting that estrogens suppress free radical production and protect striatal neurons against oxidative stress, providing another mechanism of estrogen neuroprotection in PD [64, 65].

Recent studies in both animals and humans have provided additional evidence supporting a potentially beneficial protective role for estrogen in AD. The mechanisms of estrogen protection in AD are not clear. At the molecular level, estrogen has been shown to enhance activation of the survival factors, protein kinase B, BDNF [66, 67], while inducing phosphorylation and deactivation of glycogen synthase kinase (GSK3B) and Bcl-2 associated agonist of cell death (BAD), involved in death signaling pathways in neurons [67, 68].

Progestins have also been found to exert neuroprotective effects similar to those of estrogens. Progesterone stimulates the neurological and functional recovery after spinal and brain traumas [56, 69] and exerts neuroprotection in cerebral ischemia [70, 71].

4.2. Effects of androgens

The effects of androgens on the nervous system have been far less characterized than those produced by estrogens and progestins. Androgens also exhibit a wide array of neuroprotective effects in motoneurons, including supporting cell survival, axonal regeneration, and dendritic maintenance [72]. Testosterone influences neuroplastic changes in nuclei of the limbic system, particularly in the amygdala, bed nucleus of the stria terminalis, and the hippocampus [73, 74]; it exerts neuroprotective effects by stimulating neuron survival and regeneration after a nerve injury by actions mediated via the androgen receptor [75, 76]. It has been observed to have a protective effect on apoptosis in cell cultures of human neurons. This effect is mediated directly by androgen receptors, without testosterone aromatization to estradiol [77]. Testosterone replacement in gonadectomized male adult mice reverses the pathological changes in the spine morphology of hippocampal CA1 pyramidal neurons. The dendritic spines are specialized to receive synaptic inputs, and a change in spine morphology is correlated with the strength and maturity of each synapse [78]. Similar data were obtained in experimental motoneuron damage, with the use of DHT reducing the atrophy of adjacent dendrites [79]. Recent findings suggest that one of the mechanisms of the neuroprotective effects of physical training is the increased DHT production in the hippocampus providing evidence for androgenic mediation of neurogenesis by androgen receptors [80].

Androgens may regulate the production and the levels of Aβ, by a classic genomic mechanism and rapid non-genomic signaling or via aromatization to estradiol and activation of estrogen pathways [81, 82]. Testosterone can attenuate the toxicity of Aβ in cultured hippocampal neurons via a rapid, estrogen-independent mechanism [83]. DHT increases Aβ-catabolizing enzyme neprilysin in cultured neurons by an AR-dependent mechanism, which promotes Aβ degradation, thereby decreasing Aβ levels in AD [84].

4.3. Effects of steroid precursors

Precursors of estrogens, progestins, and androgens (pregnenolone and DHEA) also affect neuronal functions. When administered in vivo, pregnenolone reduces histopathological changes, protects neural tissues from secondary lesions, and promotes the recovery of motor functions after spinal cord injury [85, 86]. DHEA is one of the first neurosteroids identified in rat brains. Neuroprotective effects induced by DHEA and its sulfate DHEAS, defined as primary in their biological action, have been documented [87]. Both steroids contribute to the differentiation and survival of neurons in cell cultures [88]; have a protective effect on hippocampal neurons against the toxic effects of glutamate [89]; stimulate the growth of neuritis of the cortical neurons of embryonic rat brains [90]; affect apoptosis, catecholamine synthesis, and secretion; and have exhibited anti-oxidant, anti-inflammatory, and anti-glucocorticoid effects [87].

Studies suggest that these are different mechanisms for DHEA and DHEAS effects. It is assumed that DHEAS mediates its effects via $GABA_A$ receptors, probably by metabolizing DHEAS into a $GABA_A$ receptor agonist, such as androsterone or androstanediol [91]. The neuroprotective effect of DHEAS to NMDA receptor-induced cytotoxicity is probably mediated by the σ1 receptor, while DHEA inhibits NMDA-induced nitric oxide (NO) production and NO synthase activity by NMDA receptor, modulating calcium/NO signaling pathway [92]. Concentrations of DHEA and of its sulfate are also important with respect to the final effect. Low concentrations of these steroids may be neuroprotective, while high concentrations of DHEA are ineffective or neurotoxic and lead to the inhibition of complex I of the mitochondrial respiratory chain [93].

4.4. Interaction between steroids and neurotrophins

Recently, researchers have studied the relationship between the gonadal steroids, adrenal steroids, and BDNF focusing on intersexual differences and incidence of mental diseases [94]. BDNF belongs to the neurotrophin family and plays an important role in the survival, differentiation, and outgrowth of select peripheral and central neurons during development. BDNF impacts significantly on neuronal survival, acting in the adult brain through a variety of cell types, which include neurons, astrocytes, oligodendrocytes, microglia, and endothelial cells. It is essential for the process of learning and improvement of cognitive function via activation of the TrkB receptor [95]. Our previous data demonstrated that the negative effect of the anticonvulsant lacosamide on the processes of learning and memory is related to suppressed expression of BDNF/TrkB ligand receptor system in the hippocampus of rats [96]. Sex steroid hormones and neurotrophic factors are involved in the neuroendocrine control of reproduction as well as in brain adaptation during reproductive aging. There is a great body of evidence showing the role BDNF plays in the pathogenesis of neurodegenerative diseases. Low post-mortem parietal cortex BDNF levels have been found in patients with mild cognitive impairment [97] and AD [97, 98].

Research shows that BDNF mRNA and protein expression levels in the brain cognitive regions are affected in a region-specific manner when hormone replacement therapy is administered. BDNF mRNA levels have been reported to be significantly reduced in almost all hippocampal layers and the cortex in 28-week ovariectomized rats [99]. Estradiol replacement therapy reverses this effect in the hippocampus, suggesting a regional divergence in ovarian steroid requirements for BDNF expression. After gonadectomy, BDNF mRNA levels are significantly reduced at postnatal day 7 in male rat pups, but after treatment with estradiol benzoate, the levels were similar to those in intact animals. The authors demonstrated that ERα and BDNF were localized in the same cells (pyramidal cells of the CA3 sub-region and to a lesser extent in CA1) within the developing hippocampus [100].

Estrogens have been implicated in the increase of hippocampal BDNF mRNA and protein levels in exercising animals. The exercise effect on BDNF upregulation was reduced after 7 weeks of estrogen deprivation. Exercise in combination with long-term estrogen replacement increased the BDNF protein above the effects of estrogen replacement alone [101].

Androgens also have a bearing on the BDNF expression; some of their effects on the nervous system are most likely to be realized through influencing the production of this neurotrophin.

Testosterone administration was shown to increase BDNF protein levels in motoneurons of spinal nucleus of the bulbocavernosus of castrated male rats [102]. Gonadectomy induces a significant decrease in the protein levels of BDNF and its downstream target post-synaptic density protein 95 (PSD-95) in the hippocampal CA1 area, which is reversed by testosterone replacement [78]. Knowledge of the interactions between BDNF and sex steroids could be essential for the understanding of the BDNF role in brain development, adaptation during aging, and the pathogenesis of neurodegenerative diseases.

5. Conclusion

The functions of the sex hormones exceed the limits of reproduction in that they regulate vital neuronal and glial features. The chronic effects of neurosteroids are due to both genomic (classical intracellular steroid receptors) and non-genomic rapid effects (ion channels and membrane receptors) in the brain.

Some of the hypothetical models of estrogen neuroprotection include complex mechanisms, which converge upon regulation of mitochondria function–preserved ATP levels via increased oxidative phosphorylation and increased antiapoptotic proteins of Bcl family. Estrogen stimulates the astrocytes to release protective growth factors and has an anti-inflammatory effect associated with suppression of microglia and inflammatory cytokines. It suppresses free radical production and protects striatal neurons against oxidative stress, providing another mechanism for neuroprotection in PD. The female sex steroids promote cell survival via protein kinase B activation and BDNF upregulation; they inactivate GSK3B and BAD, involved in neuronal death signaling pathways in AD. The androgens also have neuroprotective effects in motoneurons, including supporting neuron survival, axonal regeneration, and dendritic maintenance. Testosterone can attenuate the toxicity of Aβ and decreases Aβ levels in AD.

Despite the growing amount of research on sex hormones and neurosteroids in recent years and the ongoing discovery of biochemical mechanisms of action, their role in neurodegenerative processes remains uncertain. Further elucidation of the cellular and molecular mechanisms responsible for the effects of neurosteroids on the normal function of neuronal and glial cells would provide important insights related to the development of new therapeutic strategies aimed at delaying the onset and slowing the progression of cognitive dysfunctions and neurodegenerative diseases.

Author details

Slavi Delchev[1]* and Katerina Georgieva[2]

*Address all correspondence to: sldel@abv.bg

1 Department of Anatomy, Histology and Embryology, Faculty of Medicine, Medical University – Plovdiv, Plovdiv, Bulgaria

2 Department of Physiology, Faculty of Medicine, Medical University – Plovdiv, Plovdiv, Bulgaria

References

[1] Miller WL, Auchus RJ. The molecular biology, biochemistry, and physiology of human steroidogenesis and its disorders. Endocrine Reviews. 2011;**32**:81-151

[2] Stoffel-Wagner B. Neuroactive steroid metabolism in the human brain. European Journal of Endocrinology. 2001;**145**:669-679

[3] Molina P. Endocrine Physiology. 4th ed. New York: McGraw-Hill Medical Companies; 2013. p. 1-13 129-162, 187-248

[4] Charlier TD, Cornil CA, Patte-Mensah C, Meyer L, Mensah-Nyagan AG, Balthazart J. Local modulation of steroid action: Rapid control of enzymatic activity. Frontiers in Neuroscience. 2015;**9**:83. DOI: 10.3389/fnins.2015.00083

[5] Baulieu EE. Neurosteroids: A novel function of the brain. Psychoneuroendocrinology. 1998;**23**(8):963-987

[6] Miller WL, Bose HS. Early steps in steroidogenesis: Intracellular cholesterol trafficking. Journal of Lipid Research. 2011;**52**:2111-2135

[7] Guennoun R, Fiddes RJ, Gouezou M, Lombes M, Baulieu EE. A key enzyme in the biosynthesis of neurosteroids, 3 beta-hydroxysteroid dehydrogenase/delta 5-delta 4-isomerase (3 beta-HSD), is expressed in rat brain. Brain Research. Molecular Brain Research. 1995; **30**:287-300

[8] Porcu P, Barron AM, Frye CA, Walf AA, Yang SY, He XY, Morrow AL, Panzica GC, Melcangi RC. Neurosteroidogenesis today: Novel targets for neuroactive steroid synthesis and action and their relevance for translational research. Journal of Neuroendocrinology. 2016;**28**(2):12351. DOI: 10.1111/jne.12351

[9] Agis-Balboa RC, Pinna G, Zhubi A, Maloku E, Veldic M, Costa E, Guidotti A. Characterization of brain neurons that express enzymes mediating neurosteroid biosynthesis. Proceedings of the National Academy of Sciences. 2006;**103**(39):14602-14607

[10] Novac N, Heinzel T. Nuclear receptors: Overview and classification. Current Drug Targets. Inflammation and Allergy. 2004;**3**(4):335-346

[11] Heemers HV, Tindall DJ. Androgen receptor (AR) coregulators: A diversity of functions converging on and regulating the AR transcriptional complex. Endocrine Reviews. 2007;**28**:778-808

[12] Drengler SM, Handa RJ, Jones KJ. Effects of axotomy and testosterone on androgen receptor mRNA expression in hamster facial motoneurons. Experimental Neurology. 1997;**146**:374-379

[13] Garcia-Ovejero D, Veiga S, Garcia-Segura LM. Doncarlos LL, Glial expression of estrogen and androgen receptors after rat brain injury. The Journal of Comparative Neurology. 2002;**450**:256-271

[14] Jones KJ, Coers S, Storer PD, Tanzer L, Kinderman NB. Androgenic regulation of the central glia response following nerve damage. Journal of Neurobiology. 1999;**40**:560-573

[15] Ishunina TA, Fisser B, Swaab DF. Sex differences in androgen receptor immunoreactivity in basal forebrain nuclei of elderly and Alzheimer patients. Experimental Neurology. 2002;**176**:122-132

[16] Welshons WV, Lieberman ME, Gorski J. Nuclear localization of unoccupied oestrogen receptors. Nature. 1984;**307**:747-749

[17] Kuiper GG, Enmark E, Pelto-Huikko M, Nilsson S, Gustafsson JA. Cloning of a novel receptor expressed in rat prostate and ovary. Proceedings of the National Academy of Sciences of the United States of America. 1996;**93**:5925-5930

[18] Pfaff DW, Schwartz-Giblin S, McCarthy MM, Kow LM. Cellular and molecular mechanisms of female reproductive behaviors. In: Neill JD, editor. Physiology of Reproduction. Amsterdam: Elsevier; 2006. p. 107-220

[19] Micevych PE, Mermelstein PG. Membrane estrogen receptors acting through metabotropic glutamate receptors: An emerging mechanism of estrogen action in brain. Molecular Neurobiology. 2008;**38**:66-77

[20] Zuloaga DG, Yahn SL, Pang Y, Quihuis AM, Oyola MG, Reyna A, Thomas P, Handa RJ, Mani SK. Distribution and estrogen regulation of membrane progesterone receptor-beta in the female rat brain. Endocrinology. 2012;**153**:4432-4443

[21] Szego CM, Davis JS. Adenosine 3,5-monophosphate in rat uterus: Acute elevation by estrogen. Proceedings of the National Academy of Sciences. 1967;**58**:1711-1718

[22] Kelly MJ, Moss RL, Dudley CA. Differential sensitivity of preopticseptal neurons to microelectrophoresed estrogen during the estrous cycle. Brain Research. 1976;**114**:152-157

[23] Ervin KS, Lymer JM, Matta R, Clipperton-Allen AE, Kavaliers M, Choleris E. Estrogen involvement in social behavior in rodents: Rapid and long-term actions. Hormones and Behavior. 2015;**74**:53-76

[24] Balthazart J, Ball GF. Is brain estradiol a hormone or a neurotransmitter? Trends in Neurosciences. 2006;**29**:241-249

[25] Saldanha CJ, Remage-Healey L, Schlinger BA. Synaptocrine signaling: Steroid synthesis and action at the synapse. Endocrine Reviews. 2011;**32**:532-549

[26] Remage-Healey L. Frank Beach Award winner: Steroids as neuromodulators of brain circuits and behavior. Hormones and Behavior. 2014;**66**:552-560

[27] Rudolph LM, Cornil CA, Mittelman-Smith MA, Rainville JR, Remage-Healey L, Sinchak K, Micevych PE. Actions of steroids: New neurotroansmitters. The Journal of Neuroscience. 2016;**36**(45):11449-11458

[28] Valadez-Cosmes P, Vazquez-Martínez ER, Cerbon M, Camacho-Arroyo I. Membrane progesterone receptors in reproduction and cancer. Molecular and Cellular Endocrinology. 2016;**434**:166-175

[29] Zhou Y, Watters JJ, Dorsa DM. Estrogen rapidly induces the phosphorylation of the cAMP response element binding protein in rat brain. Endocrinology. 1996;**137**:2163-2166

[30] Boulware MI, Weick JP, Becklund BR, Kuo SP, Groth RD, Mermelstein PG. Estradiol activates group I and II metabotropic glutamate receptor signaling, leading to opposing influences on cAMP response element-binding protein. The Journal of Neuroscience. 2005;**25**:5066-5078

[31] Schwartz N, Verma A, Bivens CB, Schwartz Z, Boyan BD. Rapid steroid hormone actions via membrane receptors. Biochimica et Biophysica Acta. 2016;**1863**:2289-2298

[32] Clark S, Rainville J, Zhao X. Estrogen receptor-mediated transcription involves the activation of multiple kinase pathways in neuroblastoma cells. The Journal of Steroid Biochemistry and Molecular Biology. 2014;**139**:45-53

[33] Cornil CA, Ball GF, Balthazart J. Functional significance of the rapid regulation of brain estrogen action: Where do the estrogens come from? Brain Research. 2006;**1126**:2-26

[34] Schumacher M, Balthazart J. Testosterone-induced brain aromatase is sexually dimorphic. Brain Research. 1986;**370**:285-293

[35] Fusani L, Hutchison JB, Gahr M. Testosterone regulates the activity and expression of aromatase in the canary neostriatum. Journal of Neurobiology. 2001;**49**:1-8

[36] Sedlácek M, Korínek M, Petrovic M, Cais O, Adamusová E, Chodounská H, Vyklický LJ. Neurosteroid modulation of ionotropic glutamate receptors and excitatory synaptic transmission. Physiological Research. 2008;**57**:S49-S57

[37] Hosie AM, Wilkins ME, Smart TG. Neurosteroid binding sites on GABA(A) receptors. Pharmacology & Therapeutics. 2007;**116**:7-19

[38] Wang JM, Johnston PB, Ball BG, Brinton RD. The neurosteroid allopregnanolone promotes proliferation of rodent and human neural progenitor cells and regulates cell-cycle gene and protein expression. The Journal of Neuroscience. 2005;**25**:4706-4718

[39] Lambert JJ, Belelli D, Peden DR, Vardy AW, Peters JA. Neurosteroid modulation of $GABA_A$ receptors. Progress in Neurobiology. 2003;**71**:67-80

[40] Plassart-Schiess E, Baulieu EE. Neurosteroids: Recent findings. Brain Research. Brain Research Reviews. 2001;**37**:133-140

[41] González SL, López-Costa JJ, Labombarda F, González Deniselle MC, Guennoun R, Schumacher M, De Nicola AF. Progesterone effects on neuronal ultrastructure and expression of microtubule-associated protein 2 (MAP2) in rats with acute spinal cord injury. Cellular and Molecular Neurobiology. 2009;**29**:27-39

[42] Schwarz JM, McCarthy MM. Steroid-induced sexual differentiation of the developing brain: Multiple pathways, one goal. Journal of Neurochemistry. 2008;**105**:1561-1572

[43] Amateau SK, Alt JJ, Stamps CL, McCarthy MM. Brain estradiol content in newborn rats: Sex differences, regional heterogeneity, and possible de novo synthesis by the female telencephalon. Endocrinology. 2004;**145**:2906-2917

[44] McCarthy MM, Schlenker EH, Pfaff DW. Enduring consequences of neonatal treatment with antisense oligodeoxynucleotides to estrogen receptor messenger ribonucleic acid on sexual differentiation of rat brain. Endocrinology. 1993;**133**:433-439

[45] Engler-Chiurazzi EB, Singh M, Simpkins JW. From the 90's to now: A brief historical perspective on more than two decades of estrogen neuroprotection. Brain Research. 2016;**1633**:96-100

[46] Wise PM, Dubal DB, Wilson ME, Rau SW. Estradiol is a neuroprotective factor in in vivo and in vitro models of brain injury. Journal of Neurocytology. 2000;**29**:401-410

[47] Garcia-Segura LM, Azcoitia I, Doncarlos LL. Neuroprotection by estradiol. Progress in Neurobiology. 2001;**63**:29-60

[48] Hara Y, Waters EM, McEwen BS, Morrison JH. Estrogen effects on cognitive and synaptic health over the lifecourse. Physiological Reviews. 2015;**95**(3):785-807

[49] Ledoux VA, Smejkalova T, May RM, Cooke BM, Woolley CS. Estradiol facilitates the release of neuropeptide Y to suppress hippocampus-dependent seizures. The Journal of Neuroscience. 2009;**29**(5):1457-1468

[50] Green PS, Perez EJ, Calloway T, Simpkins JW. Estradiol attenuation of beta-amyloid-induced toxicity: A comparison of MTT and calcein AM assays. Journal of Neurocytology. 2000;**29**:419-423

[51] Zhang L, Rubinow DR, Xaing G, Li BS, Chang YH, Maric D, Barker JL, Ma W. Estrogen protects against beta-amyloid-induced neurotoxicity in rat hippocampal neurons by activation of Akt. Neuroreport. 2001;**12**:1919-1923

[52] Brann DW, Dhandapani K, Wakade C, Mahesh VB, Khan MM. Neurotrophic and neuroprotective actions of estrogen: Basic mechanisms and clinical implications. Steroids. 2007;**72**(5):381-405

[53] Nixon E, Simpkins JW. Neuroprotective effects of nonfeminizing estrogens in retinal photoreceptor neurons. Investigative Ophthalmology & Visual Science. 2012;**53**(8):4739-4747

[54] Nilsen J, Brinton RD. Mitochondria as therapeutic targets of estrogen action in the central nervous system. Current Drug Targets. CNS and Neurological Disorders. 2004;**3**(4): 297-313

[55] Schumacher M, Weill-Engerer S, Liere P, Robert F, Franklin RJ, Garcia-Segura LM, Lambert JJ, Mayo W, Melcangi RC, Parducz A, Suter U, Carelli C, Baulieu EE, Akwa Y. Steroid hormones and neurosteroids in normal and pathological aging of the nervous system. Progress in Neurobiology. 2003;**71**(1):3-29

[56] Brotfain E, Gruenbaum SE, Boyko M, Kutz R, Zlotnik A, Klein M. Neuroprotection by estrogen and progesterone in traumatic brain injury and spinal cord injury. Current Neuropharmacology. 2016;**14**(6):641-653

[57] Callier S, Morissette M, Grandbois M, Pélaprat D, Di Paolo T. Neuroprotective properties of 17beta-estrogen, progesterone, and raloxifene in MPTP C57Bl/6 mice. Synapse. 2001;**41**:131-138

[58] Ramirez AD, Liu X, Menniti FS. Repeated estradiol treatment prevents MPTP-induced dopamine depletion in male mice. Neuroendocrinology. 2003;**77**:223-231

[59] Shughrue PJ. Estrogen attenuates the MPTP-induced loss of dopamine neurons from the mouse SNc despite a lack of estrogen receptors (ERalpha and ERbeta). Experimental Neurology. 2004;**190**:468-477

[60] Gardiner SA, Morrison MF, Mozley PD, Mozley LH, Brensinger C, Bilker W, Newberg A, Battistini M. Pilot study on the effect of estrogen replacement therapy on brain dopamine transporter availability in healthy, postmenopausal women. The American Journal of Geriatric Psychiatry. 2004;**12**:621-630

[61] Currie LJ, Harrison MB, Trugman JM, Bennett JP, Wooten GF. Postmenopausal estrogen use affects risk for Parkinson disease. Archives of Neurology. 2004;**61**:886-888

[62] Kishi Y, Takahashi J, Koyanagi M, Morizane A, Okamoto Y, Horiguchi S, Tashiro K, Honjo T, Fujii S, Hashimoto N. Estrogen promotes differentiation and survival of dopaminergic neurons derived from human neural stem cells. Journal of Neuroscience Research. 2005;**79**:279-286

[63] Díaz NF, Díaz-Martínez NE, Camacho-Arroyo I, Velasco I. Estradiol promotes proliferation of dopaminergic precursors resulting in a higher proportion of dopamine neurons derived from mouse embryonic stem cells. International Journal of Developmental Neuroscience. 2009;**27**(5):493-500

[64] Wallace DR, Dodson S, Nath A, Booze RM. Estrogen attenuates gp120- and tat1-72-induced oxidative stress and prevents loss of dopamine transporter function. Synapse. 2006;**59**:51-60

[65] Dye RV, Miller KJ, Singer EJ, Levine AJ. Hormone replacement therapy and risk for neurodegenerative diseases. International Journal of Alzheimer's Disease. 2012;**2012**:258454. DOI: 10.1155/2012/258454

[66] Singh M. Ovarian hormones elicit phosphorylation of Akt and extracellular-signal regulated kinase in explants of the cerebral cortex. Endocrine. 2001;**14**(3):407-415

[67] Ishrat T, Sayeed I, Atif F, Hua F, Stein DG. Progesterone is neuroprotective against ischemic brain injury through its effects on the phosphoinositide 3-kinase/protein kinase B signaling pathway. Neuroscience. 2012;**210**:442-450

[68] Goodenough S, Schleusner D, Pietrzik C, Skutella T, Behl C. Glycogen synthase kinase 3beta links neuroprotection by 17beta-estrogen to key Alzheimer processes. Neuroscience. 2005;**132**:581-589

[69] Thomas AJ, Nockels RP, Pan HQ, Shaffrey CI, Chopp M. Progesteron is neuroprotective after acute experimental spinal cord trauma in rats. Spine. 1999;**24**:2134-2138

[70] Jiang N, Chopp M, Stein DG, Feldblum S. Progesterone is neuroprotective after transient middle cerebral artery occlusion in male rats. Brain Research. 1996;**735**:101-107

[71] Wali B, Ishrat T, Stein DG, Sayeed I. Progesterone improves long-term functional and histological outcomes after permanent stroke in older rats. Behavioural Brain Research. 2016;**305**:46-56

[72] Little CM, Coons KD, Sengelaub DR. Neuroprotective effects of testosterone on the morphology and function of somatic motoneurons following the death of neighbouring motoneurons. The Journal of Comparative Neurology. 2009;**20**:359-372

[73] De Vries GJ, Wang Z, Bullock NA, Numan S. Sex differences in the effects of testosterone and its metabolites on vasopressin messenger RNA levels in the bed nucleus of the stria terminalis of rats. The Journal of Neuroscience. 1994;**14**:1789-1794

[74] McHenry J, Carrier N, Hull E, Kabbaj M. Sex differences in anxiety and depression: Role of testosterone. Frontiers in Neuroendocrinology. 2014;**35**(1):42-57

[75] Tanzer L, Jones KJ. Gonadal steroid regulation of hamster facial nerve regeneration: Effects of dihydrotestosterone and estradiol. Experimental Neurology. 1997;**146**:258-264

[76] Jones KJ, Brown TJ, Damaser M. Neuroprotective effects of gonadal steroids on regenerating peripheral motoneurons. Brain Research Reviews. 2001;**37**:372-382

[77] Hammond J, Le Q, Goodyer C, Gelfand M, Trifiro M, LeBlanc A. Testosterone-mediated neuroprotection through the androgen receptor in human primary neurons. Journal of Neurochemistry. 2001;**77**:1319-1326

[78] Li M, Masugi-Tokita M, Takanami K, Yamada S, Kawata M. Testosterone has sublayer-specific effects on dendritic spine maturation mediated by BDNF and PSD-95 in pyramidal neurons in the hippocampus CA1 area. Brain Research. 2012;**1484**:76-84

[79] Cai Y, Chew C, Muñoz F, Sengelaub DR. Neuroprotective effects of testosterone metabolites and dependency on receptor action on the morphology of somatic motoneurons following the death of neighboring motoneurons. Developmental Neurobiology. 2016;**29**. DOI: 10.1002/dneu.22445

[80] Okamoto M, Hojo Y, Inoue K, Matsui T, Kawato S, McEwen BS, Soya H. Mild exercise increases dihydrotestosterone in hippocampus providing evidence for androgenic mediation of neurogenesis. Proceedings of the National Academy of Sciences of the United States of America. 2012;**109**(32):13100-13105

[81] Pike CJ, Carroll JC, Rosario ER, Barron AM. Protective actions of sex steroid hormones in Alzheimer's disease. Frontiers in Neuroendocrinology. 2009;**30**(2):239-258

[82] Bates KA, Harvey AR, Carruthers M, Martins RN. Androgens, andropause and neurodegeneration: Exploring the link between steroidogenesis, androgens and Alzheimer's disease. Cellular and Molecular Life Sciences. 2005;**62**(3):281-292

[83] Pike CJ, Nguyen TV, Ramsden M, Yao M, Murphy MP, Rosario ER. Androgen cell signaling pathways involved in neuroprotective actions. Hormones and Behavior. 2008;**53**(5): 693-705

[84] Pike CJ. Testosterone attenuates beta-amyloid toxicity in cultured hippocampal neurons. Brain Research. 2001;**919**:160-165

[85] Guth L, Zhang Z, Roberts E. Key role for pregnenolone in combination therapy promotes recovery after spinal cord injury. Proceedings of the National Academy of Sciences of the United States of America. 1994;**91**:12308-12312

[86] Popovich PG, Tovar CA, Wei P, Fisher L, Jakeman LB, Basso DM. A reassessment of a classic neuroprotective combination therapy for spinal cord injured rats: LPS/pregnenolone/indomethacin. Experimental Neurology. 2012;**233**(2):677-685

[87] Maninger N, Wolkowitz OM, Reus V, Epel ES, Mellon SH. Neurobiological and neuropsychiatric effects of dehydroepiandrosterone (DHEA) and DHEA sulfate (DHEAS). Frontiers in Neuroendocrinology. 2009;**30**(1):65-91

[88] Bologa L, Sharma J, Roberts E. Dehydroepiandrosterone and its sulfated derivative reduce neuronal death and enhance astrocytic differentiation in brain cell cultures. Journal of Neuroscience Research. 1987;**17**:225-234

[89] Cardounel A, Regelson W, Kalimi M. Dehydroepiandrosterone protects hippocampal neurons against neurotoxin-induced cell death: Mechanism of action. Soc. Experimental Biology and Medicine. 1999;**222**:145-149

[90] Compagnone NA, Mellon SH. Dehydroepiandrosterone: A potential signalling molecule for neocortical organization during development. Proceedings of the National Academy of Sciences of the United States of America. 1998;**95**:4678-4683

[91] Lapchak PA, Chapman DF, Nunez SY, Zivin JA. Dehydroepiandrosterone sulfate is neuroprotective in a reversible spinal cord ischemia model: Possible involvement of GABA(A) receptors. Stroke. 2000;**31**:1953-1956

[92] Kurata K, Takebayashi M, Morinobu S, Yamawaki S. beta-estradiol, dehydroepiandrosterone, and dehydroepiandrosterone sulfate protect against N-methyl-daspartate-induced neurotoxicity in rat hippocampal neurons by different mechanisms. The Journal of Pharmacology and Experimental Therapeutics. 2004;**311**:237-245

[93] Safiulina D, Peet N, Seppet E, Zharkovsky A, Kaasik A. Dehydroepiandrosterone inhibits complex I of the mitochondrial respiratory chain and is neurotoxic in vitro and in vivo at high concentrations. Toxicological Sciences. 2006;**93**:348-356

[94] Pluchino N, Russo M, Santoro AN, Litta P, Cela V, Genazzani AR. Steroid hormones and BDNF. Neuroscience. 2013;**239**:271-279

[95] Sohrabji F, Lewis DK. Estrogen-BDNF interactions: Implications for neurodegenerative diseases. Frontiers in Neuroendocrinology. 2006;**27**:404-414

[96] Shishmanova M, Koeva Y, Peychev L, Georgieva K. Suspected role of BDNF in the suppressive effects of lacosamide on cognitive functions in rats. Eur Neurophychopharmacol. 2016;**26**:S245-S246

[97] Peng S, Wuu J, Mufson EJ, Fahnestock M. Precursor form of brain derived neurotrophic factor and mature brain-derived neurotrophic factor are decreased in the pre-clinical stages of Alzheimer's disease. Journal of Neurochemistry. 2005;**93**:1412-1421

[98] Michalski B, Fahnestock M. Pro-brain-derived neurotrophic factor is decreased in parietal cortex in Alzheimer's disease. Brain Research. Molecular Brain Research. 2003;**111**: 148-154

[99] Singh M, Meyer EM, Simpkins JW. The effect of ovariectomy and estradiol replacement on brain-derived neurotrophic factor messenger ribonucleic acid expression in cortical and hippocampal brain regions of female Sprague-Dawley rats. Endocrinology. 1995;**136**:2320-2324

[100] Solum DT, Handa RJ. Estrogen regulates the development of brain-derived neurotrophic factor mRNA and protein in the rat hippocampus. The Journal of Neuroscience. 2002;**22**(7):2650-2659

[101] Berchtold NC, Kesslak JP, Pike CJ, Adlard PA, Cotman CW. Estrogen and exercise interact to regulate brain-derived neurotrophic factor mRNA and protein expression in the hippocampus. The European Journal of Neuroscience. 2001;**14**:1992-2002

[102] Verhovshek T, Cai Y, Osborne MC, Sengelaub DR. Androgen regulates brain derived neurotrophic factor in spinal motoneurons and their target musculature. Endocrinology. 2010;**151**:253-261

2

17β-Estradiol as a Neuroprotective Agent

Katalin Prokai-Tatrai and Laszlo Prokai

Abstract

The pathophysiology of neurodegeneration in the central nervous system is complex and multifactorial in nature and yet to be fully understood. Broad-spectrum neuro protective agents with multiple mechanisms of action rather than a single druggable target are, therefore, highly desirable. The main human estrogen, 17β-estradiol, can also be considered a neurosteroid as it forms de novo in the central nervous system, and it possesses beneficial effects against practically all critical contributors to neu rodegeneration to collectively thwart both the initiation and the progression of neu ronal cell death. This chapter details the main aspects of the hormone's genomic and non-genomic actions important to protect the highly vulnerably neurons of the central nervous system, as well as translational efforts to successfully realize its powerful neu roprotective potential in clinical setting while ensuring both therapeutic safety and efficacy.

Keywords: antioxidant, brain, bioprecursor prodrug, broad-spectrum neuroprotectant, brain-selective estrogen therapy, cell death, 10β,17β-dihydroxyestra-1,4-dien-3-one (DHED), estrogens, genomic and non-genomic estrogenic actions, neuroprotection, *para*-quinol, Prokai antioxidant cycle, stroke, translational research

1. Introduction

The steroid hormone 17β-estradiol (E2, **Figure 1**) is the main human estrogen that is not only involved in sexual maturation and reproduction but also has a myriad of important roles throughout the body affecting, for example, the cardiovascular system, lipid metabolism and brain health [1–4]. Therefore, E2 cannot only be considered as just a "female hormone." In humans, the other two endogenously formed estrogens are estrone (E1, **Figure 1**) and the lesser-known estriol (E3, **Figure 1**) that is the 16-hydroxy derivate of E2 and formed mostly during gestation by the placenta. E1 becomes the predominant estrogen in women after

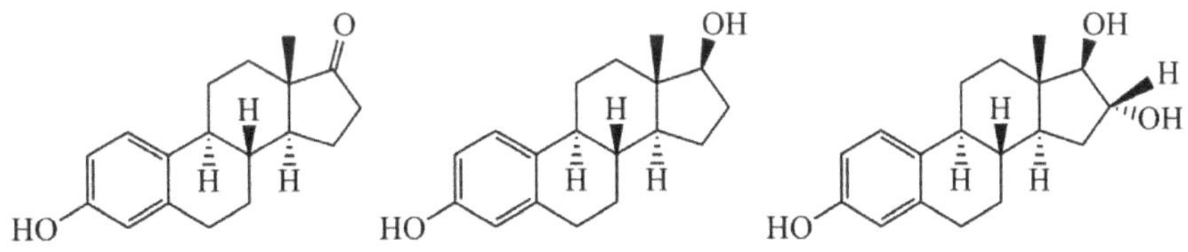

Figure 1. Chemical structure of human estrogens: estrone (E1), 17β-estradiol (E2) and estriol (E3).

menopause, when it is synthesized largely in subcutaneous fat from androstenedione. The unique structure of estrogens among steroids arises from the presence of the aromatic A-ring (**Figure 1**).

E2 is now also considered as one of the neurosteroids, as its regioselective local formation in the brain has been established [5–8]. Indeed, with today's modern analytical instrumentations and using validated bioassays that are devoid of the limitations of immunoassays [9], brain E2 level even in ovariectomized animals (i.e., in animals without gonadal E2 source) can be measured [10, 11]. It has been hypothesized that this *de novo* central formation of E2 due to the lack of gonadal E2 sources, for example, as in case of ovariectomy, is essentially a compensatory mechanism to protect the estrogen-deprived brain that cannot receive the hormone from the circulation any more, although plasma estrogen levels do not directly correlate with that of brain [12, 13]. Additionally, *de novo* synthesis of E2 with a presumed role of neuroprotection in the developing mammalian brain has also been shown [14].

Independent of the *loci* of estrogen's gonadal or extra-gonadal biosynthesis from cholesterol *via* a number of enzyme-catalyzed steps, the final process is the oxidation of the 10-methyl group of testosterone, followed by elimination and subsequent aromatization into E2 by aromatase. This step is the one that has been controlled by aromatase inhibitors in clinical practice to prevent the reoccurrence of estrogen-dependent malignancies [15].

Among estrogens and estrogenic compounds, E2 also is the best-known estrogen to be used as a powerful neuroprotective agent in various *in vitro* and preclinical animal models of neurodegeneration impacting the central nervous system (CNS) [16–20]. It is important to emphasize, though, that E2 has a large array of other beneficial effects in the CNS, including regulating body temperature, enhancing cognition and memory and ameliorating neuropsychiatric conditions in both females and males [7, 11, 21–23]. While the brain is undoubtedly the most frequently studied part of the CNS in the context of neuroprotection [24–26], the utility of E2 in protecting the eye (retina and optic nerve) [27–29] and spinal cord [30–32] have also been explored with promising outcomes.

Altogether, extensive basic science investigations brought about convincing data on the plethora of mechanisms by which E2 promotes neuronal survival and protects neurons against a wide variety of stressors addressing, thereby, practically all proposed critical contributors to neurodegeneration such as inflammation, oxidative stress, excitotoxicity and collapse of mitochondrial membrane potential. Clinical and epidemiological observations also suggest that in humans the better outcome after neurotrauma (e.g., traumatic brain and spinal cord injuries) in premenopausal females compared with age-matched men, at least in part, is due to the protective role of endogenous estrogens against neuronal injuries [33, 34].

2. Mechanistic overview of neuroprotection by estrogens

The broad-spectrum protective mechanism of E2 on injured neurons is the end result of well-orchestrated and synergistic combination of genomic and non-genomic actions of the hormone that allows for prevention of both the initiation and progression of neuronal cell death. This implicates a significant translational value for the hormone upon restricting its action to the CNS, as detailed in the following section.

2.1. Genomic pathways in E2 neuroprotection

Estrogen receptors (ERs) are expressed throughout the brain [35, 36] indicating their role in various CNS functions including neuroprotection. ER density is higher in the hypothalamus than in extrahypothalamic areas with overlapping expression of the two isoforms ERα and ERβ [35, 36]. In some brain regions, ERα or ERβ may also be co-localized in cells [37]. However, ERβ is highly expressed in the cortex [38] and hippocampus [39, 40]. Consequently, estrogen impacts the function of extrahypothalamic areas that are not involved in sex maturation and reproduction [41].

The two ERs have similar affinities to endogenous estrogens [42]. Just like many other members of the nuclear receptor superfamily of proteins, they elicit their genomic effect through gene transcription [43]. The sequence of the classical ligand-dependent genomic mechanism of estrogens' neuroprotective action is summarized in **Figure 2**. After E2 (or in general, an estrogen) distributes into the neuron and reaches the nucleus, it is ligated to its cognate receptor. The ligated ERs form homo- (ERα/ERα or ERβ/ERβ) or heterodimers (ERα/ERβ) that bind to the estrogen-response element (ERE) of the nuclear DNA. Transcriptional activation is enabled by

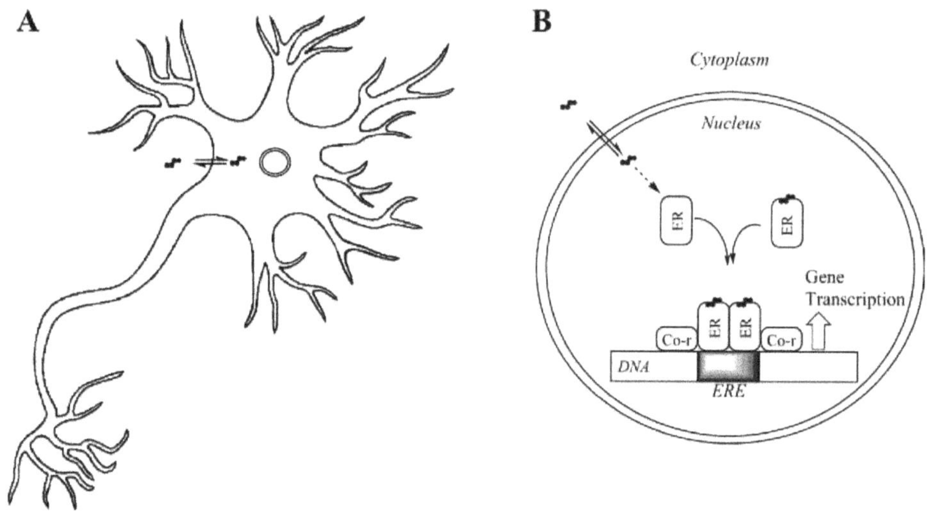

Figure 2. A simplified model for the ligand-dependent genomic mechanism of E2 neuroprotection. After E2 distributes into the neuron (A) and enters the nucleus, it binds to the cognate receptor followed by dimerization of the ligated ER that binds, together with co-regulators, to the nuclear DNA's ERE, which results in the transcription of the corresponding gene (B). E2, ER, co-regulator (Co-r) and the nuclear DNA are symbolized by the filled steroid shape, rounded rectangles and elongated rectangle showing an ERE (shaded area), respectively.

a constitutively active and a ligand-dependent function located at the amino-terminus and in the carboxy-terminal ligand-binding domain of ERs, respectively [44]. The DNA-bound dimers recruit co-regulator proteins [45], which can participate in and also recruit many enzymatic and structural proteins permitting the modulation of chromatin structure to facilitate or block gene expression [46]. Additionally, ERE-independent mechanisms have also been shown [47].

Neuroprotective target genes for E2 that directly support vital neuronal functions include neurotrophic factors such as the brain-derived neurotrophic factor [48]. Additional target genes are involved in apoptosis to remove unneeded, damaged or potentially deleterious cells [49] playing thereby a central role in development and homeostasis. Through the apoptosis-associated genomic mechanism, E2 has been shown to rescue neurons through the induction of anti-apoptotic proteins such as Bcl-2 [50] or suppression of apoptotic proteins such as the Bcl-2-associated X protein [50, 51]. Induction of several gene products that maintain cellular architecture such as neurofilament, tau and microtubulin-associated proteins and many additional genomic pathways potentially associated with E2's neuroprotection have also been described [52].

2.2. Modulation of intracellular signaling by E2

E2 also rapidly induces numerous cellular responses, which cannot be explained by a delayed genomic effect. ERs have been shown to be present in membrane compartments and in the cytoplasm [53, 54]. Specifically, ERα and ERβ are also found as homo or heterodimers at the cell membrane; they are membrane-associated but not actually embedded in the membrane. In addition, a G protein-coupled estrogen receptor (GPER) is localized mainly to intracellular membranes, including the endoplasmic reticulum and Golgi apparatus, under steady-state conditions [55]. G protein-coupled receptors such as GPER can actually signal from intracellular locations [56] and activation results in intracellular Ca^{2+}-mobilization and synthesis of phosphatidylinositol 3,4,5-triphosphate in the nucleus, which could impact gene transcription indirectly. The mitogen-activated protein kinase (MAPK) cascade [57] and the cyclic-AMP-responsive element-binding protein signaling pathway [58, 59] also respond rapidly to E2 and have been implicated in its neuroprotective effects.

An E2-ER complex can also function through cytoplasmic signaling to provide neuroprotection [60]. For example, ERs have been shown to bind in a ligand-dependent manner to the p85 alpha regulatory subunit of phosphatidylinositol 3-kinase (PI3K) [61, 62]. Therefore, stimulation with E2 increases ER-associated PI3K activity, leading to the activation of protein kinase B/Akt and endothelial nitric oxide synthase. However, modulation of intracellular pathways may occur though the binding of E2 to ERs, or independently of ligand binding [63, 64]. A representative of the non-genomic mechanism involving the modulation of intracellular signaling through ERs is summarized schematically in **Figure 3**.

E2 has been proposed to influence neurotransmission directly by binding to various transmembrane ion channels [65, 66]. Localization of ERβ to the mitochondria has also been shown [67], implicating E2 in the regulation of mitochondrial structure and function in the brain [68]. In addition to estrogen potentially influencing bioenergetics through long-lasting nuclear-associated processes, rapid mitochondria-intrinsic signaling mechanisms that promote the

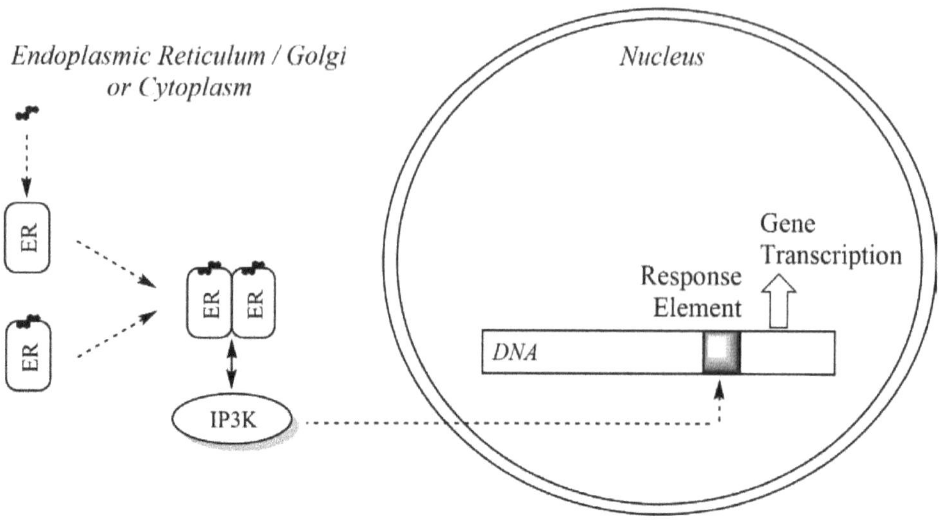

Figure 3. An example of non-genomic action of E2 involving interaction with intracellular signaling pathways through ERs. As in **Figure 2**, E2, ER and the nuclear DNA are represented by the filled steroid shapes, rounded rectangles and elongated rectangle indicating a regulated gene promoter (shaded area), respectively, while the ER-interacting protein (↔) such as PI3K is shown by a shaded oval.

maintenance of this organelle's integrity could contribute therefore to the neuroprotective action of E2. Essentially, the hormone could minimize mitochondrial dysfunctions, which accompany neurotrauma, aging and neurodegenerative diseases [69]. However, continued research is needed to fully understand molecular details about the apparently complex interactions between ERs and cellular signaling pathways in the context of neuroprotective mechanisms.

2.3. Anti-inflammatory action

The influence of E2 on neuroinflammation, a process commonly accompanying neurotrauma and neurodegenerative diseases [70–72], has been well established. Direct action on microglia and astrocytes (the cellular component of the neuroimmune system) and response to peripheral blood cells' infiltration to the brain have been implicated as major contributors to the observed anti-inflammatory action of the hormone often impacting the cerebral vasculature [73, 74]. For example, E2 can suppress chemokine-mediated induction of the cyclooxygenase-2 (COX-2) pathway in cerebral blood vessels thereby preventing migration of microglia into the brain after an inflammatory challenge [75]. Although inflammatory processes in the brain are usually associated with microglia and astrocytes, expression of the COX-2 gene in neurons and possible mechanisms by which E2 down-regulates this inflammation-associated gene have been shown recently [76]. Specifically, ERβ contributes to neuronal expression of COX-2, and E2 leads to increased recruitment of histone deacetylase 1 (HDAC1), switch-independent 3A (Sin3A) and a concomitant reduction of nuclear factor-κ B (NF-κ B) p65 occupancy and histone 4 acetylation levels. The hormone also prevents the activation of microglia and the recruitment of peripheral monocytes induced by a toxic stimulus. This effect involves ERα activation and reduces the expression of pro-inflammatory mediators and E2 have also shown to prevent morphological changes occurring in microglia during inflammatory response [77]. Decrease of microglial superoxide production and phagocytic activity by both an ER- and

MAPK-dependent pathway have also been reported among the anti-inflammatory effects of E2 [78]. In addition, the hormone inhibits pro-inflammatory gene expression by controlling intracellular localization of NF-κ B [79].

2.4. Antioxidant effects

Oxidative stress-induced damage has been linked to brain aging [80], neurodegenerative diseases [81] and neurotrauma [25, 26]. From a long time, therapeutic antioxidant interventions have been proposed to reduce the detrimental impact of oxidative stress [82]. E2's ER-independent antioxidant effects are mainly due to its ability to attenuate free-radical reactions [83], although indirect mechanisms such as up regulation of antioxidant enzymes [84, 85] and chelation of redox-active metal ions [86] have been reported. The neuroprotective effect of the hormone through direct oxidative stress reduction has been recognized in part by structure-activity relationship studies [87–89]. Acute E2 neuroprotection in ischemic brain [90] or against damage by ionizing radiation [91] may be largely conferred through antioxidant mechanisms.

The quintessential feature of estrogens as neuroprotective antioxidants is their phenolic A-ring [83, 92, 93]. Because of its lipophilicity, E2 concentrates in lipid-rich regions of the cell such as cellular membranes [94]. Therefore, it is likely that estrogens act in vivo as a highly localized antioxidant [83]. The mechanism of direct oxyradical-scavenging by E2 functioning as a phenolic antioxidant is shown schematically in **Figure 4**.

The process involves H-atom transfer that causes an interruption of free-radical chain reactions, such as lipid peroxidation (R = LOO, where L represents a lipid). Estrogens, indeed, reduce lipid peroxidation in cells and tissues of the CNS [95]. However, the chain-breaking reaction leaves behind a radical product (phenoxyl radical) whose fate has to be explained in consideration of an efficient antioxidant action observed both *in vitro* and *in vivo*. Indeed, phenolic antioxidants can be regenerated from the corresponding phenoxyl radicals by a reaction with ascorbic acid (vitamin C) [96] or through glutathione-dependent free-radical reductase [97]; therefore, a continuous antioxidant cycle is established by E2.

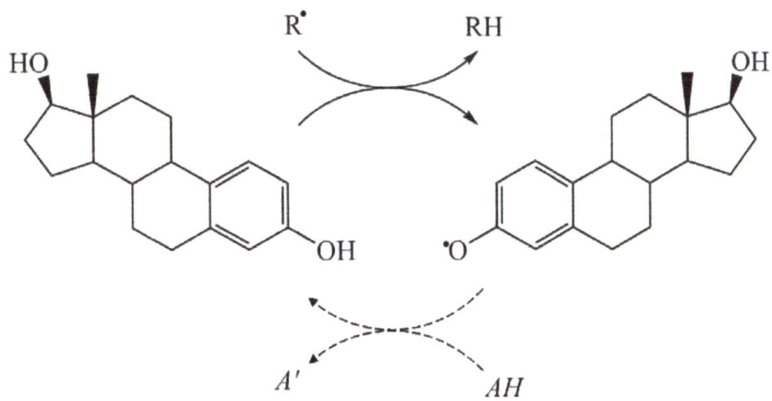

Figure 4. E2's effect through the classical phenolic antioxidant mechanism. The solid arrows represent the chain-breaking H-atom transfer, such as lipid peroxidation, while the dashed arrows indicate the conversion of the E2-derived phenoxyl radical back to the phenolic compound by an endogenous reductant (AH) such as ascorbic acid or glutathione.

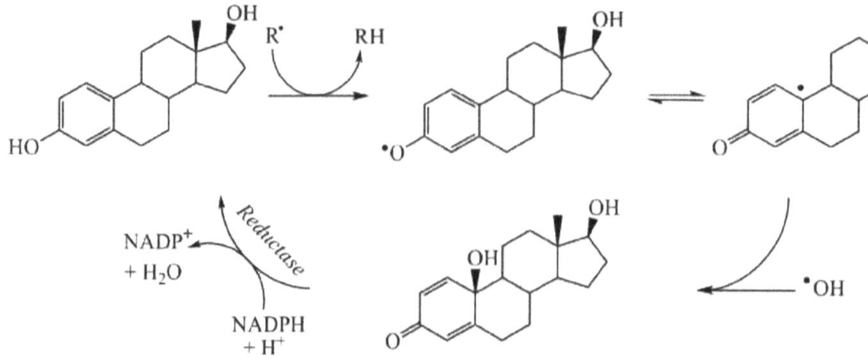

Figure 5. The Prokai antioxidant cycle for E2 through the formation of a *para*-quinol (10β,17β-dihydroxyestra-1,4-dien-3-one, DHED) as an intermediate, which is reduced to the parent hormone by enzyme-catalyzed reduction involving NADPH as cofactor.

Our laboratory pioneered in recognizing a complementary novel neuroprotective antioxidant cycle that involves a *para*-quinol as a molecular intermediate of oxyradical scavenging and, then, NADPH-mediated enzyme-catalyzed reductive aromatization [98–100] to regenerate E2, as shown in **Figure 5**. We wish to name this previously unrecognized antioxidant cycle for simple phenolic antioxidants as the "Prokai antioxidant cycle." The enzyme activity driving the reductive phase of the cycle is observed predominantly in neuronal tissue [101]. Beyond its mechanistic significance regarding oxidative stress-reducing effect, this discovery has prompted a strategy for brain-selective estrogen therapy using a prodrug approach detailed in the following section.

3. CNS-selective estrogen neurotherapy

The pathophysiology of neurodegeneration in the central nervous system is complex and multifactorial in nature [102]. Therefore, it is not surprising that an agent like E2 can provide robust protection against a myriad of neuronal insults owing to its broad-spectrum activity resulting from well-orchestrated genomic and non-genomic actions, as detailed in Section 2. The need for clinical therapeutic interventions that can be used to target multiple parallel mechanisms of neuronal injury has been repeatedly expressed [101–103]. We argue that, despite profound dichotomy between basic science and clinical studies, E2 is ideally suited to be developed as a broad-spectrum neuroprotectant if its action can be restricted to the CNS, that is, to the site of action to avoid undesirable peripheral hormonal burdens. Since neurotrauma triggers a cascade of biochemical events leading to further damages decreasing thereby the chance of appreciable functional recovery [17, 20, 102, 103], chronic pharmacotherapeutic interventions should be considered in the context of translational research. This, on the other hand, brings about critical considerations for safety and efficacy, which highlights the need for brain-selective (or in general CNS-selective) neurotherapy, considering both a preventative and a curative modality.

When estrogen neurotherapy is considered, however, one cannot ignore the (in)famous Women's Health Initiative (WHI) study [104]. This was a placebo-controlled, randomized trial of hormone "replacement" therapy in postmenopausal women that indicated detrimental consequences of estrogen and progesterone supplementations, among others, for brain health, propagating thereby a dogma that all estrogens (and progestins) are "created equal." The fact is that WHI did not use human hormones and, thus, did not study the effect of hormone replacement *per se* in aging women. On the contrary, conjugated equine estrogens (CEE) and a synthetic progestin were used for women with intact uterus. CEE is a complex mixture of over 60 different estrogens from pregnant mares' urine, and it only contains a small amount of E2: the main constituents are the sulfate esters of B-ring saturated and unsaturated estrogens [105]. The pharmacokinetic and toxicology profiles of these non-human estrogens are different from those of E2; therefore, direct comparison between E2 and CEE is fundamentally unjustified [106, 107]. Accordingly, the beneficial central effects of E2, including robust neuroprotection based on clinical, epidemiological and basic science observations should not be undermined in view of the confusion brought about by the WHI studies.

Nevertheless, an E2-based neurotherapy cannot be realized in clinical settings until E2's actions are restricted to the site of action assuring therapeutic safety and efficacy. Currently approved E2 dosage forms expose the entire body to the hormone through the circulation, potentially leading to detrimental side-effects including cardiovascular problems and the development of certain type of cancers upon chronic administration that is required for long-term neuroprotection and functional recovery after neurotrauma. Feminization (e.g., gynecomastia) is also a critical negative aspect of estrogen therapy, especially in case of children and males.

Early attempts to restrict E2's actions to the brain upon systemic administration included the so-called chemical delivery system, which was conceptually a complex prodrug approach carrying a 1,4-dihydrotrigonellyl promoiety and is capable to usher the hormone through the blood brain barrier (BBB). Once in the brain, the prodrug is oxidized analogously to that of NADP(H) $\rightleftharpoons$ $NADP^+$, locking thereby the oxidized prodrug into the brain before it releases E2 [108]. This approach does result in significantly increased brain-enhanced delivery of the hormone compared to that of simple prodrugs of E2; however, it still results in sufficient increase in circulating E2 that can produce unwanted peripheral hormonal burdens [10, 109]. Prodrugs are inert precursors of their corresponding biologically active parent drugs and they traditionally carry auxiliary bioreversible "promoiety(ies)" that are removed enzymatically (rarely *via* chemical reaction, such as pH-dependent hydrolysis) in the body [108].

An important development in achieving a true CNS-selective estrogen therapy has been achieved by our laboratory [101] and was derived from our previous discovery of a novel antioxidant cycle for estrogens we call the Prokai antioxidant cycle for simple phenolic antioxidants [98–100], and detailed in Section 2. We recognized that 10β,17β-dihydroxyestra-1,4-dien-3-one (DHED, **Figures 5** and **6**), which is chemically a *para*-quinol (not to be mistaken for quinones involved in E2-induced carcinogenesis through redox cycling [99]), can be reductively rearomatized to the parent E2 and, thus, could serve as a bioprecursor prodrug for E2. The lesser-known bioprecursor prodrugs do not carry auxiliary promoiety(ies) [108] because the bioreversible chemical manipulation is carried out within the drug molecule itself [101, 110]. Therefore, creation of bioprecursor prodrugs, such as DHED, requires significantly greater innovation than that of simple prodrugs; moreover, potential toxicity issues that may arise from the release of the "promoity(ies)" from simple prodrugs is eliminated with bioprecursor prodrugs. Indeed, we have established that CNS-specific and NADPH-dependent

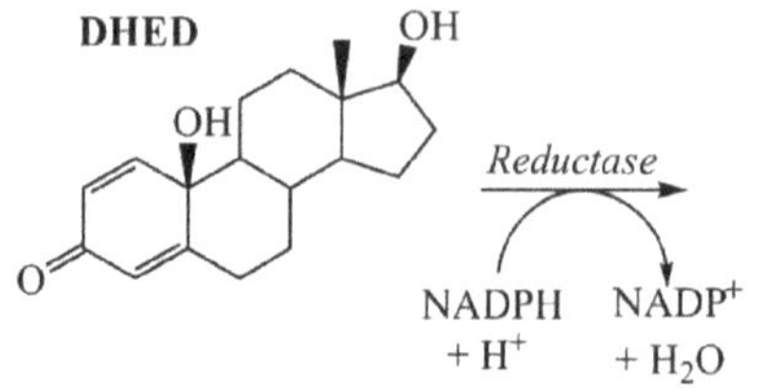

Figure 6. Schematic illustration of DHED bioprecursor prodrug's CNS-selective enzymatic metabolism to E2 *via* an NADPH-dependent reductase.

dehydrogenase/reductase metabolized DHED to E2 (**Figure 6**), while prodrug activation did not occur in the periphery. This is an unprecedented and distinguishing feature of DHED in the context of translational research [101]. With a series of *in vitro* and *in vivo* studies, we showed that with DHED, for the first time, E2's actions can be restricted to the brain independently of the route and duration of DHED administration and, therefore, it can be used (at least in preclinical settings) for the efficacious treatment of estrogen-responsive and centrally regulated maladies and injuries, including neurodegeneration brought about by ischemic stroke, without hormonal burdens for the rest of the body [101].

The transient middle cerebral artery occlusion (tMCAO) model followed by reperfusion is one the most frequently used preclinical animal models for testing an agent for its ability to act as a neuroprotectant, that is, to reduce infarct volume and aid in functional recovery [20, 24, 101, 111]. As **Figure 7** shows, a dose-dependent reduction of infarct volumes and neurological deficits was observed in DHED-treated animals. Moreover, about 10-times higher systemic E2 (i.e., the parent drug that is formed in the brain from DHED) dose was needed to achieve the same neuroprotection indicating the profound ability of the bioprecursor prodrug to enter into the brain from the circulation and, then, produce E2 within the brain, and only in

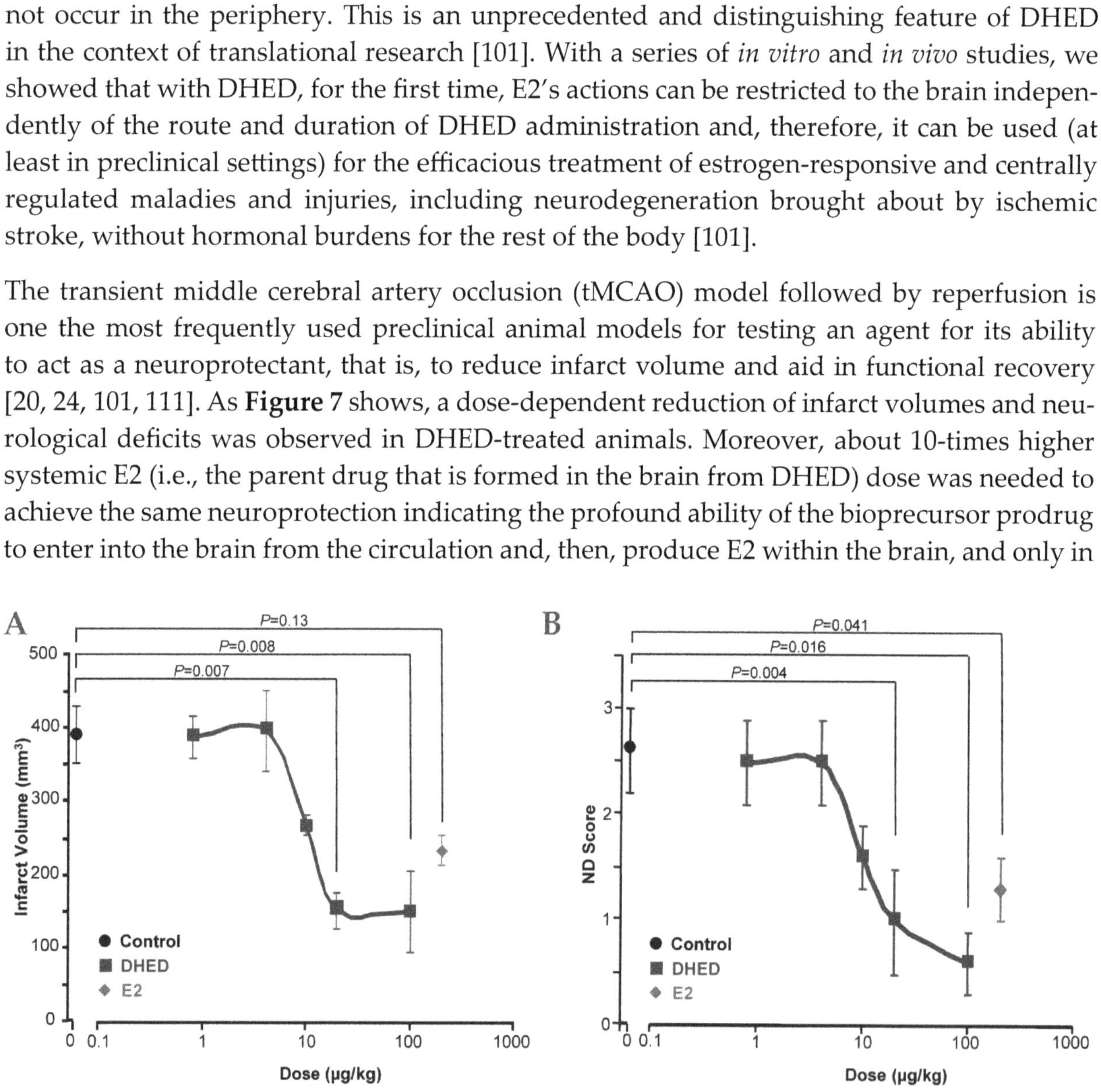

Figure 7. Dose-dependent (A) brain infarct volumes and (B) neurological deficit (ND) scores in rats treated with DHED 1 h before tMCAO followed by 24-h reperfusion [101]. The control groups received E2 (200 μg/kg, s.c., approximately representing ED50, equivalent to 50% of the maximum effect) or vehicle alone. ©Reproduced with permission by the American Association for the Advancement of Science.

the brain. In the context of translational research, it is noteworthy that the capacity to generate E2 from DHED is not lost in an injured brain, as neuroprotection was highly preserved post-stroke and, again, no hormonal exposure to the rest of the body was observed [101].

4. Conclusion

As neurotrauma and neurodegeneration in the CNS are complex and multifactorial in nature requiring therefore broad-spectrum therapeutic interventions, E2 is an attractive lead agent to address unmet medical needs in this field. The powerful antioxidant action of E2 against oxidative stress owing to its phenolic A-ring is unique among neurosteroids with potential neuroprotective roles; therefore, non-genomic mechanisms contribute significantly to the overall neuroprotection. This chapter presented an overview of our current knowledge on the well-orchestrated genomic and non-genomic events by which E2 could beneficially counteract the initiation and/or progression of neuronal cell death. However, there has been incongruency between basic science and clinical studies in terms of estrogen therapy impacting the brain because most researchers ignore the requirement to confine E2's actions into the CNS upon systemic administration to ensure therapeutic safety and efficacy. We highlighted here a novel and unique bioprecursor prodrug approach our laboratory pioneered for brain-selective delivery of E2 without exposing the rest of the body to unwanted hormonal burden.

Acknowledgements

The project was supported in part by the National Institutes of Health for the authors, in particular grant numbers NS044765, AG031535, MH100700, HD078077 & CA215550 to L.P. and AG031421 & EY027005 to K.P.-T. and by the Robert A. Welch Foundation (endowment BK-0031 to L.P.).

Author details

Katalin Prokai-Tatrai* and Laszlo Prokai

*Address all correspondence to: katalin.prokai@unthsc.edu

Department of Pharmacology and Neuroscience, University of North Texas Health Science Center, Fort Worth, TX, USA

References

[1] Turgeon JL, Carr MC, Maki PM, Mendelsohn ME, Wise PM. Complex actions of sex steroids in adipose tissue, the cardiovascular system, and brain: Insights from basic science and clinical studies. Endocrine Reviews. 2006;**27**:575-605. DOI: 10.1210/er.2005-0020

[2] Fink G, Sumner BEH, Rosie R, Grace O, Quinn JP. Estrogen control of central neurotransmission: Effect on mood, mental state, and memory. Cellular and Molecular Neurobiology. 1996;**16**:325-344. DOI: 10.1007/bf02088099

[3] Mauvais-Jarvis F, Clegg DJ, Hevener AL. The role of estrogens in control of energy balance and glucose homeostasis. Endocrine Reviews. 2013;**34**:309-338. DOI: 10.1210/er.2012-1055

[4] Gruber CJ, Tschugguel W, Schneeberger C, Huber JC. Production and actions of estrogens. New England Journal of Medicine. 2002;**346**:340-352. DOI: 10.1056/NEJMra000471

[5] Baulieu EE. Neurosteroids: A novel function of the brain. Psychoneuroendocrinology. 1998;**23**:963-987

[6] Cui J, Shen Y, Li R. Estrogen synthesis and signaling pathways during aging: From periphery to brain. Trends in Molecular Medicine. 2013;**19**:197-209. DOI: 10.1016/j.molmed.2012.12.007

[7] Barakat R, Oakley O, Kim H, Jin J, Ko CJ. Extra-gonadal sites of estrogen biosynthesis and function. BMB Reports. 2016;**49**:488-496. DOI: 10.5483/BMBRep.2016.49.9.141

[8] Simpson ER. Sources of estrogen and their importance. Journal of Steroid Biochemistry & Molecular Biology. 2003;**86**:225-230. DOI: 10.1016/S0960-0760(03)00360-1

[9] Stanczyk FZ, Cho MM, Endres DB, Morrison JL, Patel S, Paulson RJ. Limitations of direct estradiol and testosterone immunoassay kits. Steroids. 2003;**68**:1173-1178. DOI: 10.1016/j.steroids.2003.08.012

[10] Prokai-Tatrai K, Szarka S, Nguyen V, Sahyouni F, Walker C, White S, Talamantes T, Prokai L. "All in the mind?" brain-targeting chemical delivery system of 17β-estradiol (Estredox) produces significant uterotrophic side effect. Pharmaceutical and Analytical Acta. 2013;**S7**:002. DOI: 10.4172/2153-2435.S7-002

[11] Merchenthaler I, Lane M, Sabnis G, Brodie A, Nguyen V, Prokai L, Prokai-Tatrai K. Treatment with an orally bioavailable prodrug of 17β-estradiol alleviates hot flushes without hormonal effects in the periphery. Scientific Reports. 2016;**6**:30721. DOI: 10.1038/srep30721s

[12] Mc Cullough LD, Blizzard K, Simpson ER, Öz OK, Hurn PD. Aromatase cytochrome P450 and extragonadal estrogen play a role in ischemic neuroprotection. Journal of Neuroscience. 2003;**23**:8701-8705

[13] Carswell HV, Dominiczak AF, Garcia-Segura LM, Harada N, Hutchison JB, Macrae IM. Brain aromatase expression after experimental stroke: Topography and time course. The Journal of Steroid Biochemistry and Molecular Biology. 2005;**96**:89-91. DOI: 10.1016/j.jsbmb.2005.02.016

[14] McCarthy MM. Estradiol and the developing brain. Physiological Reviews. 2008;**88**:91-134. DOI: 10.1152/physrev.00010.2007

[15] Behan LA, Amir E, Casper RF. Aromatase inhibitors for prevention of breast cancer in postmenopausal women: A narrative review. Menopause. 2015;**22**:342-350. DOI: 10.1097/GME.0000000000000426

[16] Tschiffely AE, Schuh RA, Prokai-Tatrai K, Prokai L, Ottinger MA. A comparative evaluation of treatments with 17β-estradiol and its brain-selective prodrug in a double-transgenic mouse model of Alzheimer's disease. Hormons and Behavior. 2016;**83**:39-44. DOI: 10.1016/j.yhbeh.2016.05.009

[17] Raghava N, Das BC, Ray SK. Neuroprotective effects of estrogen in CNS injuries: Insights from animal models. Neuroscience and Neuroeconomics. 2017;**6**:15-29. DOI: 10.2147/NAN.S105134

[18] Zhu Y, Zhang QG, Zhang WL, Li N, Dai YX, Tu JY, Yang F, Brann DW, Wang RM. Protective effect of 17beta-estradiol upon hippocampal spine density and cognitive function in an animal model of vascular dementia. Scientific Reports. 2017;**7**:42660. DOI: 10.1038/srep42660

[19] Fiocchetti M, Ascenzi P, Marino M. Neuroprotective effects of 17β-estradiol rely on estrogen receptor membrane initiated signals. Frontiers in Physiology. 2012;**3**:73. DOI: 10.3389/fphys.2012.00073

[20] Toung TJK, Traystman RJ, Hurn PD. Estrogen-mediated neuroprotection after experi mental stroke in male rats. Stroke. 1998;**29**:1666-1670. DOI: 10.1161/01.STR.29.8.1666

[21] Gillies GE, McArthur S. Estrogen actions in the brain and the basis for differential action in men and women: A case for sex-specific medicines. Pharmacological Reviews. 2010;**62**:155-198. DOI: 10.1124/pr.109.002071

[22] Maggi A, Ciana P, Belcredito S, Vegeto E. Estrogens in the nervous system: Mechanisms and nonreproductive functions. Annual Review of Physiology. 2004;**66**:291-313. DOI: 10.1146/annurev.physiol.66.032802.154945

[23] Cornil CA, Ball GF, Balthazart J. Rapid control of male typical behaviors by brain-derived estrogens. Frontiers in Neuroendocrinology. 2012;**33**:425-446. DOI: 10.1016/j.yfrne.2012.08.003

[24] Carpenter RS, Iwuchukwu I, Hinkson CL, Reitz S, Lee W, Kukino A, Zhang A, Pike MM, Ardelta AA. High-dose estrogen treatment at reperfusion reduces lesion volume and accelerates recovery of sensorimotor function after experimental ischemic stroke. Brain Research. 2016;**15**:200-213. DOI: 10.1016/j.brainres.2016.01.058

[25] Manzanero S, Santro T, Arumugam TV. Neuronal oxidative stress in acute ischemic stroke: Sources and contribution to cell injury. Neurochemistry International. 2013;**62**:712-718. DOI: 10.1016/j.neuint.2012.11.009

[26] Cornelius C, Crupi R, Calabrese V, Graziano A, Milone P, Pennisi G, Radak Z, Calabrese EJ, Cuzzocrea S. Traumatic brain injury: Oxidative stress and neuroprotection. Antioxidants & Redox Signaling. 2013;**19**:836-853. DOI: 10.1089/ars.2012.4981

[27] Prokai-Tatrai K, Xin H, Nguyen V, Szarka S, Blazics B, Prokai L, Koulen P. 17β-estradiol eye drops protect the retinal ganglion cell layer and preserve visual function in an in vivo model of glaucoma. Molecular Pharmaceutics. 2013;**5**:3253-3261. DOI: 10.1021/mp400313u

[28] Russo R, Cavaliere F, Watanabe C, Nucci C, Bagetta G, Corasaniti MT, Sakurada S, Morrone LA. 17β-Estradiol prevents retinal ganglion cell loss induced by acute rise of intraocular pressure in rat. Progress in Brain Research. 2008;**173**:583-590. DOI: 10.1016/S0079-6123(08)01144-8

[29] Nonaka A, Kiryu J, Tsujikawa A, Yamashiro K, Miyamoto K, Nishiwaki H, Mandai M, Honda Y, Ogura Y. Administration of 17β-estradiol attenuates retinal ischemia-reperfusion injury in rats. Investigative Ophthalmology & Visual Science. 2000;**41**:2689-2696

[30] Chaovipoch P, Jelks KA, Gerhold LM, West EJ, Chongthammakun S, Floyd CL. 17beta-estradiol is protective in spinal cord injury in post- and pre-menopausal rats. Journal of Neurotrauma. 2006;**23**:830-852. DOI: 10.1089/neu.2006.23.830

[31] Samantaray S, Das A, Matzelle DC, Yu SP, Wei L, Varma A, Ray SK, Banik NL. Administration of low dose estrogen attenuates persistent inflammation, promotes angiogenesis, and improves locomotor function following chronic spinal cord injury in rats. Journal of Neurochemistry. 2016;**37**:604-617. DOI: 10.1111/jnc.13610

[32] Sribnick EA, Samantaray S, Das A, Smith J, Matzelle DD, Ray SK, Banik NL. Postinjury estrogen treatment of chronic spinal cord injury improves locomotor function in rats. Journal of Neuroscience Research. 2010;**88**:1738-1750. DOI: 10.1002/jnr.22337

[33] Datto JP, Yang J, Dietrich WD, Pearse DD. Does being female provide a neuroprotective advantage following spinal cord injury? Neural Regeneration Research. 2015;**10**:1533-1536. DOI: 10.4103/1673-5374.165213

[34] Roof RL, Hall ED. Gender differences in acute CNS trauma and stroke: Neuroprotective effects of estrogen and progesterone. Journal of Neurotrauma. 2000;**17**:367-388

[35] Shughrue PJ, Lane MV, Merchenthaler I. Comparative distribution of estrogen receptor-alpha and -beta mRNA in the rat central nervous system. Journal of Comparative Neurology. 1997;**388**:507-525. DOI: 10.1002/(SICI)1096-9861(19971201)388:4<507::AID-CNE1>3.0.CO;2-6

[36] Shughrue PJ, Scrimo PJ, Merchenthaler I. Estrogen binding and estrogen receptor characterization (ER alpha and ER beta) in the cholinergic neurons of the rat basal forebrain. Neuroscience. 2000;**96**:41-49. DOI: 10.1016/S0306-4522(99)00520-5

[37] Shughrue PJ, Scrimo PJ, Merchenthaler I. Evidence for the colocalization of estrogen receptor-beta mRNA and estrogen receptor-alpha immunoreactivity in neurons of the rat forebrain. Endocrinology. 1998;**139**:5267-5270. DOI: 10.1210/endo.139.12.6525

[38] Zhang JQ, Cai WQ, Zhou DS, Su BY. Distribution and differences of estrogen receptor beta immunoreactivity in the brain of adult male and female rats. Brain Research. 2002;**935**:73-80. DOI: 10.1016/S0006-8993(02)02460-5

[39] Milner TA, Ayoola K, Drake CT, Herrick SP, Tabori NE, McEwen BS, Warrier S, Alves SE. Ultrastructural localization of estrogen receptor beta immunoreactivity in the rat hippocampal formation. The Journal of Comparative Neurology. 2005;**491**:81-95. DOI: 10.1002/cne.20724

[40] Mitterling KL, Spencer JL, Dziedzic N, Shenoy S, McCarthy K, Waters EM, McEwen BS, Milner TA. Cellular and subcellular localization of estrogen and progestin receptor immunoreactivities in the mouse hippocampus. The Journal of Comparative Neurology. 2010;**518**:2729-2743. DOI: 10.1002/cne.22361

[41] Hara Y, Waters EM, McEwen BS, Morrison JH. Estrogen effects on cognitive and synaptic health over the lifecourse. Physiological Reviews. 2015;**95**:785-807. DOI: 10.1152/physrev.00036.2014

[42] Pike ACW, Brzozowski AM, Hubbard REA. Structural biologist's view of the oestrogen receptor. Journal of Steroidal and Molecular Biochemistry. 2000;**74**:261-268. DOI: 10.1016/S0960-0760(00)00102-3

[43] Puzianowska-Kuznicka M, Pawlik-Pachucka E, Owczarz M, Budzinska M, Polosak J. Small-molecule hormones: Molecular mechanisms of action. International Journal of Endocrinology. 2013;**2013**:601246. DOI: 10.1155/2013/601246

[44] Nilsson S, Makela S, Treuter E, Tujague M, Thomsen J, Andersson G, Enmark E, Pettersson K, Warner M, Gustafsson JA. Mechanisms of estrogen action. Physiological Reviews. 2001;**81**:1535-1565

[45] Tetel MJ, Acharya KD. Nuclear receptor coactivators: Regulators of steroid action in brain and behaviour. Journal of Neuroendocrinology. 2013;**25**:1209-1218. DOI: 10.1111/jne.12065

[46] Sovell WM. Nucleosome dynamics: HMGB1 facilitates nucleosome restructuring and collaborates in estrogen-responsive gene expression. AIMS Genetics. 2016;**3**:252-279. DOI: 10.3934/genet.2016.4.252

[47] Hall JM, Couse JF, Korach KF. The multifaceted mechanisms of estradiol and estrogen receptor signaling. Journal of Biological Chemistry. 2001;**276**:36869-36872. DOI: 10.1074/jbc.R100029200

[48] Carbone DL, Handa RJ. Sex and stress hormone influences on the expression and activity of brain-derived neurotrophic factor. Neuroscience. 2013;**239**:295-303. DOI: 10.1016/j.neuroscience.2012.10.073

[49] Hail N, Carter BZ, Konopleva M, Andreeff M. Apoptosis effector mechanisms: A requiem performed in different keys. Apoptosis. 2006;**11**:889-904. DOI: 10.1007/s10495-006-6712-8

[50] Sharma K, Mehra RD. Long-term administration of estrogen or tamoxifen to ovariectomized rats affords neuroprotection to hippocampal neurons by modulating the expression of Bcl-2 and Bax. Brain Research. 2008, 2008;**14**(1204):1-15. DOI: 10.1016/j.brainres.2008.01.080

[51] Sribnick EA, Ray SK, Nowak MW, Li L, Banik NL. 17 beta-estradiol attenuates glutamate-induced apoptosis and preserves electrophysiologic function in primary cortical neurons. Journal of Neuroscience Research. 2004;**76**:688-696. DOI: 10.1002/jnr.20124

[52] Segura-Uribe JJ, Pinto-Almazdan R, Coyoy-Salgado A, Fuentes-Venado CE, Guerra-Araiza C. Effects of estrogen receptor modulators on cytoskeletal proteins in the central nervous system. Neural Regeneration Research. 2017;**12**:1231-1240. DOI: 10.4103/1673-5374.213536

[53] Levin ER. Extranuclear steroid receptors are essential for steroid hormone actions. Annual Review of Medicine. 2015;**66**:271-280. DOI: 10.1146/annurev-med-050913-021703

[54] Boonyaratanakornkit V. Scaffolding proteins mediating membrane-initiated extra-nuclear actions of estrogen receptor. Steroids. 2011;**76**:877-844. DOI: 10.1016/j.steroids.2011.02.017

[55] Revankar CM, Cimino DF, Sklar LA, Arterburn JB, Prossnitz ER. A transmembrane intracellular estrogen receptor mediates rapid cell signaling. Science. 2005;**307**:1625-1630

[56] Platta HW, Stenmark H. Endocytosis and signaling. Current Opinion in Cell Biology. 2011;**23**:393-403. DOI: 10.1016/j.ceb.2011.03.008

[57] Sawe N, Steinberg G, Zhao H. Dual roles of the MAPK/ERK1/2 cell signaling pathway after stroke. Journal of Neuroscience Research. 2008;**86**:1659-1669. DOI: 10.1002/jnr.21604

[58] Carlstrom L, Ke ZJ, Unnerstall JR, Cohen RS, Pandey SC. Estrogen modulation of the cyclic AMP response element-binding protein pathway—Effects of long-term and acute treatments. Neuroendocrinology. 2001;**74**:227-243. DOI: 10.1159/000054690

[59] Yune TY, Park HG, Lee JY, Oh TH. Estrogen-induced bcl-2 expression after spinal cord injury is mediated through phosphoinositide-3-kinase/Akt-dependent CREB activation. Journal of Neurotrauma. 2008;**25**:1121-1131. DOI: 10.1089/neu.2008.0544

[60] Manavathi B, Kumar R. Steering estrogen signals from the plasma membrane to the nucleus: Two sides of the coin. Journal of Cellular Physiology. 2006;**207**:594-604. DOI: 10.1002/jcp.20551

[61] Simoncini T, Hafezl-Moghadam A, Brazil DP, Ley K, Chin WW, Liao JK. Interaction of oestrogen receptor with the regulatory subunit of phosphatidylinositol-3-OH kinase. Nature. 2000;**407**:538-541

[62] Malyala A, Zhang C, Bryant DN, Kelly MJ, Ronneklev OK. PI3K signaling effects in hypothalamic neurons mediated by estrogen. Journal of Comparative Neurology. 2008;**506**:895-911. DOI: 10.1002/cne.21584

[63] Coleman KM, Smith CL. Intracellular signaling pathways: Nongenomic actions of estrogens and ligand-independent activation of estrogen receptors. Frontiers in Bioscience. 2001;**6**:D1379-D1391. DOI: 10.2741/Coleman

[64] Grissom EM, Daniel JM. Evidence for ligand-independent activation of hippocampal estrogen receptor-alpha by IGF-1 in hippocampus of ovariectomized rats. Endocrinology. 2016;**157**:3149-3156. DOI: 10.1210/en.2016-1197

[65] Wang Q, Cao J, Hu F, RZ L, Wang J, Ding HX, Gao R, Xiao H. Effects of estradiol on voltage-gated sodium channels in mouse dorsal root ganglion neurons. Brain Research. 2013;**1512**:2-8. DOI: 10.1016/j.brainres.2013.02.047

[66] Kow LM, Pataky S, Dupre C, Phan A, Martin-Alguacil N, Pfaff DW. Analyses of rapid estrogen actions on rat ventromedial hypothalamic neurons. Steroids. 2016;**111**:100-112. DOI: 10.1016/j.steroids.2016.03.010

[67] Yang S, Liu R, Perez EJ, Wen Y, Stevens SM Jr, Valencia T, Brun-Zinkernagel AM, Prokai L, Will Y, Dykens J, Koulen P, Simpkins JW. Mitochondrial localization of estrogen receptor beta. Proceedings of the National Academy of Sciences of the United States of America. 2004;**101**:4130-4135. DOI: 10.1073/pnas.0306948101

[68] Susanne A, Victor MB, Beyer C. Estrogen and the regulation of mitochondrial structure and function in the brain. Journal of Steroid Biochemistry and Molecular Biology. 2012;**131**:2-9. DOI: 10.1016/j.jsbmb.2012.01.012

[69] Velarde MC. Pleiotropic actions of estrogen: A mitochondrial matter. Physiological Genomics. 2013;**46**:103-109. DOI: 10.1152/physiolgenomics.00155.2012

[70] Jose Perez-Alvarez M, Wandosell F. Stroke and neuroinflamation: Role of sexual hormones. Current Pharmaceutical Design. 2016;**22**:1334-1349. DOI: 10.2174/138161282210160304112834

[71] Simon DW, McGeachy MJ, Bayir H, Clark RSB, Loane DJ, Kochanek PM. The far-reaching scope of neuroinflammation after traumatic brain injury. Nature Reviews Neurology. 2017;**11**:171-191. DOI: 10.1038/nrneurol.2017.13

[72] Hong H, Kim B, Im HI. Pathophysiological role of neuroinflammation in neurodegenerative diseases and psychiatric disorders. International Neurology Journal. 2016;**20**:S2-S7. DOI: 10.5213/inj.1632604.302

[73] Miller VM, Duckles SP. Vascular actions of estrogens: Functional implications. Physiological Reviews. 2008;**60**:210-241. DOI: 10.1124/pr.107.08002

[74] Duckles SP, Krause DN. Mechanisms of cerebrovascular protection: Oestrogen, inflammation and mitochondria. Acta Physiologica. 2011;**203**:149-154. DOI: 10.1111/j.1748-1716.2010.02184.x

[75] Ospina JA, Brevig HN, Krause DN, Duckles SP. Estrogen suppresses IL-1 beta-mediated induction of COX-2 pathway in rat cerebral blood vessels. American Journal of Physiology. 2004;**286**:H2010-H2019. DOI: 10.1152/ajpheart.00481.2003

[76] Stacey W, Bhave S, Uht RM. Mechanisms by which 17β-Estradiol (E2) suppress neuronal cox-2 gene expression. PLoS One. 2016;**11**:e0161430. DOI: 10.1371/journal.pone.0161430

[77] Pozzi S, Benedusi V, Maggi A, Vegeto E. Estrogen action in neuroprotection and brain inflammation. Annals of the New York Academy of Sciences. 2006;**1089**:302-323. DOI: 10.1196/annals.1386.035

[78] Bruce-Keller AJ, Keeling JL, Keller JN, Huang FF, Camondola S, Mattson MP. Antiinflammatory effects of estrogen on microglial activation. Endocrinology. 2000; **141**:3646-3656. DOI: 10.1210/en.141.10.3646

[79] Ghisletti S, Meda C, Maggi A, Vegeto E. 17 β-estradiol inhibits inflammatory gene expression by controlling NF-κ B intracellular localization. Molecular and Cellular Biology. 2005;**25**:2957-2968. DOI: 10.1128/MCB.25.8.2957-2968.2005

[80] Krishnan V, Khurana S, Tai TC. Oxidative stress in aging—Matters of the heart and mind. International Journal of Molecular Sciences. 2013;**14**:17897-17925. DOI: 10.3390/ijms140917897

[81] Radi E, Formichi P, Battisti C, Federico A. Apoptosis and oxidative stress in neurodegenerative diseases. Journal of Alzheimer's Disease. 2014;**42**:S125-S152. DOI: 10.3233/JAD-132738

[82] Halliwell B, Gutteridge JMC. Lipid peroxidation, oxygen radicals, cell damage, and antioxidant therapy. The Lancet. 1984;**323**:1396-1397. DOI: 10.1016/S0140-6736(84)91886-5

[83] Prokai L, Prokai-Tatrai K, Perjesi P, Simpkins JW. Mechanistic insights into the direct antioxidant effects of estrogens. Drug Development Research. 2005;**66**:118-125. DOI: 10.1002/ddr.20050

[84] Borras C, Gambini J, Gomez-Cabrera MC, Sastre J, Pallardo FV, Mann GE, Vina J. 17β-Oestradiol up-regulates longevity-related, antioxidant enzyme expression via the ERK1 and ERK2[MAPK]/NFκB cascade. Aging Cell. 2005;**4**:113-118. DOI: 10.1111/j.1474-9726.2005.00151.x

[85] Stakhiv TM, Mesia-Vela S, Kauffman FC. Phase II antioxidant enzyme activities in brain of male and female ACI rats treated chronically with estradiol. Brain Research. 2006;**1104**:80-91. DOI: 10.1016/j.brainres.2006.05.093

[86] Ruiz-Larrea B, Leal A, Martin C, Martinez R, Lacort M. Effects of estrogens on the redox chemistry of iron: A possible mechanism of the antioxidant action of estrogens. Steroids. 1995;**60**:780-783. DOI: 10.1016/0039-128X(95)00119-B

[87] Behl C, Skutella T, Lezoualc'h F, Post A, Widmann M, Newton CJ, Holsboer F. Neuroprotection against oxidative stress by estrogens: Structure-activity relationship. Molecular Pharmacology. 1997;**51**:535-541

[88] Prokai L, Simpkins JW. Structure-nongenomic neuroprotection relationship of estrogens and estrogen-derived compounds. Pharmacology & Therapeutics. 2007;**114**:1-12. DOI: 10.1016/j.pharmthera.2007.01.006

[89] Prokai L, Rivera-Portalatin NM, Prokai-Tatrai K. Quantitative structure-activity relationships predicting the antioxidant potency of 17β-estradiol-related polycyclic phenols to inhibit lipid peroxidation. International Journal of Molecular Sciences. 2013;**14**:1443-1454. DOI: 10.3390/ijms14011443

[90] Kii N, Adachi N, Liu KY, Arai T. Acute effects of 17β-estradiol on oxidative stress in ischemic rat striatum. Journal of Neurosurgical Anesthesiology. 2005;**17**:27-32

[91] Caceres LG, Uran SL, Zubilete MAZ, Romero JI, Capani F, Guelman LR. An early treatment with 17-beta-estradiol is neuroprotective against the long-term effects of neonatal ionizing radiation exposure. Journal of Neurochemistry. 2011;**118**:626-635. DOI: 10.1111/j.1471-4159.2011.07334.x

[92] Prokai L, Oon SM, Prokai-Tatrai K, Abboud K, Simpkins JW. Synthesis and biological evaluation of 17β-alkoxyestra-1,3,5(10)-trienes as potential neuroprotectants against oxidative stress. Journal of Medicinal Chemistry. 2001;**44**:110-114. DOI: 10.1021/jm000280t

[93] Prokai-Tatrai K, Prokai L, Simpkins JW, Jung ME. Phenolic compounds protect cultured hippocampal neurons against ethanol-withdrawal induced oxidative stress. International Journal of Molecular Sciences. 2009;**10**:1173-1187. DOI: 10.3390/ijms10041773

[94] Liang Y, Belford S, Tang F, Prokai L, Simpkins JW, Hughes JA. Membrane fluidity effects of estratrienes. Brain Research Bulletin. 2001;**54**:661-668. DOI: 10.1016/S0361-9230(01)00483-X

[95] Vedder H, Anthens N, Stumm G, Wurz C, Behl C, Krieg JC. Estrogen hormones reduce lipid peroxidation in cells and tissues of the central nervous system. Journal of Neurochemistry. 1999;**72**:2531-2538. DOI: 10.1046/j.1471-4159.1999.0722531.x

[96] Packer JE, Slater TF, Wilson RL. Direct observation of a free radical interaction between vitamin E and vitamin C. Nature. 1978;**278**:737-738

[97] McCay PB, Brueggemann G, Lai EK, Powell SR. Evidence that α-tocopherol functions cyclically to quench free radicals in hepatic microsomes. Annals of the New York Academy of Sciences. 1989;**570**:32-45. DOI: 10.1111/j.1749-6632.1989.tb14906.x

[98] Prokai L, Prokai-Tatrai K, Perjesi P, Zharikova AD, Perez EJ, Liu R, Simpkins JW. Quinol-based cyclic antioxidant mechanism in estrogen neuroprotection. Proceedings of the National Academy of Sciences of the United States of America. 2003;**100**:11741-11746. DOI: 10.1073/pnas.2032621100

[99] Rivera-Portalatin NM, Vera-Serrano JL, Prokai-Tatrai K, Prokai L. Comparison of estrogen-derived ortho-quinone and para-quinol concerning induction of oxidative stress. Journal of Steroid Biochemistry and Molecular Biology. 2007;**105**:71-75. DOI: 10.1016/j.jsbmb.2006.11.025

[100] Prokai-Tatrai K, Perjesi P, Rivera-Portalatin NM, Simpkins JW, Prokai L. Mechanistic investigations on the antioxidant action of a neuroprotective estrogen derivative. Steroids. 2008;**73**:280-288. DOI: 10.1016/j.steroids.2007.10.011

[101] Prokai L, Nguyen V, Szarka S, Garg P, Sabnis G, Bimonte-Nelson HA, McLaughlin KJ, Talboom JS, Conrad CD, Shughrue PJ, Gould TD, Brodie A, Merchenthaler I, Koulen P, Prokai-Tatrai K. The prodrug DHED selectively delivers 17β-estradiol to the brain for treating estrogen-responsive disorders. Science Translational Medicine. 2015;**7**(297):297ra113. DOI: 10.1126/scitranslmed.aab1290

[102] Krishnamurthy K, Laskowitz DT. Chapter 5: Cellular and molecular mechanisms of secondary neuronal injury following traumatic brain injury. In: Laskowitz D, Grant G, editors. Translational Research in Traumatic Brain Injury. Boca Raton: CRC Press/ Taylor and Francis Group; 2016 Available from: https://www.ncbi.nlm.nih.gov/books/NBK32671

[103] Diaz-Arrastia R, Kochanek PM, Bergold P, Kenney K, Marx CE, Grimes CJ, Loh LT, Adam LT, Oskvig D, Curley KC, Salzer W. Pharmacotherapy of traumatic brain injury: State of the science and the road forward: Report of the Department of Defense Neurotrauma Pharmacology Workgroup. Journal of Neurotrauma. 2014;**31**:135-158. DOI: 10.1089/neu.2013.3019

[104] Clark JH. A critique of Women's health initiative studies (2002-2006). Nuclear Receptor Signaling. 2006;**4**:e023. DOI: 10.1621/nrs.04023

[105] Levy MJ, Boyne MT, Rogstad S, Skanchy DJ, Jiang X, Vidavsky IG. Marketplace analysis of conjugated estrogens: Determining the consistently present steroidal content with LC-MS. AAPS Journal. 2015;**17**:1438-1445. DOI: 10.1208/s12248-015-9805-x

[106] Prokai-Tatrai K, Prokai L. Impact of metabolism on the safety of estrogen therapy. Annals of the New York Academy of Sciences. 2005;**1052**:243-257. DOI: 10.1196/annals.1347.018

[107] Zhang F, Chen Y, Pisha E, Shen L, Xiong Y, van Breemen RB, Bolton JL. The major metabolite of equilin, 4-hydroxyequilin, autoxidizes to an o-quinone which isomerizes to the potent cytotoxin 4-hydroxyequilenin-o-quinone. Chemical Research in Toxicology. 1999;**12**:204-213. DOI: 10.1021/tx980217v

[108] Prokai L, Prokai-Tatrai K, Bodor N. Targeting drugs to the brain by redox chemical delivery systems. Medicinal Resesearch Reviews. 2000;**20**:367-416. DOI: 10.1002/1098-1128(200009)20:5<367::AID-MED3>3.0.CO;2-P

[109] Sarkar DK, Friedman SJ, Yen SS, Frautschy SA. Chronic inhibition of hypothalamic-pituitary-ovarian axis and body weight gain by brain-directed delivery of estradiol-17β in female rats. Neuroendocrinology. 1989;**50**:204-210. DOI: 10.1159/000125223

[110] Prokai-Tatrai K, Rivera-Portalatin NM, Rauniyar N, Prokai L. A facile microwave-assisted synthesis of p-quinols by lead(IV)acetate oxidation. Letters in Organic Chemistry. 2007;**4**:265-267. DOI: 10.2174/157017807781024200

[111] Etgen AM, Jover-Mengual T, Zukina RS. Neuroprotective actions of estradiol and novel estrogen analogs in ischemia: Translational implications. Frontiers in Neuroendocrinology. 2011;**32**:336-352. DOI: 10.1016/j.yfrne.2010.12.005

3

Dehydroepiandrosterone (DHEA) and DHEA Sulfate: Roles in Brain Function and Disease

Tracey A. Quinn, Stephen R. Robinson and David Walker

Abstract

Among the neuroactive steroids, dehydroepiandrosterone (3b-hydroxyandrost-5-ene-17-one, [DHEA]) and its sulfated metabolite DHEA sulfate (DHEAS) have been shown to be potent modulators of neural function, including neurogenesis, neuronal growth and differentiation, and neuroprotection. Highlighting the potential health significance of DHEA and DHEAS in humans, serum concentrations decrease steadily with age, with lowest concentrations present at the time many diseases of aging and neurodegeneration become apparent. This temporal association has led to the suggestion that pathology associated with cognitive decline, age-related neurological disorders such as Alzheimer's disease, dementia, amyotrophic lateral sclerosis (ALS), and adult onset schizophrenia may, in part at least, be attributed to decreased secretion of DHEA. Animal studies suggest neuroprotective functions for DHEA and DHEAS through reduction of glutamate-induced excitotoxicity. Reduced myelin loss and reactive gliosis after spinal cord injury by DHEA treatment also suggest a role for DHEA in the treatment of white matter pathologies such as multiple sclerosis. In this chapter, we discuss the physiologi cal roles of DHEA and DHEAS in the central nervous system (CNS), their potential as neuroprotective hormones with reference to documented effects on excitotoxicity and oxidative stress, and their anti-glucocorticoid actions during chronic stress. The potential for metabolic derivatives of DHEA, such as estrogens and testosterone on brain function, and their contribution to neurodevelopment and neurodegenerative conditions are also discussed.

Keywords: adrenal zona reticularis, adrenarche, adrenopause, aging, Alzheimer's disease, amyotrophic lateral sclerosis, androgens, C19 steroids, glucocorticoids, neurocognitive decline, neurogenesis, neuroprotection, estrogens, schizophrenia, steroid biosynthesis

1. Introduction

Dehydroepiandrosterone (DHEA) is the principal carbon (C)-19 steroid produced by the adrenal gland in humans and mammals [1]. DHEA and its sulfated derivative DHEAS are multifunctional steroids with actions in a wide variety of physiological systems, with effects on the brain [2], immune systems [3], and somatic growth and development [4, 5]. Although DHEA and DHEAS were identified more than 50 years ago, there remains some uncertainty as to their physiological significance, full mechanisms of action [6–9], and their roles in human disease.

In humans, DHEA is a crucial precursor of sex steroid biosynthesis and exerts indirect endocrine and intracrine actions following conversion to androgens and estrogens. In addition, DHEA acts as a neurosteroid via its effects on neurotransmitter receptors in the brain. The potential health significance of DHEA in humans is highlighted by the observation that serum concentrations decrease steadily with age, approaching lowest concentrations around the time at which many diseases of aging, particularly neurocognitive decline, become apparent. The age-related decline in DHEA levels [10] has led to the suggestion that this is associated with a decrease in cognitive function as well as the increased rates of neuronal degeneration and dysfunction that occur during aging [11, 12]. Other studies have reported altered DHEA serum concentrations in patients with conditions such as schizophrenia [13], dementia [14], and Alzheimer's disease (AD) [13, 15–18]. Due to these associations, DHEAS has been widely publicized both in the lay press [19, 20] and in the scientific literature [21, 22] for their putative anti-aging and neuroprotective effects. This has sparked controversial speculation that DHEA treatment might be a remedy for neuropsychiatric and neurodegenerative disorders [7, 23–27] and, even more optimistically, that it is a hormone with the potential to increase the life span [28].

As promising as these speculations may seem, there are many contradictions about the roles of DHEA in normal and degenerative brain function. This is especially evident when comparing preclinical and clinical data. For example, studies in animals show a myriad of neuroprotective and trophic effects of DHEAS in development and disease, while clinical studies show inconsistent, and sometimes highly conflicting, results. Clinical studies of neurodegenerative diseases have variously reported increased or decreased DHEAS concentrations in serum, cerebrospinal fluid, and brain tissue, leading to doubt as to the role of DHEA in the neuropathology of aging. It has been suggested that the incongruity in measured DHEAS concentrations may lie in the methodological differences used to sample DHEAS; however, it is possible that these changes are indicative of a more nuanced and multifaceted role. There is consistent evidence that DHEA is neuroprotective with respect to oxidative stress, neuroinflammation, and excitotoxicity, and thus it is possible that DHEA assists the defense of the brain and has a beneficial effect on cognition in healthy brains. Therefore, it is the aim of this review to briefly discuss the physiology of DHEA and its synthesis and secretion during development and aging and to discuss the relationship between alterations in DHEA concentrations and cognition. We further discuss the possible role of DHEAS in a variety of disease states, including AD, and acute illnesses such as schizophrenia, with focus on the fact that these conditions are characterized by imbalances in oxidative stress, neuroinflammation, and excitotoxicity.

2. The physiology of DHEA

In humans, DHEA is one of the most abundant hormones synthesized and secreted by the adrenal cortex. This C19 steroid displays an episodic and diurnal rhythm of synthesis and release that parallels that of cortisol [29, 30]. The major synthetic pathways for DHEA and DHEAS are shown in **Figure 1**. The *de novo* synthesis of DHEA from cholesterol depends on the presence and activity of the mitochondrial enzyme steroidogenic acute regulatory protein (StAR), the microsomal enzyme cytochrome P450 enzyme 17α-hydroxylase /17,20 lyase (P450c17), and the accessory hemoprotein cytochrome b5 (Cytb5) [32]. Importantly, P450c17 and Cytb5 need to be colocalized, because the function of Cytb5 is to selectively enhance the 17,20-lyase activity of P450c17 [33–35].

DHEAS is the precursor of approximately 50% of androgens in adult men, 75% of active estrogens in premenopausal women, and almost 100% of active estrogens after menopause [36]. DHEA has a 3- to 10-fold predominance of androgenic over estrogenic activity [37], and although a small portion of the circulating pool of DHEA is of gonadal origin in men and women, the majority of DHEA, and virtually all DHEAS, is produced by the adrenal cortex [1]. However, DHEA is also synthesized in the brain, from cholesterol and other hormonal precursors, primarily by astrocytes and oligodendrocytes; indeed, much higher concentrations of DHEAS are found in the brain than in the serum, suggesting that the DHEAS is primarily synthesized *in situ*, rather than being transported across the blood-brain barrier [38].

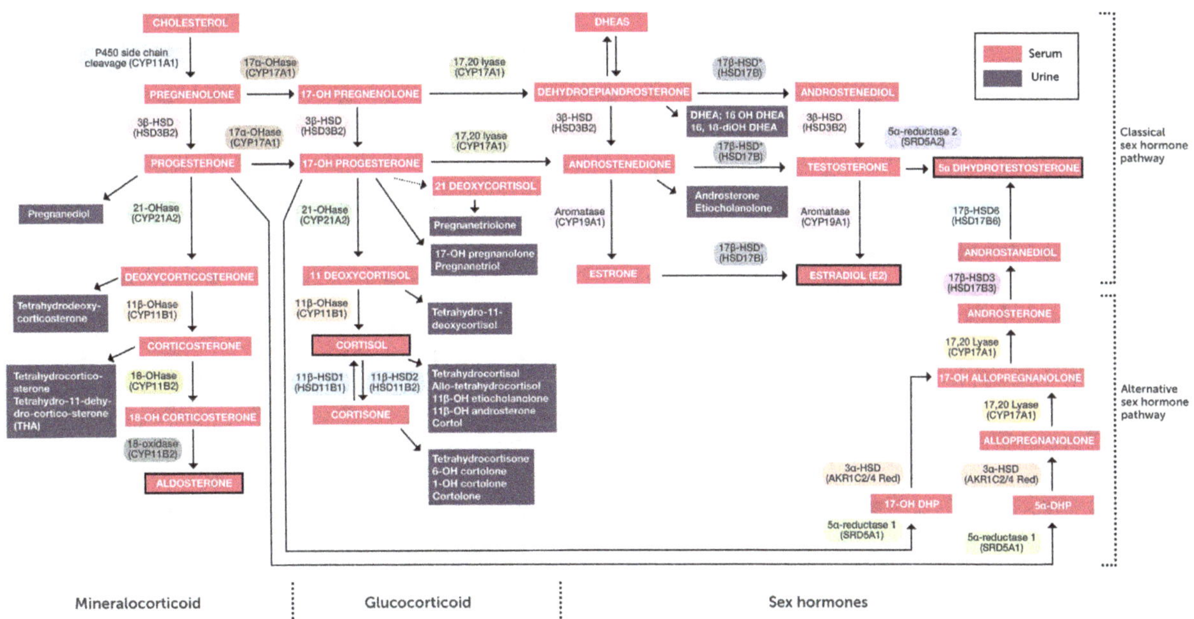

Figure 1. The complete steroid pathway showing the formation of DHEA from pregnenolone and 17OH-pregnenolone, and its reversible sulfation, and disposition via androstenes to estradiol and 5α-dihydrotestosterone. Steroid metabolites identified in serum and urines are shown in light gray boxes and dark gray boxes, respectively. From Greaves et al. [31].

The specific receptors that bind DHEA as a ligand have been of great interest for over 20 years. The biological actions of DHEA and its metabolites are mediated through androgen receptors or estrogen receptors, which belong to the nuclear receptor steroid-receptor subfamily [39]. DHEA has been found to exert both agonistic and antagonistic effects on the androgen receptor, and it acts as an agonist at both the estrogen receptor-α and estrogen receptor-β sites, with a binding preference for estrogen receptor-β [40, 41]. In the brain, DHEA is thought to affect neuronal excitability by modulating the *N*-methyl-D-aspartate (NMDA) [42–44] and sigma receptors [45], and as a positive allosteric modulator of the Gamma-aminobutyric acid type A ($GABA_{A)}$ receptor [46–49]. In addition to this, DHEA has been shown to be a selective antagonist of the glucocorticoid receptor (GR) [50].

2.1. DHEA and DHEAS synthesis during development and aging

In humans, the patterns of DHEA synthesis and secretion change markedly throughout life. In the last months of gestation, the fetal adrenal can synthesize and release considerable amounts of DHEA and DHEAS, which together with estrogen and progesterone produced by the placenta play pivotal roles in the maintenance and endocrine control of pregnancy [51]. Although the plasma concentrations of DHEAS remain high in the newborn, they decrease quickly as the fetal zone of the adrenal gland involutes after birth. From 1 to 6 years of age, the adrenal gland secretes very low concentrations of DHEAS and androstenedione [52]. However at approximately 7–8 years of age, the adrenal zona reticularis increases the production of DHEAS and androstenedione, all of which are C_{19} steroids that exert androgenic activity in several tissues by converting into potent androgens [36]. This pre-pubertal phenomenon is known as adrenarche, a biochemical, endocrine, and morphological event hypothesized to have evolved only in humans and higher primates. From an evolutionary point of view, adrenarche may be related to the highly coordinated events associated with human growth and organ maturation, particularly of the brain [53–55].

Following the onset of adrenarche, plasma concentrations of DHEAS differ between the sexes, with levels of DHEAS being about 2-fold higher in males than in females (**Figure 2**). This difference may reflect secretion of these androgens by the testes [10, 57], but it has also been proposed that the higher concentration of DHEAS in men may be attributable to steroid sulfatase, which degrades androgens. The gene for steroid sulfatase is located on the X chromosome, and in having only one copy of the gene, men may have less steroid sulfatase and consequently higher DHEAS concentrations [58].

Maximal plasma concentrations of DHEAS normally occur at 20–30 years of age (**Figure 2**), followed by a progressive decline in adrenal production in both males and females, until serum concentrations of DHEAS return to pre-adrenarche levels in persons over 80 years of age [59, 60]. The magnitude of this decline is such that serum levels of DHEAS in elderly adults are only around 10–20% of those in young adults [1, 61]. The diminution in adrenal androgens with aging is often termed 'adrenopause.' It has been suggested that adrenopause is associated with a generalized reduction in the 17,20 lyase activity of P450c17 in the zona reticularis of the adrenal gland [62]. Interestingly, it has been shown that the zona reticularis of older men is reduced in size when compared to the adrenals of young men [63], suggesting that at least part of the age-associated

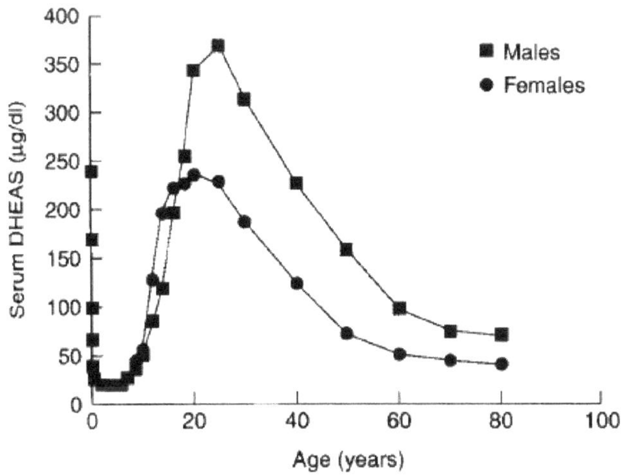

Figure 2. Concentrations of serum DHEAS as a function of age in females and males. Values are high in cord blood and immediately after birth, fall in the first months of life as the fetal adrenal zone involutes, and remain low until the onset of adrenarche at about age 8 years in girls and age 9 years in boys. Peak DHEAS concentrations are usually higher in males than in females. In both sexes, the concentrations of DHEAS decline slowly during the adult years. From Miller [56].

decrease in adrenal androgens might relate to a reduction in the number of DHEA-secreting cells in the zona reticularis itself. Although the underlying mechanisms regarding this change must be further elucidated, the temporal association between falling DHEA concentrations and the onset of age-related diseases has led many investigators to suggest that some age-related neurological disorders such as AD and dementia may be partly attributable to the decrease in systemic DHEA concentrations [11].

2.2. DHEA and cognition

The gradual decline in serum concentrations from the peak at 20–30 years of age has led to speculations that low DHEA concentrations could have a negative effect on cognitive function in later life. It has been hypothesized that rise in DHEA concentrations from 6 to 8 years until 20–30 years of age might be associated with the extended period of cortical maturation in humans [55]. While numerous animal studies have shown that DHEA can modulate cognitive performance, the outcomes of such studies in humans are less clear. For example, one study reported that DHEA supplementation improves cognitive performance in young men [64], whereas other studies detected no benefit in an older group who were predominantly male and were HIV-1 seropositive [65]. DHEA supplementation does not appear to improve cognition in the elderly [66].

A study evaluating the cognitive domains of working memory, executive function, and word processing speed in men and women aged between 60 and 88 years with low serum DHEAS concentrations found a positive association between serum DHEAS and working memory [67]. However, the relationship was sex-specific, with a trend toward a better executive function in men only. Other studies in males have shown that increased endogenous androgen concentrations (following cessation of chemical castration in males) resulted in improved performance on the Cambridge Cognitive Examination (part of the Cambridge Examination for Mental Disorders of the Elderly, a global measure of cognition and memory) and verbal recall tests [68]. A study in a population of older healthy women (aged 21–77 years) further indicated that women with high serum concentrations of DHEAS had increased performance on a variety of cognitive tests, including better verbal, visual, and spatial abilities; working memory; attention; concentration; and accuracy [69]. In older men and women in an Italian cohort, low DHEAS levels were significant predictors of accelerated decline in Mini-Mental State Examination score during the 3-year follow-up period [70]. Despite these associations, Mazat et al. [71] reported no significant role for serum DHEAS concentrations as a predictor of cognitive decline in an elderly population, while other studies conducted in frail elderly patients and nursing home residents found an inverse relationship between DHEAS levels and cognitive abilities [72, 73].

While the reasons for the conflicting data on DHEAS and cognition require further investigation, the changes in cognition are likely to be reflective of interactions with both the GABAergic and glutamatergic pathways, and possibly through the mediator brain-derived neurotrophic factor (BDNF). Neurosteroids have contrasting effects on $GABA_A$ receptors, which when activated result in chloride entry into the cell, hyperpolarization, and reduced membrane excitability [48]. Reduced metabolites of progesterone and deoxycorticosterone have an agonistic effect on $GABA_A$ receptors, resulting in chloride ion movement into the cell. In contrast, DHEAS is a $GABA_A$ antagonist and thus increases the likelihood of membrane depolarization [48, 74]. Animal studies have shown that acute exposure to DHEAS may facilitate basal synaptic transmission in the CA1 region of the hippocampus through the non-competitive potentiation of $GABA_A$ receptors [75–77]. In terms of learning and memory, studies have shown that acute administration of DHEAS facilitates primed-burst potentiation, but not the induction of long-term potentiation [78], whereas long-term potentiation is stimulated by the chronic administration of DHEAS [79].

In addition to $GABA_A$ receptor modulation, neurosteroids have been found to interact in a structure-specific manner with glutamatergic NMDA receptors. DHEAS potentiates the neuronal response to NMDA in the rat hippocampus [80]. These steroids also act as non-selective sigma-1 receptor antagonists [81], thus suppressing the activity of NMDA receptors, which are central to the process of excitotoxicity [82]. In addition, DHEAS may reduce the cytoplasmic Ca^{2+}-induced loss of mitochondrial membrane potential by preventing Ca^{2+} influx into the mitochondrial matrix [83]. The neuroprotective effect of DHEA against NMDA-induced excitotoxicity may also involve the calcium/nitric oxide signaling pathway, since DHEA has been shown to inhibit NMDA-induced nitric oxide synthase activity and the production of nitric oxide in primary cultures of hippocampal neurons [84].

The potential of DHEAS to modulate the activity of NMDA receptors through a variety of mechanisms is likely to underpin their capacity to protect neurons from excitotoxicity when high levels of extracellular glutamate are present. Of note, glutamate excitotoxicity has been implicated in AD [85] (discussed further below), where a reduction in neurosteroid production may compromise the intrinsic defense mechanisms of the central nervous system (CNS). Another possible mechanism by which DHEAS could promote neurogenesis and neuronal survival in the CNS is through the mediation of the neurotrophin BDNF [86, 87].

BDNF is expressed in several areas of the CNS and is necessary for cell proliferation and differentiation [88, 89]. In addition, BDNF plays a vital role in neural plasticity, enhances long-term potentiation, and promotes learning and memory [90, 91]. As such, a mutation or deletion of the BDNF gene in mice results in learning deficits and long-term potentiation impairment [92, 93], as well as decreased learning and memory in behavioral paradigms [90]. In humans, low plasma BDNF is associated with impairments in memory and general cognitive function in aging women [94].

A recent study investigated the effect of DHEA on cognition and learning in a rat model of vascular dementia [86] and found that DHEA treatment significantly preserved working and reference memory, which was accompanied by a significant increase in the levels of acetylcholine, norepinephrine, and dopamine in the brain. Of note was a significant increase in the hippocampal expression of BDNF after DHEA treatment [86]. In a rodent model, Naert et al., [95] showed that DHEAS treatment can lead to biphasic increases in BDNF in the hippocampus and amygdala, but decreased BDNF concentrations in the hypothalamus. It is interesting to note that glucocorticoids are also involved in BDNF regulation [27, 96], where stress has been found to decrease the expression of BDNF, leading to neuronal atrophy and degeneration in the hippocampus and the cortex, a process that may be common to both development and aging [97, 98]. These findings are important, considering, that BDNF expression is also altered in acute psychiatric disorders such as major depression [99, 100] and schizophrenia [101], as well as in neurodegenerative diseases such as AD [102].

2.3. DHEA and AD

AD is a chronic neurodegenerative disorder characterized by progressive memory loss and cognitive deterioration. It is the most common form of dementia, affecting about 50 million people worldwide [103], with the majority of cases in the elderly population, which presents global health and economic challenges [104]. Currently, there are no disease-modifying therapies available to treat AD [105], and it represents a major unmet need in neurological research and patient management. The neuropathological hallmarks of AD include neurofibrillary tangles, which are formed when the neuronal cytoskeletal protein tau becomes hyperphosphorylated and precipitates, and also amyloid plaques, which are abnormal deposits of extracellular protein that accumulate after cleavage of the β-amyloid precursor protein [106]. Other degenerative changes include cerebral amyloid angiopathy, glial inflammatory responses, and synaptic loss. These processes ultimately lead to neuronal atrophy, white matter loss, and a reduction in the volumes of the entorhinal, temporal, and frontal cortices as well as the hippocampus [107], followed by devastating clinical sequelae and resultant morbidity and mortality [108].

Sporadic AD is the predominant form of the disease, present in more than 95% of patients, and it usually occurs after 65 years of age [109]. The etiology of sporadic AD is multifactorial and may be associated with a number of risk factors including advancing age [110, 111], increased oxidative stress [112, 113], autoimmunity [114], and excess glucocorticoids [115–117]. Although serum DHEA levels decrease with age, the majority of studies have reported that serum DHEAS levels in AD patients are even lower than in age-matched healthy controls. For instance, Yanase et al. [18] found that patients with AD or cerebrovascular dementia had lower concentrations of serum DHEAS and a lower DHEAS/DHEA ratio when compared to controls. Several other clinical studies have reported lower serum concentrations of DHEAS in patients with AD [14, 118–120], a reduction paralleled by decreases in the brain and cerebral spinal fluid [121, 122]. For instance, Weill-Engerer and colleagues [108] reported that not only are brain levels of DHEAS significantly lower in AD, but also the lower levels are inversely correlated with the presence of phosphorylated tau and β-amyloid. A few studies have not detected differences in serum DHEAS concentrations between AD patients and controls [120, 123], and there is one report that serum DHEAS levels are increased in mild-moderate AD [124]. The reasons for these differences between studies have not yet been elucidated.

In contrast to the majority of studies, Naylor and colleagues [125] reported that cerebral spinal fluid levels of DHEA are significantly elevated in AD, as are tissue levels in the temporal cortex, with the extent of elevation being correlated with disease severity, as assessed by the burden of β-amyloid plaques. Similarly, Brown and colleagues [126] reported increased DHEA concentrations in the brains and cerebral spinal fluid of patients with AD when compared with controls, even though mean serum concentrations of DHEA did not differ. Interestingly, in this study, DHEA concentrations were highest in the hippocampus of AD patients, a region that does not express P450c17. Brown and colleagues speculated that the higher concentrations of DHEA in the hippocampus may have been produced by an as-yet-unknown pathway that involved the oxidation of an unknown precursor. This speculation has been given support by the finding that the addition of redox-active ferrous iron to serum samples causes a significant increase in the amount of detectable DHEA [127]. It is also supported by the demonstration that oxidative stress associated with the presence of β-amyloid treatment induces DHEA synthesis in human and rodent cells *in vitro* [126–129]. In this context, it is interesting that the brain regions containing the higher concentrations of DHEA [126] also have higher burdens of neuritic plaques and β-amyloid immunoreactivity, features that are generally associated with AD progression [130]. It may be significant that DHEA protects HT-22 cells (an immortalized mouse hippocampal cell line) against amyloid β protein toxicity in a dose-dependent manner [131].

Another link to the pathogenesis and progression of AD comes from the anti-inflammatory properties of DHEA [132]. Hence, the local production of DHEA in the AD brain may function, at least in part, to reduce the level of inflammation that would otherwise be injurious to neurons if left unchecked. Serum levels of DHEAS have been shown to negatively correlate with serum interleukin-6 (IL-6), to inhibit IL-6 secretion from human mononuclear cells [133], and to inhibit cytokine-stimulated, NF-κB–mediated transcription, partly through an anti-oxidant property [134]. Interestingly, elevated levels of IL-6 are consistently detected in the brains of AD patients, but not in the brains of non-demented elderly persons [135]. Several studies have suggested that an increase of circulating IL-6 in AD patients indicates immune activation and may be related to the pathophysiology of AD [136–138].

Perhaps the most intriguing link between DHEA and AD comes from its association with systemic stress and glucocorticoid production, which has lead to the hypothesis that chronic stress is an important factor in AD pathogenesis [139]. Epidemiological evidence supports a role for stress in AD because elderly individuals prone to psychological distress are more likely to develop the disorder than age-matched, nonstressed individuals [117]. Cortisol is the most prominent stress-related glucocorticoid in human serum. Serum cortisol levels are elevated in patients with AD [140], as are the levels of urinary cortisol [141]. It is pertinent that the overactivation of $GABA_A$ receptors plays a central role in anxiety disorders and consequently these receptors are the principal targets of anxiolytic drugs for the treatment of affective disorders [142]. Since DHEAS antagonizes $GABA_A$ receptors, they are thought to act as endogenous anxiolytics, and hence a reduction in the availability of DHEAS in aging or AD could contribute to increased anxiety and stimulate the chronic production of cortisol.

Animal experiments have shown that excess concentrations of glucocorticoids during prolonged periods of stress can have deleterious effects on the brain, especially in aged animals, and particularly affecting the hippocampus [143]. Glucocorticoids exert several actions on the brain, including the stimulation of glutamatergic neurotransmission via the stimulation of glucocorticoid receptors (GR), which if left unchecked can lead to excitotoxicity. Several studies have shown that DHEA can protect against the effects of glucocorticoid-mediated neurotoxicity [144, 145]. The neuroprotective effects of DHEA have been modeled *in vivo* where the toxic effects of corticosterone in the dentate gyrus of male rats were suppressed by low concentrations of DHEA [146]. The protection conferred by DHEA may be via downregulating the expression of glucocorticoid receptors [147]. In cultured HT-22 cells, DHEA augmentation suppresses the nuclear localization of the GR in response to glutamate toxicity, as assessed by immunohistochemistry [131]. Thus, inhibition of GR translocation into the nucleus is a possible mechanism of DHEA's anti-glucocorticoid effects. DHEA administration reduces GR expression in hippocampal cells in the mouse [131] and reduces glucocorticoid receptors by 50% in the rat liver [145]. Furthermore, DHEA may act as a GR antagonist and can attenuate the translocation of stress-activated protein kinase-3 in rat hippocampal primary cultures [148].

DHEA may also attenuate the neurotoxic effects of cortisol by reducing the regeneration of active glucocorticoids. The 7α-hydroxylated metabolite of DHEA (7α-hydroxy-DHEA) has antiglucocorticoid effects in target tissues by competition with 11-keto glucocorticoids for access to 11β-hydroxysteroid dehydrogenase-1 [149]. Enzyme kinetic data from yeast-expressed human 11β- hydroxysteroid dehydrogenase imply that 7α-hydroxysteroid substrates are preferred to cortisone by this enzyme [150]. Therefore, in tissues such as the brain, 7α-hydroxy-DHEA may act as an endogenous inhibitor of 11β- hydroxysteroid dehydrogenase, thereby reducing the regeneration of active glucocorticoids [151]. 7α-hydroxy-DHEA may have more potent bioactivity and stronger neuroprotective and antiglucocorticoid effects than DHEA itself [152]. Interestingly, some investigators have hypothesized that the degree of metabolism of DHEA to 7α-hydroxy-DHEA is related to the pathology of AD [122, 151, 153, 154]. This is evident in the study by Yau et al. [151], which found that gene expression for cytochrome P4507b (which converts DHEA into 7α-hydroxy-DHEA) was significantly decreased in hippocampal dentate neurons from patients with AD when compared to controls [151]. Another study found lower plasma 7α-hydroxy-DHEA concentrations in patients with AD when compared to controls [154].

Taken together, the preceding observations are generally supportive of the view that DHEAS levels in serum are reduced in AD when compared to those in healthy age-matched controls.

Given that DHEAS reduces oxidative stress and neuroinflammation, protects against glutamate excitotoxicity, and minimizes the negative effects of cortisol on the brain, the reduced levels of serum DHEAS are likely to increase the vulnerability of the brain to these factors. While limited evidence suggests that the brain may compensate by increasing the local production of DHEAS, this may not be sufficient to slow the pathogenesis of the disease.

2.4. DHEA in schizophrenia

In addition to neurodegenerative diseases, there is evidence that low levels of circulating DHEA with normal levels of glucocorticoids (cortisol) place the developing brain at risk for a range of acute neuropsychiatric disorders, including major depressive disorder, bipolar disorder, and anxiety [155–158]. It is further hypothesized that abnormalities of the hypothalamic-pituitary-adrenal (HPA) axis play a central role in the pathogenesis and etiology of schizophrenia [159–161]. Low ratios of DHEA to cortisol have been noted in patients with schizophrenia and are positively associated with the severity of depression, state and trait anxiety, anger, and hostility [155]. DHEA augmentation in affected patients has been seen to attenuate the severity of some negative symptoms associated with this mental illness, including lack of volition and drive, and social withdrawal [16, 162].

Previous studies have found evidence of abnormal dopaminergic activity [163] and deficits in GABAergic and glutamatergic activity [164] in the brain tissue of patients with schizophrenia. Neuroactive steroids such as DHEA modulate the activity of these neurotransmitter systems, both directly and indirectly, and therefore may contribute to the pathophysiology of the illness [82, 165–168]. A number of studies [169] have reported elevated plasma levels of DHEA and DHEAS in severely psychotic male subjects [170, 171], medicated patients with chronic schizophrenia [172], and nonmedicated first-episode patients [170, 173] compared with controls. Elevated DHEA levels have been detected in the *post-mortem* brain tissue of schizophrenic patients in both the posterior cingulate and parietal cortex [171]. In addition to this, the levels of allopregnanolone are significantly lower in the schizophrenic parietal cortex when compared with healthy controls, whereas pregnenolone levels are significantly higher [49]. Since both of these neurosteroids are downstream metabolites of DHEA, these data suggest that DHEA is preferentially metabolized to pregnenolone in patients with schizophrenia [49]. As DHEA is a positive modulator of excitatory NMDA receptors, and allopregnanolone is a positive modulator of the inhibitory $GABA_A$ receptors, the shift in the ratio of DHEA:allopregnanolone could favor a net increase in neuronal excitation [49], similar to the alterations in brain neurotransmitter systems seen in schizophrenia patients.

As a result of the positive modulatory effects of DHEA on NMDA receptors [49], in addition to its capacity to enhance learning and memory in rodent models [174], it may be speculated that an elevation of DHEA levels reflects a compensatory process in the schizophrenic brain. It is possible that subjects with schizophrenia may be physiologically resistant to DHEA action in some manner (potentially resulting in the increased synthesis of this neurosteroid) or that there is dysregulation in a feedback system involving the HPA axis [175]. Specifically, DHEA increases following cortisol-releasing hormone [49] and adrenocorticotropic hormone [176] administration in humans, and persistent DHEA elevations may reflect a prolonged upregulation of this axis [177].

As noted earlier, DHEA can protect neurons from glutamate excitotoxicity, β-amyloid toxicity, and oxidative stress [49, 131], and furthermore, oxidative stress can lead to increased DHEA formation [84, 178]. Oxidative stressors may therefore stimulate DHEA levels in schizophrenic patients [126], in an adaptive change to other precipitating disease factors.

However, other studies have found no difference in DHEA levels between schizophrenic and control subjects [49], and some studies have reported significantly reduced plasma DHEA concentrations [179–181], particularly in the morning [180, 182, 183], as well as abnormal DHEA diurnal rhythms [184] in schizophrenics compared with matched controls. Furthermore, DHEA augmentation has been found to be effective in the management of depressive and anxiety symptoms of patients with schizophrenia [185], suggesting that higher levels of circulating DHEA in schizophrenic populations may be associated with superior functioning [16]. The inconsistency between studies is understandable in view of the wide clinical polymorphism, variability of psychometric properties (distress and anxiety), drug treatment, and clinical responsiveness of schizophrenia patients to their antipsychotic treatment [169].

It may be difficult to interpret the significance of elevated or decreased DHEA levels in the absence of concentrations of other HPA axis hormones. Dysregulation of the HPA axis described in schizophrenia [13] includes increased basal cortisol levels [186], cortisol nonsuppression on the dexamethasone suppression test [187], increased adrenocorticotropic hormone and cortisol response to the dexamethasone/cortisol releasing hormone challenge test [188], and increases in glucocorticoid receptor mRNA as observed *post-mortem* [189]. DHEA and cortisol are both cleaved from 17-hydroxypregnenolone and are adrenocorticotropic hormone regulated [190]. It is not clear, therefore, if an elevated DHEA concentration is specific to a particular disease state or due to a generalized overactivation of the HPA axis. This difference is of functional significance as DHEA possesses antiglucocorticoid properties and may protect against some of the deleterious effects of persistently elevated cortisol levels [145]. This can be clarified by determining the cortisol/DHEA ratio, which may be a more appropriate measurement than DHEA alone [191]. If the biological response to stress is impaired among schizophrenia patients, it is possible that the cortisol/DHEA ratio would be elevated as a result of stress associated with the illness [192].

There is also evidence for oligodendrocyte and myelin dysfunction in neuropathologies such as schizophrenia and bipolar affective disorder, where alterations in the cortisol/DHEA ratio have been observed [16, 17, 155]. Some key oligodendrocyte and myelination genes (such as proteolipid protein 1 and myelin-associated glycoprotein), and transcription factors that regulate the expression of these genes, are downregulated in brains of schizophrenia and bipolar subjects [193]. Together, these studies indicate that common pathophysiological pathways may govern the disease phenotypes of schizophrenia, as well as other neurodegenerative diseases that specifically involve oligodendrocytes.

3. Conclusion

A significant body of preclinical research investigating the biological actions of DHEA have shown that this steroid, and its sulfated congener DHEAS, has a multifunctional role in a variety of physiological systems, including in the developing and aging brain. A summary of the actions of DHEA relevant to the discussion above is shown in **Table 1**. The present review has highlighted the involvement of DHEAS in glutamatergic and GABAergic

DHEA	Effects/function
Receptor interactions:	Agonistic and antagonistic effects on AR, agonist at ERα and ERβ [40, 41]
	Modulates the NMDA receptor [42–44]
	Positive allosteric modulator of the GABA-A receptor [46–49]
	Nonselective sigma-1 receptor antagonist [81]
	Selective antagonist of the GR [50]
Development & regeneration:	Maintenance and endocrine control of pregnancy [51]
	Associated with human growth and organ maturation, particularly of the brain, during adrenarche [53–55]
	Promotes neurogenesis and neuronal survival in the CNS through the mediation of BDNF [86, 87]
Memory and learning:	DHEAS may facilitate basal synaptic transmission in the CA1 region of the hippocampus [75–77]
	Acute DHEAS administration facilitates primed-burst potentiation [78] and chronic administration of DHEAS stimulates LTP [79]
	DHEA treatment significantly preserves working and reference memories and increases acetylcholine, norepinephrine, and dopamine concentrations in the rat brain [86]
Neuroprotection: *Anti-excitatory actions*	Reduces the cytoplasmic Ca^{2+}-induced loss of mitochondrial membrane potential by preventing Ca^{2+} influx into the mitochondrial matrix [83]
	Inhibits NMDA-induced nitric oxide synthase activity and the production of nitric oxide in primary cultures of hippocampal neurons [84]
	Protect neurons from glutamate excitotoxicity, β-amyloid toxicity, and oxidative stress [49, 131]
Anti-inflammatory actions	Inhibits IL-6 secretion from human mononuclear cells [133]
	Inhibits cytokine-stimulated, NF-κB–mediated transcription, partly through an antioxidant property [134]
Antiglucocorticoid actions	GR antagonist and can attenuate the translocation of stress-activated protein kinase-3 in rat hippocampal primary cultures [148]
	Suppresses the nuclear localization of the GR in response to glutamate toxicity and inhibition of GR translocation into the nucleus [131]
	Downregulation of the expression of glucocorticoid receptors [147]
	Reduces the regeneration of active glucocorticoids [149]

Abbreviations: AR, androgen receptor; BDNF, brain-derived neurotrophic factor; CNS, central nervous system; DHEA, dehydroepiandrosterone; DHEAS, dehydroepiandrosterone sulfate; ER, estrogen receptor; GABA-A, Gamma-aminobutyric acid receptor A; GR, glucocorticoid receptor; IL-6, interleukin 6; LTP, long-term potentiation; NMDA, N-methyl-D-aspartate.

Table 1. Summary of functions of DHEA related to development and aging.

neurotransmission, where this neurohormone acts as an important modulator of neuronal excitability. Consequently, perturbations in the level of DHEA can affect cognition and mood. DHEAS has also been shown to respond to stress and to modulate the effects of cortisol on the brain. Reductions in the availability of DHEAS can increase the likelihood of glutamate excitotoxicity as well as exacerbate the deleterious effects of cortisol. Evidence indicates that the brain is not dependent on serum levels of DHEA as it is able to synthesis DHEAS *in situ*. Indeed, there appears to be a capacity to produce DHEA in direct response to oxidative stress. We have shown that in AD, the levels of DHEA are depleted, and the subsequent loss of protection from glutamate, cortisol, and oxidative stress may contribute to the pathogenesis of the disease. Conversely, in schizophrenia, there appears to be an elevation in the availability of DHEA, and this may act to decrease the influence of the GABAergic inhibitory pathways in favor of excitatory neurotransmission. While these emerging roles for DHEA are exciting, the present review also highlighted the discordant findings in the clinical literature, and it is clear that much remains to be learned about the contribution of DHEAS to brain function in both health and disease.

Acknowledgements

The authors are grateful for support and many discussions from Dr. Udani Ratnayake, Dr. Stacey Ellery, Dr. Margie Castillo-Melendez, and Dr. Hayley Dickinson from The Ritchie Centre, Hudson Institute of Medical Research, and from Professor Jonathan Hirst, University of Newcastle, New South Wales, Australia. Tracey Quinn received support from an Australian Post-graduate Award (APA) postgraduate scholarship for some of the studies reported above. Tracey Quinn and David Walker are grateful for funding from National Health & Medical Research Council of Australia and Cerebral Palsy Alliance. We also acknowledge generous support from the Victorian Government Infrastructure Fund to the Hudson Institute of Medical Research.

Author details

Tracey A. Quinn[1], Stephen R. Robinson[2] and David Walker[2*]

*Address all correspondence to: david.walker@rmit.edu.au

1 The Ritchie Centre, Monash University, Melbourne, Australia

2 School of Health and Biomedical Sciences, RMIT University, Melbourne, Australia

References

[1] Parker CR. Dehydroepiandrosterone and dehydroepiandrosterone sulfate production in the human adrenal during development and aging. Steroids. 1999;**64**:640-647

[2] Kroboth PD, Salek FS, Pittenger AL, Fabian TJ, Frye RF. DHEA and DHEA-S: A review. Journal of Clinical Pharmacology. 1999;**39**:327-348

[3] Chen CC, Parker Jr CR. Adrenal androgens and the immune system. Seminars in Reproductive Medicine. 2004;**22**:369-377

[4] Arquitt AB, Stoecker BJ, Hermann JS, Winterfeldt EA. Dehydroepiandrosterone sulfate, cholesterol, hemoglobin, and anthropometric measures related to growth in male adolescents. Journal of the American Dietetic Association. 1991;**91**:575-579

[5] Zemel BS, Katz SH. The contribution of adrenal and gonadal androgens to the growth in height of adolescent males. American Journal of Physical Anthropology. 1986;**71**:459-466

[6] Johnson M, Bebb R, Sirrs S. Uses of DHEA in aging and other disease states. Ageing Research Reviews. 2002;**1**:29-41

[7] Allolio B, Arlt W. DHEA treatment: Myth or reality? Trends in Endocrinology & Metabolism. 2002;**13**:288-294

[8] Eberling P, Koivisto V. Physiological importance of dehydroepiandrosterone. The Lancet. 1994;**343**:1479-1481

[9] Widstrom RL, Dillon JS. Is There a Receptor for Dehydroepiandrosterone or Dehydroepiandrosterone Sulfate?: Seminars in Reproductive Medicine. New York, NY, USA: Thieme Medical Publishers, Inc.; 2004;**22**:289-298

[10] Rainey WE, Carr BR, Sasano H, Suzuki T, Mason JI. Dissecting human adrenal androgen production. Trends in Endocrinology & Metabolism. 2002;**13**:234-239

[11] Berr C, Lafont S, Debuire B, Dartigues JF, Baulieu EE. Relationships of dehydroepiandrosterone sulfate in the elderly with functional, psychological, and mental status, and short-term mortality: A french community-based study. Proceedings of the National Academy of Sciences of the United States of America. 1996;**93**:13410-13415

[12] Krug A, Ziegler C, Bornstein S. DHEA and DHEA-S, and their functions in the brain and adrenal medulla. In: Ritsner M, Weizman A, editors. Neuroactive Steroids in Brain Function, Behavior and Neuropsychiatric Disorders. The Netherlands: Springer; 2008. p. 227-239

[13] Ritsner M, Gibel A, Maayan R, Ratner Y, Ram E, Biadsy H, Modai I, Weizman A, Ritsner M, Gibel A, Ram E, Maayan R, Weizman A. Alterations in DHEA metabolism in schizophrenia: Two-month case-control study. European Neuropsychopharmacology. 2006;**16**:137-146

[14] Aldred S, Mecocci P. Decreased dehydroepiandrosterone (DHEA) and dehydroepiandrosterone sulfate (DHEA-S) concentrations in plasma of Alzheimer's disease (AD) patients. Archives of Gerontology and Geriatrics. 2010;**51**:e16-e18

[15] Ritsner M, Maayan R, Gibel A, Weizman A. Differences in blood pregnenolone and dehydroepiandrosterone levels between schizophrenia patients and healthy subjects. European Neuropsychopharmacology. 2007;**17**:358-365

[16] Strous RD, Maayan R, Lapidus R, Stryjer R, Lustig M, Kotler M, Weizman A. Dehydroepiandrosterone augmentation in the management of negative, depressive, and anxiety symptoms in schizophrenia. Archives of General Psychiatry. 2003;**60**:133-141

[17] Gallagher P, Watson S, Smith MS, Young AH, Ferrier IN. Plasma cortisol-dehydroepiandrosterone (DHEA) ratios in schizophrenia and bipolar disorder. Schizophrenia Research. 2007;**90**:258-265

[18] Yanase T, Fukahori M, Taniguchi S, Nishi Y, Sakai Y, Takayanagi R, Haji M, Nawata H. Serum dehydroepiandrosterone (DHEA) and DHEA-sulfate (DHEA-S) in Alzheimer's disease and in cerebrovascular dementia. Endocrine Journal. 1996;**43**:119-123

[19] Wick G. Anti-aging'medicine: Does it exist? A critical discussion of 'anti-aging health products'. Experimental Gerontology. 2002;**37**:1137-1140

[20] Jaroff: New age therapy. Time 1995;**23**:52

[21] Morales AJ, Nolan JJ, Nelson JC, Yen S. Effects of replacement dose of dehydroepiandrosterone in men and women of advancing age. Journal of Clinical Endocrinology and Metabolism. 1994;**78**:1360-1367

[22] Nawata H, Yanase T, Goto K, Okabe T, Ashida K. Mechanism of action of anti-aging DHEA-S and the replacement of DHEA-S. Mechanisms of Ageing and Development. 2002;**123**:1101-1106

[23] Sands DE, Chamberlain GH. Treatment of inadequate personality in juveniles by dehydroisoandrosterone: preliminary report. British Medical Journal. 1952;**2**:66-68

[24] Strauss EB, Sands DE, Robinson AM, Tindall WJ, Stevenson WA. Use of dehydroisoandrosterone in psychiatric treatment: A preliminary survey. British Medical Journal. 1952;**2**:64-66

[25] Watson RR, Huls A, Araghinikuam M, Chung S. Dehydroepiandrosterone and diseases of aging. Drugs & Aging. 1996;**9**:274-291

[26] Bastianetto S, Ramassamy C, Poirier J, Quirion R. Dehydroepiandrosterone (DHEA) protects hippocampal cells from oxidative stress-induced damage. Molecular Brain Research. 1999;**66**:35-41

[27] Evans JG, Malouf R, Huppert F, van Niekerk JK: Dehydroepiandrosterone (DHEA) supplementation for cognitive function in healthy elderly people. Cochrane Database of Systematic Reviews 2006

[28] Olshansky SJ, Hayflick L, Carnes BA. No truth to the fountain of youth. Scientific American. 2004;**14**:98-102

[29] Rosenfeld R, Hellman L, Roffwarg H, Weitzman ED, Fukushima DK, Gallagher T. Dehydroisoandrosterone is secreted episodically and synchronously with cortisol by normal man. The Journal of Clinical Endocrinology and Metabolism. 1971;**33**:87-92

[30] Lejeune-Lenain C, Van Cauter E, Desir D, Beyloos M, Franckson J. Control of circadian and episodic variations of adrenal androgens secretion in man. Journal of Endocrinological Investigation. 1987;**10**:267

[31] Greaves RF et al. Clinical Chemistry and Laboratory Medicine. 2017;**55**(4):522-529

[32] Parker CR, Staton B, Grilliot M. Ontogeny of cytochrome b-5 and cytochrome p450c17 in the human fetal adrenal gland during normal development. Endocrine Research. 2004; **30**:541-542

[33] Kominami S, Ogawa N, Morimune R, Huang DY, Takemori S. The role of cytochrome-b5 in adrenal microsomal steroidogenesis. Journal of Steroid Biochemistry and Molecular Biology. 1992;**42**:57-64

[34] Katagiri M, Kagawa N, Waterman MR. The role of cytochrome b5 in the biosynthesis of androgens by human p450c17. Archives of Biochemistry and Biophysics. 1995; **317**:343-347

[35] Nguyen AD, Corbin CJ, Pattison JC, Bird IM, Conley AJ. The developmental increase in adrenocortical 17,20-lyase activity (biochemical adrenarche) is driven primarily by increasing cytochrome b5 in neonatal rhesus macaques. Endocrinology. 2009; **150**:1748-1756

[36] Labrie F, Bélanger A, Luu-The V, Labrie C, Simard J, Cusan L, Gomez J-L, Candas B. DHEA and the intracrine formation of androgens and estrogens in peripheral target tissues: Its role during aging. Steroids. 1998;**63**:322-328

[37] Labrie C, Flamand M, Belanger A, Labrie F. High bioavailability of dehydroepiandrosterone administered percutaneously in the rat. The Journal of Endocrinology. 1996; **150**:S107-S118

[38] Maninger N, Wolkowitz OM, Reus VI, Epel ES, Mellon SH. Neurobiological and neuropsychiatric effects of dehydroepiandrosterone (DHEA) and DHEA sulfate (DHEA-S). Frontiers in Neuroendocrinology. 2009;**30**:65-91

[39] Mangelsdorf DJ, Thummel C, Beato M, Herrlich P, Schütz G, Umesono K, Blumberg B, Kastner P, Mark M, Chambon P. The nuclear receptor superfamily: The second decade. Cell. 1995;**83**:835-839

[40] Chen F, Knecht K, Birzin E, Fisher J, Wilkinson H, Mojena M, Moreno CT, Schmidt A, Harada S-i, Freedman LP. Direct agonist/antagonist functions of dehydroepiandrosterone. Endocrinology. 2005;**146**:4568-4576

[41] Arnold JT, Blackman MR. Does DHEA exert direct effects on androgen and estrogen receptors, and does it promote or prevent prostate cancer? Endocrinology. 2005;**146**:4565-4567

[42] Holsboer F, Grasser A, Friess E, Wiedemann K. Steroid effects on central neurons and implications for psychiatric and neurological disorders. Brain Corticosteroid Receptors. 1994;**746**:345-361

[43] Baulieu EE. Neurosteroids: Of the nervous system, by the nervous system, for the nervous system. Recent Progress in Hormone Research. 1997;**52**:1-32

[44] Rupprecht R. The neuropsychopharmacological potential of neuroactive steroids. Journal of Psychiatric Research. 1997;**31**:297-314

[45] T-P S, London ED, Jaffe JH. Steroid binding at sigma receptors suggests a link between endocrine, nervous, and immune systems. Science. 1988;**240**:219-221

[46] FS W, Gibbs TT, Farb DH. Pregnenolone sulfate – A positive allosteric modulator at the N-methyl-D-aspartate receptor. Molecular Pharmacology. 1991;**40**:333-336

[47] Irwin RP, Lin SZ, Rogawski MA, Purdy RH, Paul SM. Steroid potentiation and inhibition of N-methyl-D-aspartate receptor-mediated intracellular Ca^{++} responses – structure-activity studies. Journal of Pharmacology and Experimental Therapeutics. 1994;**271**:677-682

[48] Compagnone NA, Mellon SH. Dehydroepiandrosterone: A potential signalling molecule for neocortical organization during development. Proceedings of the National Academy of Sciences of the United States of America. 1998;**95**:4678-4683

[49] Marx CE, Stevens RD, Shampine LJ, Uzunova V, Trost WT, Butterfield MI, Massing MW, Hamer RM, Morrow AL, Lieberman JA. Neuroactive steroids are altered in schizophrenia and bipolar disorder: Relevance to pathophysiology and therapeutics. Neuropsychopharmacology. 2006;**31**:1249-1263

[50] Sacco M, Valenti G, Corvi Mora P, FCW W, Ray DW. DHEA, a selective glucocorticoid receptor antagonist: Its role in immune system regulation and metabolism. Journal of Endocrinological Investigation. 2002;**25**:81-82

[51] Ishimoto H, Jaffe RB. Development and function of the human fetal adrenal cortex: A key component in the feto-placental unit. Endocrine Reviews. 2011;**32**:317-355

[52] de Peretti E, Forest MG. Pattern of plasma dehydroepiandrosterone sulfate levels in humans from birth to adulthood: Evidence for testicular production. The Journal of Clinical Endocrinology and Metabolism 1978;**47**:572-577

[53] Cutler GB, Glenn M, BUSH M, Hodgen GD, Graham CE, Loriaux DL. Adrenarche: A survey of rodents, domestic animals, and primates. Endocrinology. 1978;**103**:2112-2118

[54] Smail PJ, Faiman C, Hobson WC, Fuller GB, Winter JSD. Further studies on adrenarche in nonhuman primates. Endocrinology. 1982;**111**:844-848

[55] Campbell B. Adrenarche and the evolution of human life history. American Journal of Human Biology. 2006;**18**:569-589

[56] Miller WL. The molecular basis of premature adrenarche: An hypothesis. Acta Paediatrica. Supplementum. 1999;**433**:60-66

[57] Goto M, Hanley KP, Marcos J, Wood PJ, Wright S, Postle AD, Cameron IT, Mason JI, Wilson DI, Hanley NA. In humans, early cortisol biosynthesis provides a mechanism to safeguard female sexual development. Journal of Clinical Investigation. 2006;**116**:953-960

[58] Miller WL. Androgen synthesis in adrenarche. Reviews in Endocrine and Metabolic Disorders. 2009;**10**:3-17

[59] Bates K, Harvey AR, Carruthers M, Martins R. Androgens, andropause and neurodegeneration: Exploring the link between steroidogenesis, androgens and Alzheimer's disease. Cellular and Molecular Life Sciences. 2005;**62**:28

[60] Labrie F, Bélanger A, Cusan L, Gomez J-L, Candas B. Marked decline in serum concentrations of adrenal c19 sex steroid precursors and conjugated androgen metabolites during aging. Journal of Clinical Endocrinology & Metabolism. 1997;**82**:2396-2402

[61] Havelock JC, Auchus RJ, Rainey WE. The rise in adrenal androgen biosynthesis: Adrenarche. Seminars in Reproductive Medicine. 2004;**22**:337-347

[62] Dharia S, Slane A, Jian M, Conner M, Conley AJ, Brissie RM, Parker CR. Effects of aging on cytochrome b5 expression in the human adrenal gland. The Journal of Clinical Endocrinology and Metabolism. 2005;**90**:4357-4361

[63] Parker C, Mixon R, Brissie R, Grizzle W. Aging alters zonation in the adrenal cortex of men. The Journal of Clinical Endocrinology and Metabolism. 1997;**82**:3898-3901

[64] Alhaj HA, Massey AE, McAllister-Williams RH. Effects of DHEA administration on episodic memory, cortisol and mood in healthy young men: A double-blind, placebo-controlled study. Psychopharmacology. 2006;**188**:541-551

[65] Bradley M, McElhiney M, Rabkin J. DHEA and cognition in hiv-positive patients with non-major depression. Psychosomatics. 2012;**53**:244-249

[66] Grimley Evans J, Malouf R, Huppert FA, Van Niekerk JK. Dehydroepiandrosterone (DHEA) supplementation for cognitive function in healthy elderly people. The Cochrane Library. 2006

[67] Hildreth KL, Gozansky WS, Jankowski CM, Grigsby J, Wolfe P, Kohrt WM. Association of serum dehydroepiandrosterone sulfate and cognition in older adults: Sex steroid, inflammatory, and metabolic mechanisms. Neuropsychology. 2013;**27**:356

[68] Almeida OP, Waterreus A, Spry N, Flicker L, Martins RN. One year follow-up study of the association between chemical castration, sex hormones, beta-amyloid, memory and depression in men. Psychoneuroendocrinology. 2004;**29**:1071-1081

[69] Davis SR, Shah SM, McKenzie DP, Kulkarni J, Davison SL, Bell RJ. Dehydroepiandrosterone sulfate levels are associated with more favorable cognitive function in women. Journal of Clinical Endocrinology & Metabolism. 2008;**93**:801-808

[70] Valenti G, Ferrucci L, Lauretani F, Ceresini G, Bandinelli S, Luci M, Ceda G, Maggio M, Schwartz R. Dehydroepiandrosterone sulfate and cognitive function in the elderly: The inchianti study. Journal of Endocrinological Investigation. 2009;**32**:766-772

[71] Mazat L, Lafont S, Berr C, Debuire B, Tessier J-F, Dartigues J-F, Baulieu E-E. Prospective measurements of dehydroepiandrosterone sulfate in a cohort of elderly subjects: Relationship to gender, subjective health, smoking habits, and 10-year mortality. Proceedings of the National Academy of Sciences. 2001;**98**:8145-8150

[72] Morrison MF, Katz IR, Parmelee P, Boyce AA, TenHave T. Dehydroepiandrosterone sulfate (DHEA-S) and psychiatric and laboratory measures of frailty in a residential care population. The American Journal of Geriatric Psychiatry. 1998;**6**:277-284

[73] Breuer B, Martucci C, Wallenstein S, Likourezos A, Libow LS, Peterson A, Zumoff B. Relationship of endogenous levels of sex hormones to cognition and depression in frail, elderly women. The American Journal of Geriatric Psychiatry. 2002;**10**:311-320

[74] Demirgören S, Majewska M, Spivak CE, London E. Receptor binding and electrophysiological effects of dehydroepiandrosterone sulfate, an antagonist of the gaba a receptor. Neuroscience. 1991;**45**:127-135

[75] Park-Chung M, Malayev A, Purdy RH, Gibbs TT, Farb DH. Sulfated and unsulfated steroids modulate γ-aminobutyric acid a receptor function through distinct sites. Brain Research. 1999;**830**:72-87

[76] Majewska MD. Neuronal actions of dehydroepiandrosterone possible roles in brain development, aging, memory, and affect. Annals of the New York Academy of Sciences. 1995;**774**:111-120

[77] Meyer J, Lee S, Wittenberg G, Randall R, Gruol D. Neurosteroid regulation of inhibitory synaptic transmission in the rat hippocampus in vitro. Neuroscience. 1999;**90**:1177-1183

[78] Diamond DM, Branch BJ, Fleshner M. The neurosteroid dehydroepiandrosterone sulfate (DHEA-S) enhances hippocampal primed burst, but not long-term, potentiation. Neuroscience Letters. 1996;**202**:204-208

[79] Chen L, Dai X-N, Sokabe M. Chronic administration of dehydroepiandrosterone sulfate (DHEAs) primes for facilitated induction of long-term potentiation via $sigma_1$ (σ_1) receptor: Optical imaging study in rat hippocampal slices. Neuropharmacology. 2006;**50**:380-392

[80] Maurice T, Roman FJ, Privat A. Modulation by neurosteroids of the in vivo (+)-[3h] skf-10,047 binding to σ1 receptors in the mouse forebrain. Journal of Neuroscience Research. 1996;**46**:734-743

[81] Maurice T, Grégoire C, Espallergues J. Neuro (active) steroids actions at the neuromodulatory $sigma_1(\sigma_1)$ receptor: Biochemical and physiological evidences, consequences in neuroprotection. Pharmacology Biochemistry and Behavior. 2006;**84**:581-597

[82] Konradi C, Heckers S. Molecular aspects of glutamate dysregulation: Implications for schizophrenia and its treatment. Pharmacology & Therapeutics. 2003;**97**:153-179

[83] Kaasik A, Safiulina D, Kalda A, Zharkovsky A. Dehydroepiandrosterone with other neurosteroids preserve neuronal mitochondria from calcium overload. The Journal of Steroid Biochemistry and Molecular Biology. 2003;**87**:97-103

[84] Kurata K, Takebayashi M, Morinobu S, Yamawaki S. Beta-estradiol, dehydroepiandrosterone, and dehydroepiandrosterone sulfate protect against N-methyl-D-aspartate-induced neurotoxicity in rat hippocampal neurons by different mechanisms. Journal of Pharmacology and Experimental Therapeutics. 2004;**311**:237-245

[85] X-x D, Wang Y, Qin Z-h. Molecular mechanisms of excitotoxicity and their relevance to pathogenesis of neurodegenerative diseases. Acta Pharmacologica Sinica. 2009;**30**:379-387

[86] Sakr H, Khalil K, Hussein A, Zaki M, Eid R, Alkhateeb M. Effect of dehydroepiandrosterone (DHEA) on memory and brain derived neurotrophic factor (BDNF) in a rat model of vascular dementia. Journal of Physiology and Pharmacology. 2014;**65**:41-53

[87] Pluchino N, Russo M, Santoro A, Litta P, Cela V, Genazzani A. Steroid hormones and BDNF. Neuroscience. 2013;**239**:271-279

[88] Numakawa T, Suzuki S, Kumamaru E, Adachi N, Richards M, Kunugi H. BDNF function and intracellular signaling in neurons. Histology and Histopathology. 2010;**25**:237-258

[89] Mattson MP. Glutamate and neurotrophic factors in neuronal plasticity and disease. Annals of the New York Academy of Sciences. 2008;**1144**:97-112

[90] Lu Y, Christian K, Lu B. BDNF: A key regulator for protein synthesis-dependent LTP and long-term memory? Neurobiology of Learning and Memory. 2008;**89**:312-323

[91] Korte M, Staiger V, Griesbeck O, Thoenen H, Bonhoeffer T. The involvement of brain-derived neurotrophic factor in hippocampal long-term potentiation revealed by gene targeting experiments. Journal of Physiology-Paris. 1996;**90**:157-164

[92] Patterson SL, Abel T, Deuel TA, Martin KC, Rose JC, Kandel ER. Recombinant BDNF rescues deficits in basal synaptic transmission and hippocampal LTP in BDNF knockout mice. Neuron. 1996;**16**:1137-1145

[93] Monteggia LM, Barrot M, Powell CM, Berton O, Galanis V, Gemelli T, Meuth S, Nagy A, Greene RW, Nestler EJ. Essential role of brain-derived neurotrophic factor in adult hippocampal function. Proceedings of the National Academy of Sciences of the United States of America. 2004;**101**:10827-10832

[94] Komulainen P, Pedersen M, Hanninen T, Bruunsgaard H, Lakka TA, Kivipelto M, Hassinen M, Rauramaa TH, Pedersen BK, Rauramaa R. BDNF is a novel marker of cognitive function in ageing women: The Dr's extra study. Neurobiology of Learning and Memory. 2008;**90**:596-603

[95] Gl N, Maurice T, Tapia-Arancibia L, Givalois L. Neuroactive steroids modulate hpa axis activity and cerebral brain-derived neurotrophic factor (BDNF) protein levels in adult male rats. Psychoneuroendocrinology. 2007;**32**:1062-1078

[96] Barbany G, Persson H. Regulation of neurotrophin mRNA expression in the rat brain by glucocorticoids. European Journal of Neuroscience. 1992;**4**:396-403

[97] Roceri M, Cirulli F, Pessina C, Peretto P, Racagni G, Riva MA. Postnatal repeated maternal deprivation produces age-dependent changes of brain-derived neurotrophic factor expression in selected rat brain regions. Biological Psychiatry. 2004;**55**:708-714

[98] Murakami S, Imbe H, Morikawa Y, Kubo C, Senba E. Chronic stress, as well as acute stress, reduces BDNF mRNA expression in the rat hippocampus but less robustly. Neuroscience Research. 2005;**53**:129-139

[99] Tamatam A, Khanum F, Bawa AS. Genetic biomarkers of depression. Indian Journal of Human Genetics. 2012;**18**:20-33

[100] Karege F, Perret G, Bondolfi G, Schwald M, Bertschy G, Aubry J-M. Decreased serum brain-derived neurotrophic factor levels in major depressed patients. Psychiatry Research. 2002;**109**:143-148

[101] Toyooka K, Asama K, Watanabe Y, Muratake T, Takahashi M, Someya T, Nawa H. Decreased levels of brain-derived neurotrophic factor in serum of chronic schizophrenic patients. Psychiatry Research. 2002;**110**:249-257

[102] Connor B, Young D, Yan Q, Faull R, Synek B, Dragunow M. Brain-derived neurotrophic factor is reduced in Alzheimer's disease. Molecular Brain Research. 1997;**49**:71-81

[103] Scheltens P, Blennow K, Breteler MM, de Strooper B, Frisoni GB, Salloway S, Van der Flier WM: Alzheimer's disease. Lancet (London, England) 2016;**388**:505-517

[104] Wimo A, Jönsson L, Bond J, Prince M, Winblad B. International AD: The worldwide economic impact of dementia 2010. Alzheimer's & Dementia. 2013;**9**:1-11.e13

[105] Citron M. Alzheimer's disease: Strategies for disease modification. Nature Reviews. Drug Discovery. 2010;**9**:387-398

[106] Serrano-Pozo A, Frosch MP, Masliah E, Hyman BT. Neuropathological alterations in Alzheimer disease. Cold Spring Harbor Perspectives in Medicine. 2011;**1**:a006189

[107] Arnold SE, Hyman BT, Flory J, Damasio AR, Van Hoesen GW. The topographical and neuroanatomical distribution of neurofibrillary tangles and neuritic plaques in the cerebral cortex of patients with Alzheimer's disease. Cerebral Cortex. 1991;**1**:103-116

[108] Nuovo G, Paniccia B, Mezache L, Quiñónez M, Williams J, Vandiver P, Fadda P, Amann V. Diagnostic pathology of Alzheimer's disease from routine microscopy to immunohistochemistry and experimental correlations. Annals of Diagnostic Pathology. 2017; **28**:24-29

[109] Bekris LM, C-E Y, Bird TD, Tsuang DW. Genetics of Alzheimer disease. Journal of Geriatric Psychiatry and Neurology. 2010;**23**:213-227

[110] Hebert LE, Scherr PA, Bienias JL, Bennett DA, Evans DA. Alzheimer disease in the us population: Prevalence estimates using the 2000 census. Archives of Neurology. 2003;**60**:1119-1122

[111] Launer L, Andersen K, Dewey M, Letenneur L, Ott A, Amaducci L, Brayne C, Copeland J, Dartigues J-F, Kragh-Sorensen P. Rates and risk factors for dementia and Alzheimer's disease results from EURODEM pooled analyses. Neurology. 1999;**52**:78-78

[112] Markesbery WR. Oxidative stress hypothesis in Alzheimer's disease. Free Radical Biology and Medicine. 1997;**23**:134-147

[113] Lin MT, Beal MF. Mitochondrial dysfunction and oxidative stress in neurodegenerative diseases. Nature. 2006;**443**:787-795

[114] Sardi F, Fassina L, Venturini L, Inguscio M, Guerriero F, Rolfo E, Ricevuti G. Alzheimer's disease, autoimmunity and inflammation. The good, the bad and the ugly. Autoimmunity Reviews. 2011;**11**:149-153

[115] Green KN, Billings LM, Roozendaal B, McGaugh JL, LaFerla FM. Glucocorticoids increase amyloid-β and tau pathology in a mouse model of Alzheimer's disease. Journal of Neuroscience. 2006;**26**:9047-9056

[116] Stein-Behrens B, Mattson M, Chang I, Yeh M, Sapolsky R. Stress exacerbates neuron loss and cytoskeletal pathology in the hippocampus. Journal of Neuroscience. 1994; **14**:5373-5380

[117] Wilson R, Barnes L, Bennett D, Li Y, Bienias J, de Leon CM, Evans D: Proneness to psychological distress and risk of Alzheimer disease in a biracial community. Neurology 2005;**64**:380-382

[118] Sunderland T, Merril C, Harrington M, Lawlor B, Molchan S, Martinez R, Murphy D. Reduced plasma dehydroepiandrosterone concentrations in Alzheimer's disease. The Lancet. 1989;**334**:570

[119] Näsman B, Olsson T, Bäckström T, Eriksson S, Grankvist K, Viitanen M, Bucht G. Serum dehydroepiandrosterone sulfate in Alzheimer's disease and in multi-infarct dementia. Biological Psychiatry. 1991;**30**:684-690

[120] Leblhuber F, Windhager E, Reisecker F, Steinparz F, Dienstl E, Cuckle H, Stone R, Smith D, Wald N, Brammer M. Dehydroepiandrosterone sulphate in Alzheimer's disease. The Lancet. 1990;**336**:449-450

[121] Weill-Engerer S, David J-P, Sazdovitch V, Liere P, Eychenne B, Pianos A, Schumacher M, Delacourte A, Baulieu E-E, Akwa Y. Neurosteroid quantification in human brain regions: Comparison between Alzheimer's and nondemented patients. The Journal of Clinical Endocrinology & Metabolism. 2002;**87**:5138-5143

[122] Kim S-B, Hill M, Kwak Y-T, Hampl R, Jo D-H, Morfin R. Neurosteroids: Cerebrospinal fluid levels for Alzheimer's disease and vascular dementia diagnostics. The Journal of Clinical Endocrinology & Metabolism. 2003;**88**:5199-5206

[123] Schneider LS, Hinsey M, Lyness S. Plasma dehydroepiandrosterone sulfate in Alzheimer's disease. Biological Psychiatry. 1992;**31**:205-208

[124] Rasmuson S, Näsman B, Carlström K, Olsson T. Increased levels of adrenocortical and gonadal hormones in mild to moderate Alzheimer's disease. Dementia and Geriatric Cognitive Disorders. 2002;**13**:74-79

[125] Naylor JC, Hulette CM, Steffens DC, Shampine LJ, Ervin JF, Payne VM, Massing MW, Kilts JD, Strauss JL, Calhoun PS, Calnaido RP, Blazer DG, Lieberman JA, Madison RD, Marx CE. Cerebrospinal fluid dehydroepiandrosterone levels are correlated with brain dehydroepiandrosterone levels, elevated in Alzheimer's disease, and related to neuropathological disease stage. The Journal of Clinical Endocrinology and Metabolism. 2008;**93**:3173-3178

[126] Brown RC, Han ZQ, Cascio C, Papadopoulos V. Oxidative stress-mediated DHEA formation in Alzheimer's disease pathology. Neurobiology of Aging. 2003;**24**:57-65

[127] Rammouz G, Lecanu L, Papadopoulos V. Oxidative stress-mediated brain dehydroepiandrosterone (DHEA) formation in Alzheimer's disease diagnosis. Frontiers in Endocrinology. 2011;**2**:69

[128] Cascio C, Brown RC, Liu Y, Han Z, Hales DB, Papadopoulos V. Pathways of dehydroepiandrosterone formation in rat brain glia. The Journal of Steroid Biochemistry and Molecular Biology. 2000;**75**:177-186

[129] Brown RC, Cascio C, Papadopoulos V. Pathways of neurosteroid biosynthesis in cell lines from human brain: Regulation of dehydroepiandrosterone formation by oxidative stress and beta-amyloid peptide. Journal of Neurochemistry. 2000;**74**:847-859

[130] Gella A, Durany N. Oxidative stress in Alzheimer disease. Cell Adhesion & Migration. 2009;**3**:88-93

[131] Cardounel A, Regelson W, Kalimi M. Dehydroepiandrosterone protects hippocampal neurons against neurotoxin-induced cell death: Mechanism of action. Proceedings of the Society for Experimental Biology and Medicine. 1999;**222**:145-149

[132] Straub RH, Scholmerich J, Zietz B. Replacement therapy with DHEA plus corticosteroids in patients with chronic inflammatory diseases – substitutes of adrenal and sex hormones. Zeitschrift fur Rheumatologie. 2000;**59**(Suppl 2):Ii/108-Ii/118

[133] Straub RH, Konecna L, Hrach S, Rothe G, Kreutz M, Schölmerich J, Falk W, Lang B. Serum dehydroepiandrosterone (DHEA) and DHEA sulfate are negatively correlated with serum interleukin-6 (il-6), and DHEA inhibits il-6 secretion from mononuclear cells in man in vitro: Possible link between endocrinosenescence and immunosenescence. The Journal of Clinical Endocrinology & Metabolism. 1998;**83**:2012-2017

[134] Iwasaki Y, Asai M, Yoshida M, Nigawara T, Kambayashi M, Nakashima N. Dehydroepiandrosterone-sulfate inhibits nuclear factor-kappaB-dependent transcription in hepatocytes, possibly through antioxidant effect. The Journal of Clinical Endocrinology and Metabolism. 2004;**89**:3449-3454

[135] Hüll M, Fiebich BL, Lieb K, Strauss S, Berger M, Volk B, Bauer J. Interleukin-6-associated inflammatory processes in Alzheimer's disease: New therapeutic options. Neurobiology of Aging. 1996;**17**:795-800

[136] Singh VK, Guthikonda P. Circulating cytokines in Alzheimer's disease. Journal of Psychiatric Research. 1997;**31**:657-660

[137] Cojocaru IM, Cojocaru M, Miu G, Sapira V. Study of interleukin-6 production in Alzheimer's disease. Romanian journal of internal medicine = Revue roumaine de medecine interne. 2011;**49**:55-58

[138] Rubio-Perez JM, Morillas-Ruiz JM. A review: Inflammatory process in Alzheimer's disease, role of cytokines. The Scientific World Journal. 2012;**2012**:756357

[139] Machado A, Herrera AJ, de Pablos RM, Espinosa-Oliva AM, Sarmiento M, Ayala A, Venero JL, Santiago M, Villarán RF, Delgado-Cortés MJ: Chronic stress as a risk factor for Alzheimer's disease. Reviews in the Neurosciences 2014;**25**:785-804

[140] Lei J. Change of serum acth and cortisol levels in Alzheimer disease and mild cognition impairment. Zhonghua Yi Xue Za Zhi. 2010;**90**:2894-2896

[141] Curto M, Martocchia A, Ferracuti S, Comite F, Scaccianoce S, Girardi P, Nicoletti F, Falaschi P. Increased total urinary cortisol (TUC) and serum brain-derived neurotrophic factor (BDNF) ratio in Alzheimer disease (AD)-affected patients. Alzheimer Disease & Associated Disorders. 2017;**31**(2):173-176

[142] Nuss P. Anxiety disorders and gaba neurotransmission: A disturbance of modulation. Neuropsychiatric Disease and Treatment. 2015;**11**:165-175

[143] Sapolsky RM, Krey LC, McEWEN BS. Prolonged glucocorticoid exposure reduces hippocampal neuron number: Implications for aging. Journal of Neuroscience. 1985; **5**:1222-1227

[144] Hu Y, Cardounel A, Gursoy E, Anderson P, Kalimi M. Anti-stress effects of dehydroepiandrosterone: Protection of rats against repeated immobilization stress-induced weight loss, glucocorticoid receptor production, and lipid peroxidation. Biochem Pharmacol. 2000;**59**:753-762

[145] Kalimi M, Shafagoj Y, Loria R, Padgett D, Regelson W. Anti-glucocorticoid effects of dehydroepiandrosterone (DHEA). Molecular and Cellular Biochemistry. 1994;**131**:99-104

[146] Karishma KK, Herbert J. Dehydroepiandrosterone (DHEA) stimulates neurogenesis in the hippocampus of the rat, promotes survival of newly formed neurons and prevents corticosterone-induced suppression. European Journal of Neuroscience. 2002; **16**:445-453

[147] Saponaro S, Guarnieri V, Pescarmona GP, Silvagno F. Long-term exposure to dehydroepiandrosterone affects the transcriptional activity of the glucocorticoid receptor. The Journal of Steroid Biochemistry and Molecular Biology. 2007;**103**:129-136

[148] Kimonides VG, Spillantini MG, Sofroniew MV, Fawcett JW, Herbert J. Dehydroepiandrosterone antagonizes the neurotoxic effects of corticosterone and translocation of stress-activated protein kinase 3 in hippocampal primary cultures. Neuroscience. 1999; **89**:429-436

[149] Muller C, Hennebert O, Morfin R. The native anti-glucocorticoid paradigm. The Journal of Steroid Biochemistry and Molecular Biology. 2006;**100**:95-105

[150] Muller C, Pompon D, Urban P, Morfin R. Inter-conversion of 7alpha- and 7beta-hydroxy-dehydroepiandrosterone by the human 11beta-hydroxysteroid dehydrogenase type 1. The Journal of Steroid Biochemistry and Molecular Biology. 2006;**99**:215-222

[151] Yau J, Rasmuson S, Andrew R, Graham M, Noble J, Olsson T, Fuchs E, Lathe R, Seckl J. Dehydroepiandrosterone 7-hydroxylase cyp7b: Predominant expression in primate hippocampus and reduced expression in Alzheimer's disease. Neuroscience. 2003;**121**:307-314

[152] Morfin R, Starka L. Neurosteroid 7-hydroxylation products in the brain. International Review of Neurobiology. 2001;**46**:79-95

[153] Attal-Khemis S, Dalmeyda V, Michot JL, Roudier M, Morfin R. Increased total 7 alpha-hydroxy-dehydroepiandrosterone in serum of patients with Alzheimer's disease. The journals of gerontology Series A, Biological sciences and medical sciences. 1998;**53**: B125-B132

[154] Bicikova M, Ripova D, Hill M, Jirak R, Havlikova H, Tallova J, Hampl R. Plasma levels of 7-hydroxylated dehydroepiandrosterone (DHEA) metabolites and selected amino-thiols as discriminatory tools of Alzheimer's disease and vascular dementia. Clinical Chemistry and Laboratory Medicine. 2004;**42**:518-524

[155] Ritsner M, Maayan R, Gibel A, Strous RD, Modai I, Weizman A. Elevation of the cortisol/dehydroepiandrosterone ratio in schizophrenia patients. European Neuropsychopharmacology. 2004;**14**:267-273

[156] Goodyer I, Park R, Netherton C, Herbert J. Possible role of cortisol and dehydroepiandrosterone in human development and psychopathology. The British Journal of Psychiatry. 2001;**179**:243-249

[157] Wolkowitz OM, Reus VI. Neuropsychiatric effects of dehydroepiandros- terone (DHEA). In: Kalimi M, Regelson W, editors. Dehydroepiandros- terone (DHEA): biochemical, physiological and clinical aspects. Berlin: Walter De Gruyter, 2000;271-298

[158] Harris DS, Wolkowitz OM, Reus VI. Movement disorder, memory, psychiatric symptoms and serum DHEA levels in schizophrenic and schizoaffective patients. The World Journal of Biological Psychiatry. 2001;**2**:99-102

[159] Kunugi H, Nanko S, Murray RM. Obstetric complications and schizophrenia: Prenatal underdevelopment and subsequent neurodevelopmental impairment. The British Journal of Psychiatry. 2001;**40**:S25-S29

[160] Barker DJP. The developmental origins of adult disease. Journal of the American College of Nutrition. 2004;**23**:588S-595S

[161] Gilmore JH, Jarskog LF, Vadlamudi S. Maternal poly i:C exposure during pregnancy regulates TNF-alpha, BDNF, and NGF expression in neonatal brain and the maternal-fetal unit of the rat. Journal of Neuroimmunology. 2005;**159**:106-112

[162] Strous RD, Stryjer R, Maayan R, Gal G, Viglin D, Katz E, Eisner D, Weizman A. Analysis of clinical symptomatology, extrapyramidal symptoms and neurocognitive dysfunction following dehydroepiandrosterone (DHEA) administration in olanzapine treated schizophrenia patients: A randomized, double-blind placebo controlled trial. Psychoneuroendocrinology. 2007;**32**:96-105

[163] Raison CL, Miller AH. When not enough is too much: The role of insufficient glucocorticoid signaling in the pathophysiology of stress-related disorders. American Journal of Psychiatry. 2003;**160**:1554-1565

[164] Seeman P, Kapur S. Schizophrenia: More dopamine, more d-2 receptors. Proceedings of the National Academy of Sciences of the United States of America. 2000;**97**:7673-7675

[165] Blum BP, Mann JJ. The gabaergic system in schizophrenia. International Journal of Neuropsychopharmacology. 2002;**5**:159-179

[166] Coyle JT, Tsai G, Goff D. Converging evidence of nmda receptor hypofunction in the pathophysiology of schizophrenia. Glutamate and Disorders of Cognition and Motivation. 2003;**1003**:318-327

[167] Wassef A, Baker J, Kochan LD. Gaba and schizophrenia: A review of basic science and clinical studies. Journal of Clinical Psychopharmacology. 2003;**23**:601-640

[168] Costa E, Davis JM, Dong E, Grayson DR, Guidotti A, Tremolizzo L, Veldic M. A gabaergic cortical deficit dominates schizophrenia pathophysiology. Critical Reviews in Neurobiology. 2004;**16**:1-23

[169] MacKenzie EM, Odontiadis J, Le Melledo JM, Prior TI, Baker GB. The relevance of neuroactive steroids in schizophrenia, depression, and anxiety disorders. Cellular and Molecular Neurobiology. 2007;**27**:541-574

[170] Oades RD, Schepker R. Serum gonadal-steroid hormones in young schizophrenic-patients. Psychoneuroendocrinology. 1994;**19**:373-385

[171] Strous RD, Maayan R, Lapidus R, Goredetsky L, Zeldich E, Kotler M, Weizman A. Increased circulatory dehydroepiandrosterone and dehydroepiandrosterone-sulphate in first-episode schizophrenia: Relationship to gender, aggression and symptomatology. Schizophrenia Research. 2004;**71**:427-434

[172] Howard JS. Severe psychosis and the adrenal androgens. Integrative Physiology and Behavioral Sciences. 1992;**27**:209-215

[173] di Michele F, Caltagirone C, Bonaviri G, Romeo E, Spalletta G: Plasma dehydroepiandrosterone levels are strongly increased in schizophrenia. Journal of Psychiatric Research 2005;**39**:267-273

[174] Debonnel G, Bergeron R, deMontigny C. Potentiation by dehydroepiandrosterone of the neuronal response to N-methyl-D-aspartate in the Ca(3) region of the rat dorsal hippocampus: An effect mediated via sigma receptors. Journal of Endocrinology. 1996;**150**:S33-S42

[175] Flood JF, Morley JE, Roberts E. Memory-enhancing effects in male mice of pregnenolone and steroids metabolically derived from it. Proceedings of the National Academy of Sciences of the United States of America. 1992;**89**:1567-1571

[176] Genazzani AR, Petraglia F, Bernardi F, Casarosa E, Salvestroni C, Tonetti A, Nappi RE, Luisi S, Palumbo M, Purdy RH, Luisi M. Circulating levels of allopregnanolone in humans: Gender, age, and endocrine influences. Journal of Clinical Endocrinology and Metabolism. 1998;**83**:2099-2103

[177] Rasmusson AM, Vasek J, Lipschitz DS, Vojvodal D, Mustone ME, Shi QH, Gudmundsen G, Morgan CA, Wolfe J, Charney DS. An increased capacity for adrenal DHEA release is associated with decreased avoidance and negative mood symptoms in women with ptsd. Neuropsychopharmacology. 2004;**29**:1546-1557

[178] Kimonides VG, Khatibi NH, Svendsen CN, Sofroniew MV, Herbert J. Dehydroepiandrosterone (DHEA) and DHEA-sulfate (DHEAs) protect hippocampal neurons against excitatory amino acid-induced neurotoxicity. Proceedings of the National Academy of Sciences of the United States of America. 1998;**95**:1852-1857

[179] Brophy MH, Rush AJ, Crowley G. Cortisol, estadiol and androgens in acutely ill paranoid schizophrenics. Biological Psychiatry. 1983;**18**:583-590

[180] Harris DS, Wolkowitz OM, Reus VI. Movement disorder, psychiatric symptoms and serum DHEA levels in schizophrenic and schizoaffective patients. World Journal of Biological Psychiatry. 2001;**2**:99-102

[181] Shirayama Y, Chen ACH, Nakagawa S, Russell DS, Duman RS. Brain-derived neurotrophic factor produces antidepressant effects in behavioral models of depression. Journal of Neuroscience. 2002;**22**:3251-3261

[182] Tourney G, Hatfield L. Plasma androgens in male schizophrenics. Archives of General Psychiatry. 1972;**27**:753

[183] Oertel GW, Benes P, Schirazi M, Holzmann H, Hoffmann G. Interaction between dehydroepiandrosterone, cyclic adenosine-3′,5′-monophosphate and glucose-6-phosphate-dehydrogenase in normal and diseases subjects. Experientia. 1974;**30**:872-873

[184] Tourney G, Erb JL. Temporal variations in androgens and stress hormones in control and schizophrenic subjects. Biological Psychiatry. 1979;**14**:395-404

[185] Erb JL, Kadane JB, Tourney G, Mickelsen R, Trader D, Szabo R, Davis V. Discrimination between schizophrenic and control subjects by means of plasma dehydroepiandosterone meausurements. Journal of Clinical Endocrinology and Metabolism. 1981;**52**:181-186

[186] Cotter D, Pariante CM. Stress and the progression of the developmental hypothesis of schizophrenia. The British Journal of Psychiatry. 2002;**181**:363-365

[187] Ryan MCM, Sharifi N, Condren R, Thakore JH. Evidence of basal pituitary-AD renal overactivity in first episode, drug naive patients with schizophrenia. Psychoneuroendocrinology. 2004;**29**:1065-1070

[188] Dewan MJ, Pandurangi AK, Boucher ML, Levy BF, Major LF. Abnormal dexamethasone suppression test-results in chronic-schizophrenic patients. American Journal of Psychiatry. 1982;**139**:1501-1503

[189] Lammers CH, GarciaBorreguero D, Schmider J, Gotthardt U, Dettling M, Holsboer F, Heuser IJE. Combined dexamethasone/corticotropin-releasing hormone test in patients with schizophrenia and in normal controls. Biological Psychiatry. 1995;**38**:803-807

[190] Webster MJ, Knable MB, O'Grady J, Orthmann J, Weickert CS. Regional specificity of brain gluclocorticoid receptor mRNA alterations in subjects with schizophrenia and mood disorders. Molecular Psychiatry. 2002;**7**:985-994

[191] Young AH, Gallagher P, Porter RJ. Elevation of the cortisol-dehydroepiandrosterone ratio in drug-free depressed patients. American Journal of Psychiatry. 2002;**159**:1237-1239

[192] Hechter O, Grossman A, Chatterton RT. Relationship of dehydroepiandrosterone and cortisol in disease. Medical Hypotheses. 1997;**49**:85-91

[193] Tkachev D, Mimmack ML, Ryan MM, Wayland M, Freeman T, Jones PB, Starkey M, Webster MJ, Yolken RH, Bahn S. Oligodendrocyte dysfunction in schizophrenia and bipolar disorder. Lancet (London, England). 2003;**362**:798-805

4

Gender Differences in Frontotemporal Lobar Degeneration (FTLD) Support an Estrogenic Model of Delayed Onset

Claire V. Flaherty, Arghavan S. Zangeneh,
Marissa A. Harrison and Sanjana Marikunte

Abstract

Gender differences in frontotemporal lobar degeneration (FTLD) have been reported in the literature but not well characterized or explored. In the present work, we propose that steroid hormone estrogens delay the onset of FTLD in pre-menopausal women compared to age equivalent men, and may provide neuroprotection in the early post-menopausal period. We present a model wherein estrogens serve a regulatory role in attenuating the microglia conversion from the benign to active form in response to cell stress that might otherwise trigger an inflammatory response. Via microglia stabilization, estrogens preserve the homeostasis of both the ubiquitin-proteosome degradation system and lysosome-autophagy recycling system. Both systems have been implicated in the genetic forms of FTLD, with the latter system recognized to be associated with the majority of them.

Keywords: frontotemporal lobar degeneration (FTLD), gender differences, estrogens, autophagy, microglia, neuroprotection

1. Introduction

FTLD is second only to Alzheimer's disease as a leading cause of primary degenerative dementia in those under age 65 [1, 2]. Researchers estimate that it is responsible for one out of six cases of pre-senile dementia in post-mortem confirmed cases of individuals under age 70 [3]. FTLD symptoms range from motor and language impairment to profound behavioral changes and deficits [4, 5], including severely attenuated initiative to profound impulsivity

[6]. FTLD is characterized by three subtypes: behavioral variant frontotemporal dementia (bvFTD), semantic dementia (SD), and primary progressive aphasia agrammatic variant (PPA-agrammatic), although there remains ongoing discussion about their classification [5, 7]. As the most prevalent form of pre-senile dementia after early onset Alzheimer and vascular dementia [8], gender differences in onset and characteristics of FTLD have received little attention in comparison to older onset Alzheimer's dementia. The initial conclusions of the Women's Health Initiative Memory Study (WHIMS) associated long-term estrogen replacement in women ≥65 years of age with increased risk of senile dementia but not mild cognitive impairment (MCI) [9]. MCI, as the Alzheimer's dementia prodrome, is known to remain stable in 1/2 to 2/3 of patients, with stability largely dependent upon the absence of apolipoprotein E e4 (APOE e4) alleles [10]. Consistent with this, estrogen replacement risk of senile dementia has been shown to be dependent upon the presence of the APOE e4 gene. In their longitudinal evaluation of the cognitive status of 12,612 participants of the Nurses' Health Study (≥70 years old) over 4 years, Kang and Grodstein [11] found that participants on hormone replacement since menopause onset, who were carriers of the APOE e4 allele demonstrated a significantly worse rate of cognition decline than nonhormone users. In the absence of APOE e4, the cognitive status of participants was equivalent, regardless of hormone replacement status. While findings did not demonstrate any significant benefit from hormone replacement in this cohort, the authors point out that this was a relatively homogeneous population of highly educated female nurses. Cognitive reserve may have protected nonestrogen users from declines into dementia during the 4 year period of study.

With respect to FTD, Ratnavalli and colleagues [12] found that men were four times more likely than women to be affected by bvFTD. They posited that this may have been an artifact of their small sample size, but also referred to older research documenting higher rates of FTLD in men [13] and encouraged further exploration. Johnson and colleagues [14] also reported sex differences. They found that more men had bvFTD and SD, while more women had progressive nonfluent aphasia. They noted that this may be due to sex-specific vulnerability to neurodegeneration for women in the left frontal region and men in right frontal and bilateral temporal regions. Bede and colleagues [15] recently evidenced gender differences in amyotrophic lateral sclerosis (ALS), considered to be a motor variant of FTLD on a clinical continuum [16, 17] with characteristics of FTLD in the absence of dementia in up to 50% of cases [18].

2. The role of estrogen in the brain

Beyond their role as reproductive hormones, estrogens, specifically 17β estradiol, exert a neuroprotective role in the brain through estrogen receptors widely distributed in the male and female brain. Multiple estrogen signaling pathways are now recognized in the human brain that are involved in the protection of brain from cognitive decline, emotional dysregulation, and neurodegeneration [19]. Moreover, the neuroendocrine response to stress is gender-specific and associated with the presence of gender-specific gonadal steroids [20]. Estrogen has been shown to be involved in cortical and subcortical hypothalamic-pituitary-adrenal (HPA) function [21], with activation of HPA arousal circuitry evidenced to be regulated in adult women by the hormonal cycle [21, 22].

All three subtypes of FTLD (bvFTLD, SD, and PPA-agrammatic) are associated with alterations in arousal, characterized by apathy. Our recent findings from a national, multicenter study of nondemented ALS with cognitive impairment and/or behavioral impairment were consistent with this, while evidencing a significantly greater incidence of impulsivity and jocularity in males, as well as personal neglect in females [23]. We contend that this distinction is due to the involvement of ventromedial natural reward and dominance circuitry in the emerging neurodegenerative disease process and the role of estrogen therein (**Figures 1** and **2**).

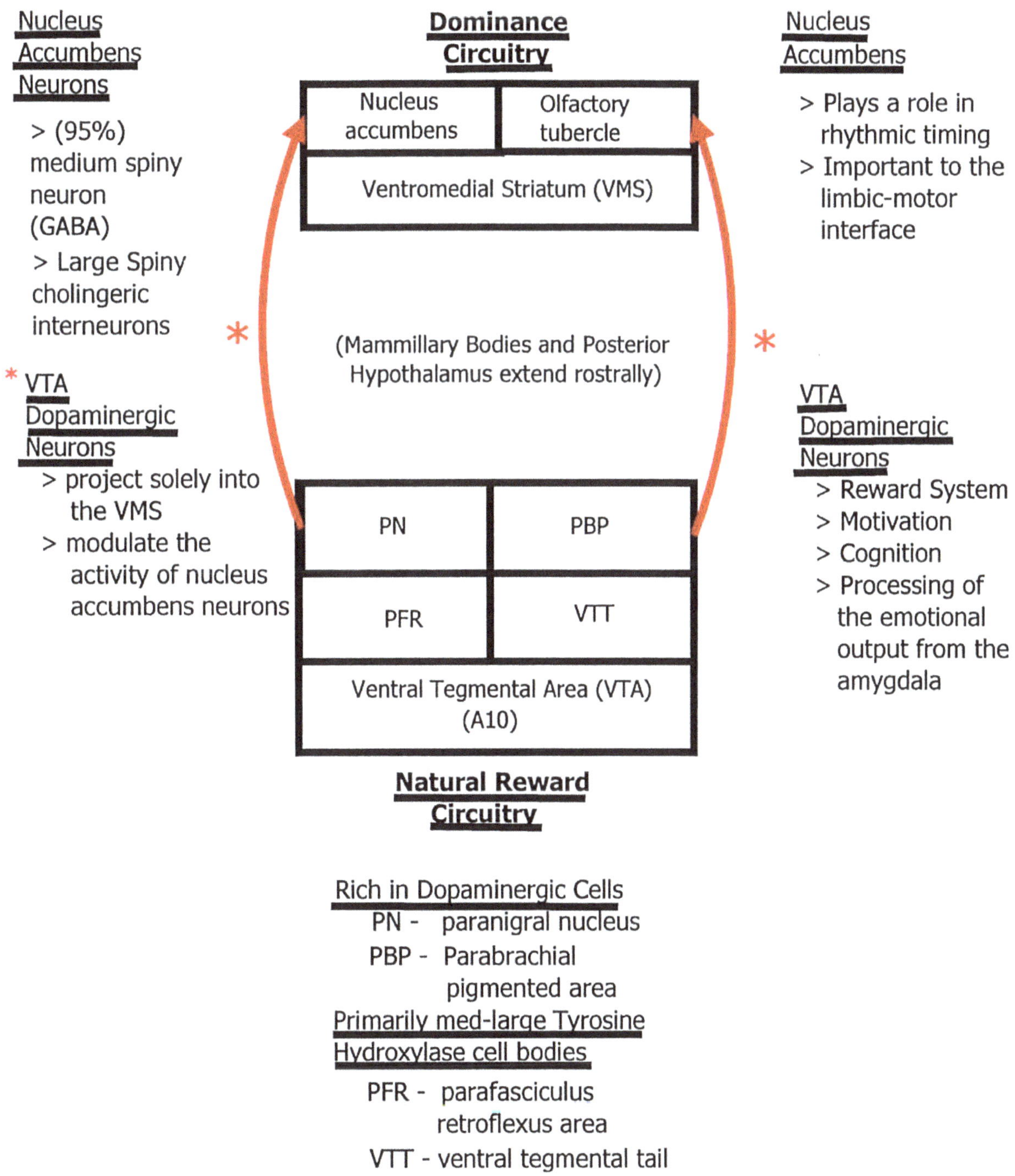

Figure 1. Mesostriatal pathway: natural reward–dominance neural system.

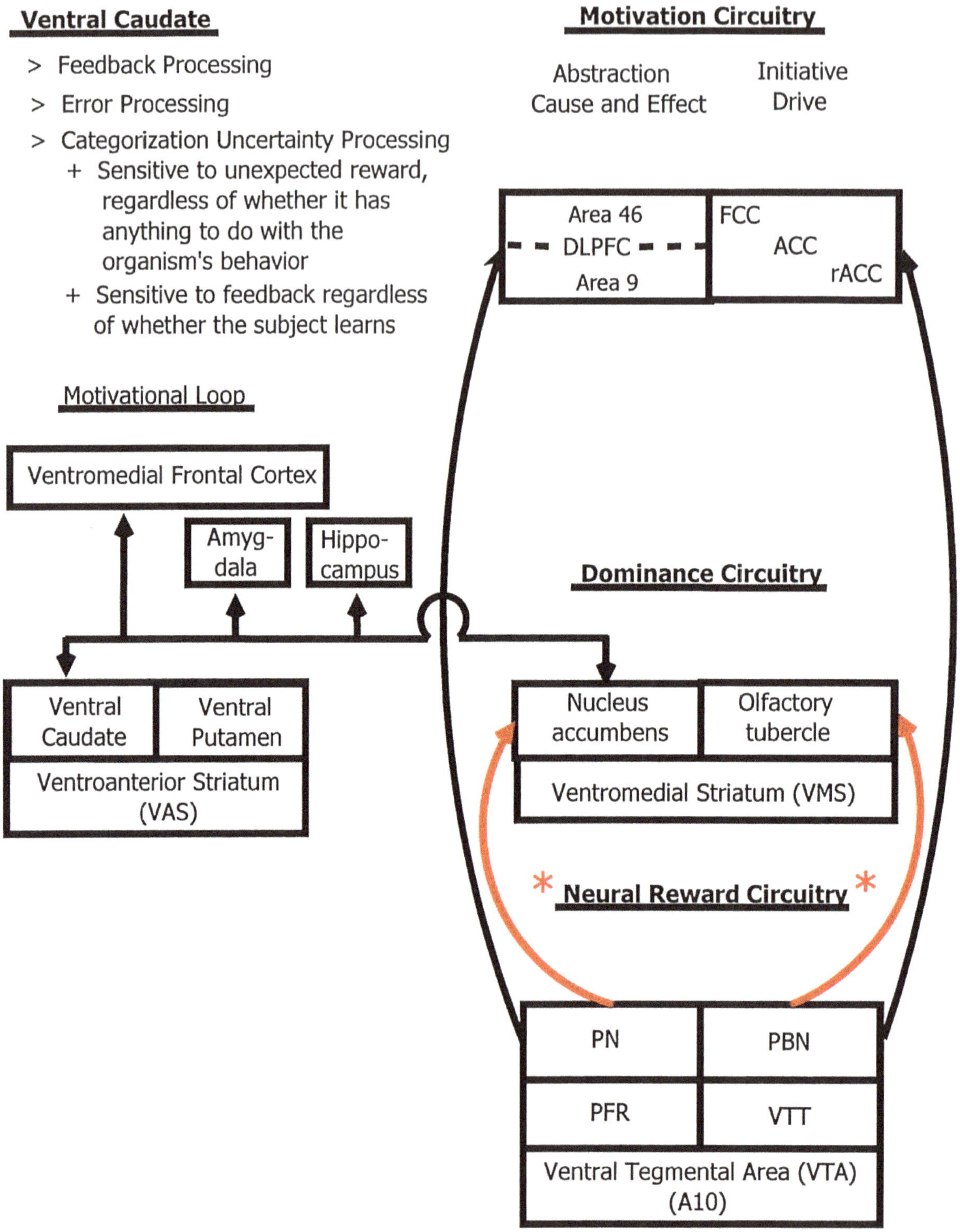

Figure 2. Mesocortical pathway: natural reward–dominance–motivation neural system; PN = paranigral nucleus, PBN = parabrachial pigmented area, PFR = parafasciculus retroflexus area, VTT = ventral tegmental tail, DLPFC = dorsolateral pre-frontal cortex, FCC = frontocingulate cortex, ACC = anterior cingulate cortex, and rACC = rostral ACC.

More recently, we evidenced greater cognitive and behavioral stability in 78 women from this cohort, based upon both site of disease onset (midbrain vs. spinal cord) and estrogen status (high vs. low).

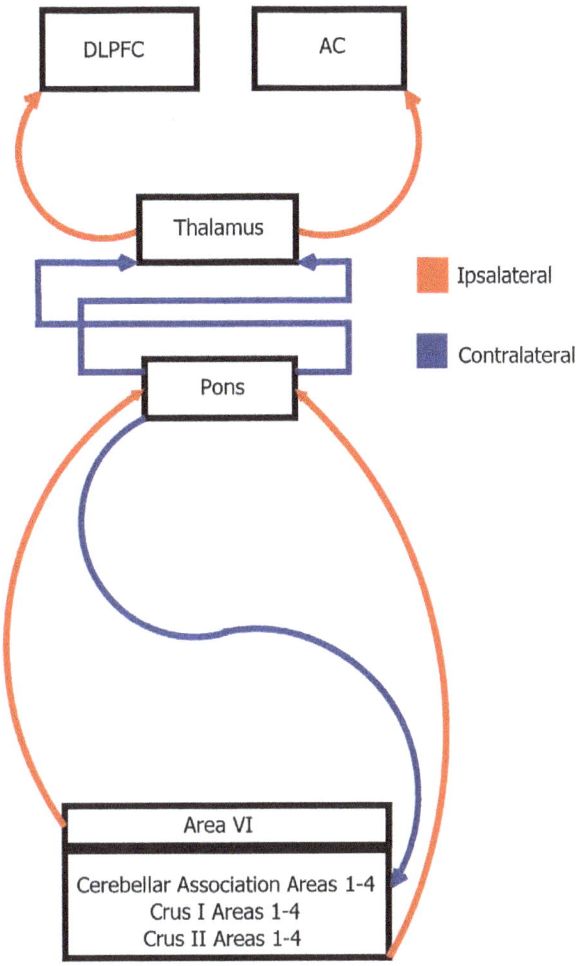

Figure 3. Cerebellar regulation of the mesocortical pathway: regulation of the natural reward-dominance-motivation neural system.

Given that midbrain onset females in our study demonstrated estrogen neuroprotection with respect to cognitive executive functions, we expanded our model of midbrain involvement in FTLD to involve the role of the cerebellum in executive functioning decline, based upon our own findings and recent imaging evidence [24] (**Figure 3**).

It has been widely established that ovarian gonadosteroidal hormones provide protection against brain injury and degeneration and provide cognitive maintenance [25–27]. Evidence of estradiol (the primary ovarian estrogen) neuroprotection comes from histopathological studies in rats [28] as well as healthy human females [29]. The release of neuroestradiol from the stalk median eminence (SME) of the hypothalamus in ovarectomized female monkeys has recently been evidenced [30]. Electrical stimulation of the medial basal hypothalamus resulted in release of both gonadotrophin releasing hormone (GnRH) and estrodial. This suggests its vital role as a neurotransmitter involved in regulation of GnRH release.

In recent neuroimaging data, the evidence of estrogen regulation of anterior cingulate cortex (ACC)-associated motivation in healthy human females was evidenced by examining the effects of estrogen on the neural correlates of emotional response inhibition. Applying an in-subject design involving 20 right-handed female subjects of average age 25.4 years, Amin and colleagues [31] combined 3.0 T functional magnetic resonance imaging (fMRI) with quantitative analysis of ovarian hormones. All participants evidenced stability of mood across the menstrual cycle. Subjects were scanned during the early follicular phase, when levels of estrogen and progesterone were low, and during the mid-luteal phase, when levels of estrogen and progesterone were high. Subjects were scanned while they were engaged in a verbal go/no-go task involving positive, negative, and neutral stimuli. This task was chosen because it was already evidenced in the literature to activate the dorsolateral prefrontal cortex (DLPFC) and the ACC. Cycle phase and condition were within-subject independent variables, while mean reaction time and accuracy of response were independent variables. During the follicular phase (low hormones), women exhibited significantly decreased activation in the bilateral ACC and some portions of the left PFC in response to positive distracters, relative to positive targets. During the luteal phase (high hormones), however, women exhibited decreased activation in the ACC in response to negative distracters and increased activation in the DLPFC in response to positive distracters. The investigators noted that the luteal phase findings were consistent with literature associating human female estrogen levels with positive affect. They further noted that their findings of negative correlation between estradiol levels and activation in response to negative distractors, relative to negative targets, were consistent with previous research [21]. This contention is further supported by more recent findings from the KEEPS longitudinal clinical trial focused on the potential for estrogen neuroprotection in 693 younger post-menopausal women of average age 52.6 years old and 1.4 years past their last menstrual period [32]. Following 4½ years, the estrogen replacement subgroups (N = 693) evidenced significant improvements in depression and anxiety in comparison to a placebo subgroup (N = 262). Cognitive status remained stable with monitoring to assess dementia incidence with aging ongoing.

3. Estrogen regulation of the stress response as a model of neuroprotection

Goldstein and colleagues [21] applied an fMRI paradigm to examine the effect of estrogen on brain regions involved in the stress response by using aversive affective stimuli in a group of 12 right-handed women, ages 36–40. Their imaging data evidenced an association between the early follicular phase (low estrogen) and significantly increased activation to neutral stimuli, relative to negative targets, in the central amygdala nuclei, paraventricular hypothalamic nuclei, peripeduncular nuclei, orbital frontal cortex, and AC gyrus (ACG). In comparison to the early follicular phase, the luteal phase (high estrogen) was associated with decreased activation in the central amygdaloid, ventromedial hypothalamic, orbital frontal, and cingulate nuclei in response to negative vs. neutral stimuli. With respect to FTLD, we propose a model whereby estrogen provides neuroprotection by mediation of the neuroimmunological and neuroendocrinological stress response (i.e., release of anti-inflammatories and stress associated hormones) (**Figure 4**).

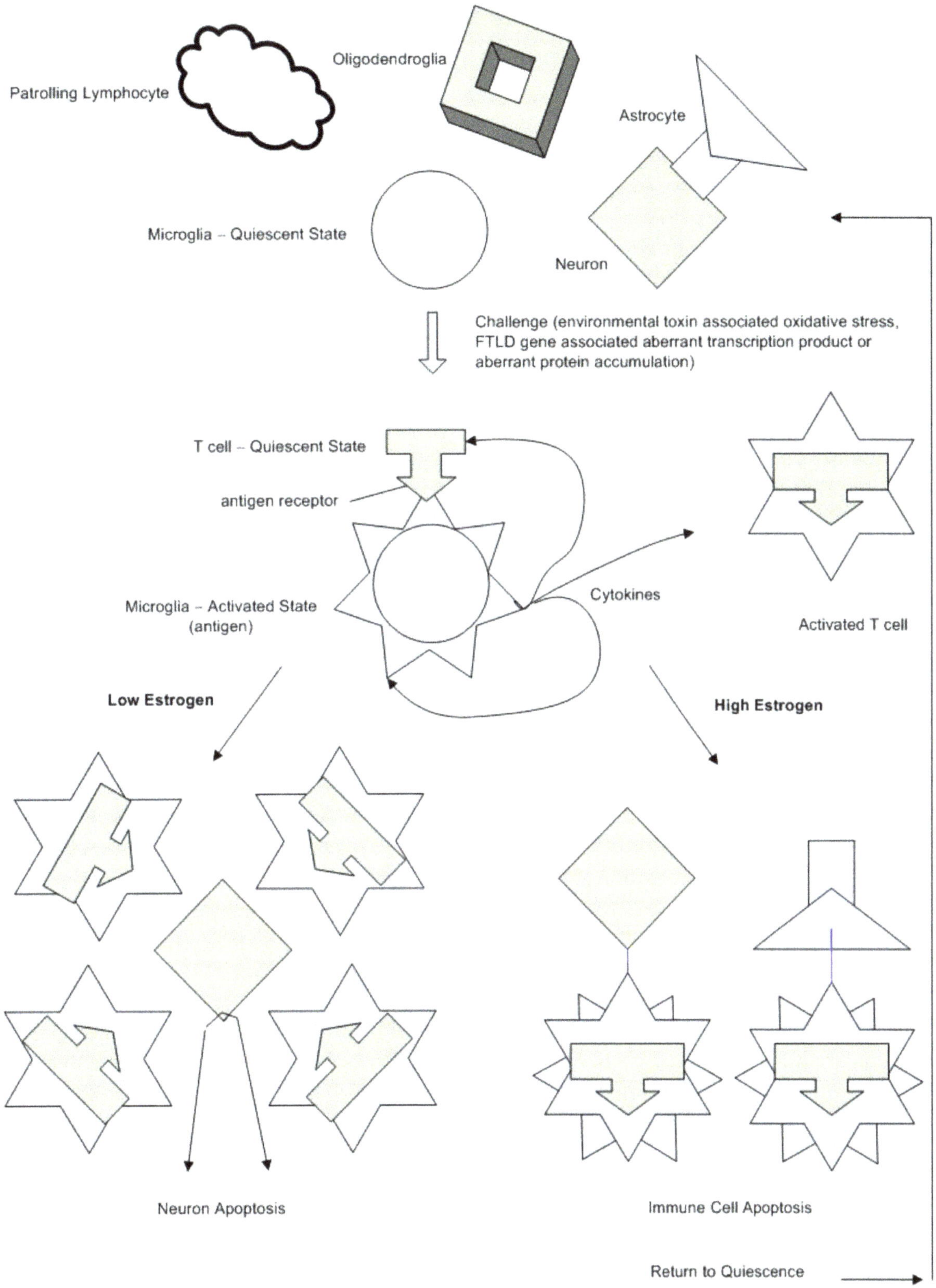

Figure 4. Estrogen binding to microglia induces feedback inhibition of the inflammatory cascade, resulting in neuroprotection. Mice models of toxic demyelination evidence estrogen induction of insulin-like growth factor 1 (IGF-1) expression by astrocytes. IGF-1 then promotes proliferation of oligodendrocyte precursors and their differentiation into mature remyelinating oligodendrocytes.

4. Lysosome and proteosome homeostasis: estrogen mitigation of the microglia inflammatory response in neurodegeneration

As disorders of aging, many neurodegenerative diseases demonstrate significant gender differences in their prevalence, symptomatology, and prognosis, implicating gonadal steroidal hormones in their pathophysiology [33, 34]. Parkinson's disease (PD) has for a long time been recognized to be more prevalent in males than in females, with a relative male to female ratio ranging from 1.4 to 3.7. Evidence suggests that levels of estrogens or progesterone or differences in their respective receptor levels could account for this gender difference [35, 36]. Particularly with respect to early onset dementia, emerging with onset of menopause or andropause, endogenous estrogen regulates brain physiology through a concerted action on diverse cell types and molecular targets [37]. Women who undergo surgical removal of the ovaries before menopause clearly demonstrate that oophorectomy is associated with an increased risk of cognitive impairment and dementia [38]. Women's Health Initiative (WHI) data, taking into consideration the time between menopause onset and hormone therapy initiation, showed beneficial effects of estrogens when therapy was initiated early after menopause, with detrimental effects associated with treatment started several years following menopause [39]. This supports the theory of estrogen as a neuroprotective agent while underscoring the limitations of the approach. Estrogen protection has a 'window-in-time': potentially effective if applied around the menopause period and maintained for a 5–10 year period of clinical effectiveness, given the absence of significant cancer or dementia risk factors [40], including the presence of the APOE e4 gene [11].

The neuroendocrine system is a powerful regulator of the inflammatory response in health and disease states [41]. In addition to regulating peripheral immune responses, steroid hormones, including glucocorticoids and gonadal steroids, support anti-inflammatory properties in the brain [42]. Steroid hormone protective actions in the nervous system range from stabilizing the blood brain barrier (BBB), alleviating brain edema, dampening pro-inflammatory/supporting anti-inflammatory processes, activating anti-apoptotic pathways, stimulating survival-promoting factors, counteracting oxidative stress, promoting respiratory chain function, and reducing glutamate excitotoxicity [43–48].

Estrogens are known to exert their actions through members of the nuclear hormone receptor superfamily, ERα [49], and the more recently identified estrogen receptor–ERβ [50–52]. Estrogen is recognized to exert an inhibitory response to neuroinflammation, with specificity of binding to microglia, resulting in the attenuation of the inflammatory response [53]. 17β-estradiol and progesterone have also been shown to mediate anti-inflammatory activity and improve neuronal survival [44, 54–56]. 17β-estradiol targets many pathways active in secondary injury; including oxidative stress, inflammation, apoptosis, and ischemia [57] (**Figure 4**).

Detecting the expression of the two estrogen receptors ERα and ERβ in cells of the monocyte-macrophage lineage, Vegeto and colleagues first evidenced the role that estrogens play in inflammatory diseases [58] with several laboratories later demonstrating that these gonadal steroid hormones act in a variety of macrophage-like cells to regulate the inflammatory response triggered by diverse inflammatory stimuli [59, 60]. In addition to having a regulatory role in the immune system, ERβ is involved in tumor suppression [61]. Thus, in recent years, pharmaceutical companies have generated selective agonists for ERα and ERβ, with ERβ research ongoing for ERβ development as a cancer preventative, as an anti-inflammatory drug and for the attenuation of neurodegenerative diseases [62].

Microglia are mediators of the innate immune defense, acting as antigens and scavenger cells during brain inflammation, acute central nervous system (CNS) injury, and neurodegeneration in the course of aging [63]. As such, they represent the resident macrophages of the CNS, comprising 5–15% of total cells in the brain [64]. As the brain-resident immunocompetent cells, microglia are critical for proper innate immune responses in the brain [42]. In the steady state, they perform housekeeping chores via autophagy [65] and may participate in postnatal neuronal development, whereas following trauma or pathogenic insult; they initiate the inflammatory response as part of the brain immune defense [66]. In the course of this, they increase their release of several inflammatory-associated substances, including reactive oxygen intermediates, nitric oxide (NO), and (inflammatory) cytokines [interleukin-1 and 6 (IL-1 and IL-6), interferon-g (IFN-g), and tumor necrosis factor-α (TNF-α)] [67].

Microglia cells express a set of classical and non-classical steroidal hormonal receptors, including ERα, ERβ, progesterone receptors (PR), glucocorticoid receptors (GR), and mineralocorticoid receptors (MR) [42, 68]. The central role of ERα and ERβ in the regulation of the microglia inflammatory response, in conjunction with the recent discovery of medial basal hypothalamic neuroestradiol, suggests the potential of estrogens to mitigate the pathogenesis and progression of neuroinflammation and neurodegeneration [69]. In particular, two gonadal steroid hormones, 17α-estradiol and progesterone, provide robust neuroprotection in a variety of experimental brain injury models [43, 54, 70, 71] and under neurodegenerative conditions [72–74]. It is possible that 17α-estradiol is an effective neuroprotective agent due to its actions as an anti-oxidant, anti-inflammatory, and anti-apoptotic steroid hormone [42, 57, 75–77].

Given the role of estrogenic steroids in modulating neurogenesis and the generation of dendritic spines and neuroprotection, Jellinck and colleagues [66] explored the question of whether microglia might serve as a regional *source* for estrogenic steroids. With respect to neuroprotection, dehydroepiandrosterone (DHEA) is considered to exert its positive influence via conversion to estrogen (estrone and estradiol). However, this conversion is slow and limited in brain cell cultures, with the exception of microglia [66]. These researchers were able to demonstrate the presence of the enzyme necessary for the rate limiting step of this conversion within microglia cells, supporting their contention that microglia are integral to regional regulation of adult estrogen-dependent brain plasticity and neuroprotection.

In the healthy CNS, microglia appear in a "resident state" with a ramified morphology (**Figure 4**). However, microglia are very susceptible to changes in the CNS milieu and become rapidly activated in response to CNS insult. Attracted by endogenous and other chemical messenger factors, microglial cells demonstrate the capacity to migrate toward the site of brain injury. Upon activation, microglia undergo morphological and functional changes such as hypertrophy and up-regulation of major histocompatibility complex (MHC) antigens. Activated cells secrete inflammatory mediators, including cytokines and chemokines [78, 79]. Microglia can also produce different types of free superoxide radicals and prostanoids [55].

As a first line of defense, activated microglia perform phagocytosis of apoptotic neuronal cell bodies via the lysozyme-autophagy recycling system. However, chronic activation of microglia with associated excess pro-inflammatory response in the aftermath of CNS insult may overwhelm this natural recycling system of the cell, resulting in cytotoxicity [80]. In the aftermath of stroke, for example, microglial activation is one of the earliest responses; requiring several hours to fully develop, while persisting for up to several days [81, 82]. The microglia inflammatory response, therefore, needs to be tightly controlled to avoid collateral damage within intact brain tissue. Estrogen appears to provide this level of regulation.

Microglia express steroid hormone receptors that include ER-α, with immunoreactivity evidenced by electron microscopy studies [35, 42, 68, 83–86]. Indeed, the neurodegenerative process of several CNS diseases, including amyotrophic lateral sclerosis, frontotemporal lobar degeneration, multiple sclerosis, Alzheimer's disease, and Parkinson's disease are associated with the activation of microglia cells, which drive the resident inflammatory response [17, 87–89]. In addition, a number of pro-inflammatory mediators are elevated in the CNS or cerebrospinal fluid of neurodegenerative disease patients [30]. Given this, it is particularly important to recognize that estrogen is understood to maintain microglia in the benign form, associated with suppression of the inflammatory response, suggesting its protective role in the aging brain against ubiquitin-proteosome mediated degradation.

Estrogen signaling is characterized by cell-specificity and dose dependent responsiveness. Divergent effects of estrogens have been reported for T cell activation [90], microglia modulation, and astroglia effects based upon different hormone concentrations [91, 92]. 17β-estradiol inhibits microglial activation following exposure to bacterial lipopolysaccharides [53], with estrogen-induced neuroprotection from autophagy lysis or proteasome degradation related to declines in TNF-α expression and NO production [43, 53]. NADPH oxidase represents one important source of free radicals in activated microglia [92], which catalyzes the reduction of oxygen to superoxide radical [93]. 17β-estradiol has been shown to decrease lipopolysaccharides-induced superoxide production and release in N-9 microglia cell lines [94].

ERα and ERβ are intracellular proteins, which activate a multitude of genomic as well as nongenomic effectors in neural cells [87]. Through the use of an estrogen receptor antagonist [ICI 182780], hormone action in microglia has been attributed to the activation of endogenous ERs, since antagonist binding was able to block the effect of estradiol, suggesting a receptor-mediated effect of the hormone [35, 53, 95, 96]. Using estrogen receptor knock out mutant mice, several investigators have described the selective involvement of ERα in the anti-inflammatory and neuroprotective activity of estradiol against neuroinflammatory and vascular pathologies of the brain [97–100]. In ICI 182780 studies, ERα appeared to be selectively involved in estradiol anti-inflammatory activity in microglia, a finding later confirmed by additional experimentation using primary cultures of microglia as well as cell lines [97, 101].

Estrogen-dependent attenuation of microglia activation has been demonstrated to involve reduced lysosome-phagocytic activity, production of reactive oxygen and nitrogen species and other factors of the inflammatory cascade [35, 94, 102–104]. The inhibitory activity of estrogens on microglia-associated neuroinflammation may prove to be a beneficial therapeutic opportunity for delaying the onset and progression of early onset neurodegenerative diseases such as FTLD, with replacement offsetting menopause associated declines.

Importantly, estradiol does not alter the inflammatory signaling cascade in microglia if it is administered after inflammatory stimuli [94, 97, 101]. Moreover, prolonged hormonal deprivation has been evidenced to affect estrogen protective activity in ischemia; resulting in a null or even pro-inflammatory response following administration of exogenous hormone [105]. Collectively, the experimental evidence indicates that the efficacy of estrogenic molecules as anti-inflammatory agents is confined to a therapeutic window and that their use should be considered only as preventive pharmacological strategies. Applied during the pre-clinical or prodrome stage, estrogen represents a therapeutic opportunity to forestall the onset and mitigate the progression of pre-senile neurodegenerative disease processes, particularly those like FTLD that typically emerge in mid-life, prior to or throughout the course of menopause and andropause. With the advent of personalized medicine, it may eventually be possible to identify genotypically high risk individuals and intervene with hormone replacement therapy while the neurodegenerative disease process remains at the sub-clinical level.

5. Estrogen interaction with cellular signaling molecules

Estrogen exerts an indirect effect on microglia through specific interactions with cellular signaling molecules. Nitric oxide synthases, a family of enzymes catalyzing the production of NO from L-arginine, are important cellular signaling molecules. The inducible isoform, inducible nitric oxide synthase (iNOS), serves a number of roles, including involvement in the immune response, with production of NO as an immune defense mechanism, due to its free radical nature. It is the proximate cause of septic shock and may function in autoimmune disease [106, 107]. In rats and microglia cell lines, the expression of iNOS and release of reactive oxygen species is reduced in certain cell types through the action of estrogen, including microglia [53, 76, 94], while expression of endothelial and neuronal subtypes of iNOS are increased [108].

After immunostimulation by lipopolysaccharides, estrogen but not progesterone has been shown to attenuate microglial superoxide release and phagocytotic activity as well as iNOS expression [94]. These effects are transmitted through an estrogen receptor-dependent activation of the MAP-kinase signaling system. Using a transient focal ischemia animal model, investigators have shown that estrogen and progesterone prevent the hypoxia-induced attraction and activation of local microglia and their morphological transition into an activated phenotype in the cortical penumbra [109]. The reduced stimulation of microglia is considered to result from diminished cytokine and interleukin expression and release in local astroglia, consequent to the close concerted communication between these two glial cell types during tissue stress. Focal ischemic mouse model experiments further evidence diminution of the penumbra of estrogen/progesterone-treated animals, along with reduction in chemokine levels, central microglia, and recruited monocytes. Ischemic mouse model data are confirmed by several other studies, which have demonstrated that these steroid hormones affect local cytokine production during brain inflammation in microglia [53, 76, 110], in astroglia [111, 112], and in unidentified cell types [113].

Mitogen-activated protein kinases (MAPKs) are involved in directing cellular responses to a diverse array of stimuli, such as mitogens, osmotic stress, heat shock, and microglia generated pro-inflammatory cytokines (e.g., TNFα, IL-6, and IL-1β) [114]. MAPKs regulate proliferation, gene expression, differentiation, mitosis, cell survival, and apoptosis [115]. Several MAPK pathways, including p42/44 MAPKs, are known to be activated by 17β estradiol [116]. Moreover, studies have evidenced the importance of activated p42/44 MAPK pathways in estrogen-mediated neuroprotection and microglia homeostasis [117]. When activated in response to inflammation, microglia release large amounts of oxygen and nitrogen radicals. Proteosomes clear oxidized and damaged proteins from cells, serving as a microglia compensatory response to activation. In the mouse model, the p42/44 MAPK pathway participates in estrogen-mediated proteasome activation, with estrogen up-regulation of proteosome activity considered to be one way estrogen potentially promotes microglial viability [117, 118].

Calcium-dependent protease with papain-like activity, or calpain, is a cytoplasmic cysteine protease that is activated by calcium [119]. Calpain is involved in neurodegeneration in a variety of injuries and diseases [120]. Calpain cleaves many substrates, including cytoskeletal proteins, axonal, and myelin proteins, and pro-apoptotic Bax causing mitochondrial cytochrome c release, activation of caspase-3, and activation of microglia [121–123]. Studies indicate that estrogen attenuates Ca^{2+} influx via modulation of L-type Ca^{2+} channels and the Na^{+}/Ca^{2+} exchanger [124]. Estrogen has also been shown to reduce calpain expression and activity, resulting in reduced axon degeneration and neuronal apoptosis in vitro [125].

Finally, estrogen is involved in regulation of microglial matrix metalloproteinases [126]. Metalloproteases secreted from microglia mediate inflammation and tissue degradation through processing of pro-inflammatory cytokines and damage to the BBB [127]. Progestins and estrogens affect matrix metalloproteinase enzyme activity in microglial cells, reducing indications of microglial inflammation [97, 126, 128].

6. Evidence of estrogenic effects in FTLD

Although few studies known to-date have focused on estrogenic effects in FTLD, indirect evidence comes from physiological studies in both normal and genetically disordered individuals. In this regard, it is notable that FTLD is associated with over a dozen genetic mutations that include the ALS-associated X linked UBQLN2 variant [129]. Neuropathologically, FTLD is primarily represented by two subtypes: one involving aberrant inclusions of microtubule protein tau, and one involving inclusions of TAR DNA binding protein [130].

6.1. Appetite regulation

Both bvFTD and SD are associated with changes in appetite and eating habits, with overeating and a preference for sweets and excessive seasonings, including salt [131–133]. Appetite is recognized to be modulated by gonadal steroid hormones, including peripheral and central mediating mechanisms [131, 134, 135]. In the healthy adult, sex differences in eating exist, regulated by the hypothalamic-pituitary-gonadal (HPG) axis. Little is known about the direct effect of testosterone on eating, while the effects of 17β-estradiol, the primary estrogen, have been well characterized. Hypothalamic centers are recognized to be intimately involved in the regulation of appetite, with extensive neuronal control reflected in their innervation by axons expressing all the major neurotransmitters [136, 137]. Hypothalamic centers are known to play a vital role in neuronal action of insulin and adipose tissue-secreted leptins. Estrogen binding (i.e., estradiol-triggered calcium influx) results in appetite suppression, with parvabumin potentially serving a protective role in the attenuation of calcium overload-associated neuronal degeneration (see Sinchack and Wagner for a detailed review) [138].

The posterior hypothalamus contains nuclei that play a critical role in regulating feeding behavior [136, 137]. Recent in vivo structural neuroimaging demonstrated a relationship between deterioration in the posterior hypothalamus and appetite disturbances in FTLD, an early sign of disease onset evident within 2 years of diagnosis [133]. Post-mortem analysis further evidenced sparse TDP-43-immunoreactive neurites within TDP-43 positive cases, with occasional intracytoplasmic inclusions in posterior hypothalamic neurons [133]. In their analysis of the differential effects of peripheral hormones vs. hypothalamic pathology on eating behavior in FTLD, Ahmed and colleagues [131] found higher levels of the hypothalamic derived satiation hormone agouti-related peptide in the serum of bvFTD and SD patients, with both groups having elevated scores on a questionnaire of eating behaviors. Atrophy of the posterior and total hypothlamus was found only for the bvFTD subgroup [131]. Interestingly, gender differences could not be examined, due to the relatively low numbers of females in both the bvFTD (4/15) and SD (8/18) subgroups, in comparison to gender matched controls (12/11).

6.2. Motivation regulation

As a bvFTD subtype, apathy is characterized by inertia and loss of volition, as well as apathy, in association with pathology within the dorsolateral convexities of the frontal lobe [139]. As an amotivational syndrome, apathy is also well recognized to be associated with disruptions to the ventral anterior cingulate cortex [139, 140]. In addition, regions known to be associated with Apathy include the medial dorsal nucleus of the thalamus, caudate nucleus, ventral medial striate (nucleus accumbens) and globus pallidus; with the cortical-striatal-thalamic-cortical circuit being the circuit most implicated in the Apathy syndrome [141]. Apathy neural circuitry is linked to the richly dopaminergic nonmotor limbic loop of the basal ganglia, with adaptive behaviors requiring a combination of reward evaluation, associative learning, and ability to develop appropriate action plans [142]. Dopamine deficiencies are often characteristic of FTLD. Clinical trials involving the use of dopaminergic psychostimulants have evidenced improvements in symptomology ranging from apathy to disinhibition and risk taking behaviors [143]. With respect to the potential for estrogen derivatives to mitigate apathy in FTLD, the responsiveness of dopamine neurons to estrogens has long been established, with inducement of dopamine synthesis and release, as well as dopamine neuron differentiation [144–147].

6.3. Turner syndrome

The overarching role of gonadal steroidal regulation of brain anatomy and physiology with respect to cognitive and affective executive functioning comes from studies of Turner syndrome, one of the most common sex chromosome-associated genetic disorders. Turner syndrome results in females from the complete or partial loss of one X chromosome, with partial loss involving the distal tip of its short arm [148, 149]. Turner syndrome individuals retain a healthy sense of desire for social interaction, while experiencing disruption in social salience in association with a right hemisphere learning disability. Turner syndrome is typically associated with early loss of ovarian function, leading to gonadal steroid deficiencies that result in pubertal delay and lack of developmental maturation. On a cognitive level, Turner Syndrome results in attentional deficits, disruptions to arithmetic reasoning, visuospatial processing, and executive functions. fMRI studies of Turner Syndrome adults provided with estrogen replacement to allow for physical maturation have implicated the parietal, amygdala and prefrontal areas in this condition, in association with tasks of working memory, as well as interpretation of facial emotional expressions, and mediation of arousal by affective stimuli. Provision of estrogen replacement to stimulate developmental maturation thus has the indirect effect of mitigating many cognitive and behavioral abnormalities also characteristic of cognitive and behavioral declines seen in emerging FTLD in females [23, 24, 150].

7. Summary

Early researchers found no evidence that FTLD affects men and women differentially [151, 152]. However, recent work has demonstrated hormonal differences in FTLD females not seen in either male FTLD or Alzheimer's patients [153]. Moreover, a multitude of genes have been identified associating FTLD characteristics with ALS, a motor variant of FTLD. ALS is known to have a greater percentage of males among patients who present with disease onset prior to mid-life and to have fMRI evidenced distinct patterns of neurophysiological change with ALS disease progression [15], up to half of whom potentially evidenced signs of FTLD associated cognitive and/or behavioral decline [18]. With respect to concerns about the association between estrogen replacement therapy and increased dementia risk in older women, raised by the results of the Woman's Health Initiative studies of the 1990s, estrogen replacement risk of senile dementia has been shown to be dependent upon the presence of the APOE e4 gene [11]. In the present effort, we present evidence that estrogen, in the absence of the APOE e4 genetic risk factor for Alzheimer's dementia, serves a neuroprotective role in females, including an association between female estrogen levels and cognitive and behavioral stability in emerging FTLD. The potential for estrogen replacement to delay disease onset in females vulnerable to FTLD, a condition typically emerging in midlife, is in need of further exploration.

Disclosure

The authors have no conflicts of interest to disclose.

Author details

Claire V. Flaherty[1]*, Arghavan S. Zangeneh[1], Marissa A. Harrison[2] and Sanjana Marikunte[3]

*Address all correspondence to: cflahertycraig@pennstatehealth.psu.edu

1 Department of Neurology, Penn State Hershey Medical Center, Hershey, PA, USA

2 Department of Psychology, Penn State Middletown, Harrisburg, PA, USA

3 Department of Biochemistry and Molecular Biology, Penn State University, PA, USA

References

[1] Snowden JS, Neary D, Mann DM. Frontotemporal dementia. British Journal of Psychiatry. 2002;**180**(2):140-143

[2] Rademakers R, Baker M, Gass J, et al. Phenotypic variability associated with progranulin haploinsufficiency in patients with the common 1477C→ T (Arg493X) mutation: An international initiative. Lancet Neurology. 2007;**6**(10):857-868

[3] Barker WW et al. Relative frequencies of Alzheimer disease, Lewy body, vascular and frontotemporal dementia, and hippocampal sclerosis in the State of Florida Brain Bank. Alzheimer Disease and Associated Disorders. 2002;**16**(4):203-212

[4] Rosen HJ et al. Behavioral features in semantic dementia vs other forms of progressive aphasias. Neurology. 2006;**67**(10):1752-1756

[5] Rascovsky K, Grossman M. Clinical diagnostic criteria and classification controversies in frontotemporal lobar degeneration. International Review of Psychiatry. 2013;**25**(2): 145-158

[6] Levenson RW, Sturm VE, Haase CM. Emotional and behavioral symptoms in neurodegenerative disease: A model for studying the neural bases of psychopathology. Annual Review of Clinical Psychology. 2014;**10**:581-606

[7] Chare L, Hodges JR, Leyton CE, et al. Journal of Neurology, Neurosurgery, and Psychiatry. 2014;**85**:866-871

[8] Vieira R, Caixeta L, Machado S, et al. Epidemiology of early-onset dementia: A review of the literature. Clinical Practice & Epidemiology in Mental Health. 2013;**9**:88-95

[9] Maki PM, Henderson VW. Hormone therapy, dementia, and cognition: The Woman's Health Initiative ten years on. Climacteric. 2012 June;**15**(3):256-262. DOI: 10.3109/13697137.2012.6660613

[10] Clem MA, Holliday RP, Pandya S, Hynan LS, Lacritz LH, Woon FL. Predictors that a diagnosis of mild cognitive impairment will remain stable 3 years later. Cognitive and Behavioral Neurology. 2017;**30**(1):8-15

[11] Kang JH, Grodstein F. Postmenopausal hormone therapy, timing of initiation, APOE and cognitive decline. Neurobiology of Aging. 2012;**33**(7):1129-1137

[12] Ratnavalli E, Brayne C, Dawson K, Hodges JR. The prevalence of frontotemporal dementia. Neurology. 2002;**58**(11):1615-1621

[13] Heston LL, White JA, Mastri AR. Pick's disease: Clinical genetics and natural history. Archives of General Psychiatry. 1987;**44**:409-411

[14] Johnson JK, Diehl J, Mendez MF, Neuhaus J, Shapira JS, Forman M, Chute DJ, et al. Frontotemporal lobar degeneration: Demographic characteristics of 353 patients. Archives of Neurology. 2005;**62**:925-930

[15] Bede P, Elamin M, Byrne S, Hardiman O. Sexual dimorphism in ALS: Exploring gender-specific neuroimaging signatures. Amyotrophic Lateral Sclerosis Frontotemporal Degeneration. 2014;**15**:235-243

[16] Park H, Chung S. New perspectives on Parkinsonism in frontotemporal lobar degeneration. Journal of Movement Disorders. 2013;**6**:1-8

[17] Snowden J, Rollinson S, Thompson JC, Harris JM, Stopford CL, Richardson AMT, et al. Distinct clinical and pathological characteristics of frontotemporal dementia associated with C9ORF72 mutations. Brain. 2012;**135**:693-708

[18] LeBlond C, Kaneb H, Dion P, Rouleau G. Dissection of genetic factors associated with amyotrophic lateral sclerosis. Experimental Neurology. 2014;**262**(B):91-101 Epub 2014 Apr 26

[19] Arevalo MA, Azcoitia I, Garcia-Segura LM. The neuroprotective actions of oestradiol and oestrogen receptors. Nature Reviews Neuroscience. 2015;**16**(1):17-29. DOI: 10.1038/nrn3856 Published online 26 November 2014

[20] Patchev V, Hayashi S, Orokasa C, Almeida O. Implications of estrogen-dependent brain organization for gender differences in hypothalamic-pituitary-adrenal regulation. The FASEB Journal. 1995;**9**:419-423

[21] Goldstein JM, Jerram M, Poldrack R, et al. Hormonal cycle modulates arousal circuitry in women using functional magnetic resonance imaging. The Journal of Neuroscience. 2005;**25**(40):9309-9316

[22] Dang TN, Dobson-Stone C, Glaros EN, et al. Endogenous progesterone levels and frontotemporal dementia: Modulation of TDP-43 and Tau levels in vitro and treatment of the A315T TARDBP mouse model. Disease Models & Mechanisms. 2013;**6**(5):1198-1204

[23] Flaherty C, Brothers A, Hoffer D, et al. VALUES: A national multicenter study demonstrating gender differences in amyotrophic lateral sclerosis with behavioral impairment. Neurodegenerative Disease Management. 2013;**3**(6):515-524

[24] Flaherty C, Kraft J, Brothers A, Harrison M, Legro RS, Manni A, Yang C, Simmons Z. For the VALUES Consortium. The relationship between oestrogen and executive functioning

in ALS females with emerging Frontotemporal Lobar Degeneration (FTLD) supports a neuroendocrine model of FTLD attenuation. Amyotrophic Lateral Sclerosis & Frontotemporal Degeneration. 2016:1-12

[25] Hoffman GE, Merchenthaler I, Zup SL. Neuroprotection by ovarian hormones in animal models of neurological disease. Endocrine. 2006;**29**(2):217-231

[26] Simpkins JW, Yang SH, Liu R, Perez E, Cai ZY, Covey DF, Green PS. Estrogen-like compounds for ischemic neuroprotection. Stroke. 2004;**35**:2648-2651

[27] Marin R, Guerra B, Alonso R, Ramirez CM, Diaz M. Estrogen activates classical and alternative mechanisms to orchestrate neuroprotection. Current Neurovascular Research. 2005;**2**:287-301

[28] Radenahmad N, Saleh F, Sawangjaroen K, et al. Young coconut juice, a potential therapeutic agent that could significantly reduce some pathologies associated with Alzheimer's disease: Novel findings. British Journal of Nutrition. 2011;**105**(5):738

[29] Radenahmad N, Saleh F, Sawangjaroen K, et al. Young coconut juice significantly reduces histopathological changes in the brain that are induced by hormonal imbalance: A possible implication to postmenopausal women. Histology and Histopathology. 2009;**24**(6):667-674

[30] Glick D, Barth S, Macleod KF. Autophagy: Cellular and molecular mechanisms. The Journal of Pathology. 2010;**221**(1):3-12

[31] Amin Z, Epperson CN, Constable RT, Canli T. Effects of estrogen variation on neural correlates of emotional response inhibition. NeuroImage. 2006;**32**(1):457-464

[32] Gleason CE, Dowling NM, Wharton W, Manson JE, Miller VM, Atwood CS, et al. Effects of hormone therapy on cognition and mood in recently postmenopausal women: Findings from the randomized, controlled KEEPS–Cognitive and Affective study. PLoS Medicine. 2015;**12**(6):e1001833. DOI: 10.1371/journal.pmed.1001833

[33] Norbury R, Cutter WJ, Compton J, et al. The neuroprotective effects of estrogen on the aging brain. Experimental Gerontology. 2003;**38**(1):109-117

[34] Johann S, Dahm M, Kipp M, Beyer C, Arnold S. Oestrogen regulates mitochondrial respiratory chain enzyme transcription in the mouse spinal cord. Journal of Neuroendocrinology. 2010;**22**(8):926-935

[35] Liu X, Fan XL, Zhao Y, et al. Estrogen provides neuroprotection against activated microglia-induced dopaminergic neuronal injury through both estrogen receptor-alpha and estrogen receptor-beta in microglia. Journal of Neuroscience Research. 2005;**81**(5):653-665

[36] Wooten G, Currie L, Bovbjerg V, Lee J, Patrie J. Are men at greater risk for Parkinson's disease than women? Journal of Neurology, Neurosurgery, and Psychiatry. 2004;**75**(4):637-639

[37] Maggi A, Ciana P, Belcredito S, Vegeto E. Estrogens in the nervous system: Mechanisms and nonreproductive functions. Annual Review of Physiology. 2004;**66**:291-313

[38] Rocca W, Bower J, Maraganore D, et al. Increased risk of cognitive impairment or dementia in women who underwent oophorectomy before menopause. Neurology. 2007;**69**(11):1074-1083

[39] Resnick SM, Maki PM, Rapp SR, et al. Effects of combination estrogen plus progestin hormone treatment on cognition and affect. Journal of Clinical Endocrinology and Metabolism. 2006;**91**(5):1802-1810

[40] Sherwin BB. Estrogen and memory in women: How can we reconcile the findings? Hormones and Behavior. 2005;**47**:371-375. PMID: 15708768

[41] Sternberg E. Neuroendocrine regulation of autoimmune/inflammatory disease. The Journal of Endocrinology. 2001;**169**(3):429-435

[42] Sierra A, Gottfried-Blackmore A, Milner TA, BS ME, Bulloch K. Steroid hormone receptor expression and function in microglia. Glia. 2008;**56**(6):659-674

[43] Herson PS, Koerner IP, Hurn PD. Sex, sex steroids and brain injury. Seminars in Reproductive Medicine. 2009;**27**(3):229-239

[44] Johann S, Beyer C. Neuroprotection by gonadal steroid hormones in acute brain damage requires cooperation with astroglia and microglia. The Journal of Steroid Biochemistry and Molecular Biology. 2012;**137**:71-81

[45] O'Donnell ME, Lam TI, Tran LQ, Foroutan S, Anderson SE. Estradiol reduces activity of the blood–brain barrier Na–K–Cl cotransporter and decreases edema formation in permanent middle cerebral artery occlusion. Journal of Cerebral Blood Flow & Metabolism. 2006;**26**(10):1234-1249

[46] Pawlak J, Brito V, Küppers E, Beyer C. Regulation of glutamate transporter GLAST and GLT-1 expression in astrocytes by estrogen. Molecular Brain Research. 2005;**138**(1):1-7

[47] Zhang Q-G, Raz L, Wang R, et al. Estrogen attenuates ischemic oxidative damage via an estrogen receptor α-mediated inhibition of NADPH oxidase activation. The Journal of Neuroscience. 2009;**29**(44):13823-13836

[48] Morale MC, Serra PA, L'Episcopo F, et al. Estrogen, neuroinflammation and neuroprotection in Parkinson's disease: Glia dictates resistance versus vulnerability to neurodegeneration. Neuroscience. 2006;**138**(3):869-878

[49] Greene GL, Gilna P, Waterfield M, et al. Sequence and expression of human estrogen receptor complementary DNA. Science. 1986;**231**(4742):1150-1154

[50] Kuiper G, Enmark E, Pelto-Huikko M, Nilsson S, Gustafsson J-A. Cloning of a novel receptor expressed in rat prostate and ovary. PNAS. 1996;**93**(12):5925-5930

[51] Ogawa S, Inoue S, Watanabe T, et al. The complete primary structure of human estrogen receptor β (hERβ) and its heterodimerization with ER α in vivo and in vitro. Biochemical and Biophysical Research Communications. 1998;**243**(1):122-126

[52] Mosselman S, Polman J, Dijkema R. ERβ: Identification and characterization of a novel human estrogen receptor. FEBS Letters. 1996;**392**(1):49-53

[53] Vegeto E, Bonincontro C, Pollio G, et al. Estrogen prevents the lipopolysaccharide-induced inflammatory response in microglia. The Journal of Neuroscience. 2001;**21**(6):1809-1818

[54] McEwen BS, Alves SE. Estrogen actions in the central nervous system. Endocrine Reviews. 1999;**20**(3):279-307

[55] Sawada H, Ibi M, Kihara T, et al. Estradiol protects mesencephalic dopaminergic neurons from oxidative stress-induced neuronal death. Journal of Neuroscience Research. 1998;**54**(5):707-719

[56] Samantaray S, Smith JA, Das A, et al. Low dose estrogen prevents neuronal degeneration and microglial reactivity in an acute model of spinal cord injury: Effect of dosing, route of administration, and therapy delay. Neurochemical Research. 2011;**36**(10):1809-1816

[57] Arevalo MA, Santos-Galindo M, Bellini MJ, Azcoitia I, Garcia-Segura LM. Actions of estrogens on glial cells: Implications for neuroprotection. BBA General Subjects. 2010; **1800**:1106-1112

[58] Vegeto E, Pollio G, Pellicciari C, Maggi A. Estrogen and progesterone induction of survival of monoblastoid cells undergoing TNF-alpha-induced apoptosis. The FASEB Journal. 1999;**13**(8):793-803

[59] Hapangama D, Kamal A, Bulmer J. Estrogen receptor β: The guardian of the endometrium. Human Reproduction Update. 2015;**21**(2):174-193

[60] Hsieh Y, Hsieh F, Chen Y, Hu C, Jeng J, Tang S, et al. Associations of estradiol levels and genetic polymorphisms of inflammatory genes with the risk of ischemic stroke. Journal of Biomedical Science. 2017;**24**:25

[61] Begam J, Jubie S, Nanjan M. Estrogen receptor agonists/antagonists in breast cancer therapy: A critical review. Bioorganic Chemistry. 2017;**71**:257-274

[62] Dey P, Ström A, Gustafsson JA. Estrogen receptor β upregulates FOXO3a and causes induction of apoptosis through PUMA in prostate cancer. Oncogene. 2014;**33**(33): 4213-4225. DOI: 10.1038/onc.2013.384 Epub 2013 Sep 30

[63] Kreutzberg GW. Microglia: A sensor for pathological events in the CNS. Trends in Neurosciences. 1996;**19**(8):312-318

[64] Lawson L, Perry V, Dri P, Gordon S. Heterogeneity in the distribution and morphology of microglia in the normal adult mouse brain. Neuroscience. 1990;**39**(1):151-170

[65] Raivich G, Bohatschek M, Kloss CU, et al. Neuroglial activation repertoire in the injured brain: Graded response, molecular mechanisms and cues to physiological function. Brain Research Reviews. 1999;**30**(1):77-105

[66] Jellinck PH, Kaufmann M, Gottfried-Blackmore A, et al. Selective conversion by microglia of dehydroepiandrosterone to 5-androstenediol—A steroid with inherent estrogenic properties. Journal of Steroid Biochemistry. 2007;**107**(3):156-162

[67] Mor G, Nilsen J, Horvath T, et al. Estrogen and microglia: A regulatory system that affects the brain. Journal of Neurobiology. 1999;**40**(4):484-496

[68] Wong AM, Rozovsky I, Arimoto JM, et al. Progesterone influence on neurite outgrowth involves microglia. Endocrinology. 2009;**150**(1):324-332

[69] Kenealy BP, Kapoor A, Guerriero KA, et al. Neuroestradiol in the hypothalamus contributes to the regulation of gonadotropin releasing hormone release. The Journal of Neuroscience. 2013;**33**(49):19051-19059

[70] Acs P, Kipp M, Norkute A, et al. 17β-estradiol and progesterone prevent cuprizone provoked demyelination of corpus callosum in male mice. Glia. 2009;**57**(8):807-814

[71] Ishrat T, Sayeed I, Atif F, Hua F, Stein DG. Progesterone and allopregnanolone attenuate blood–brain barrier dysfunction following permanent focal ischemia by regulating the expression of matrix metalloproteinases. Experimental Neurology. 2010;**226**(1):183-190

[72] Xu H, Gouras GK, Greenfield JP, Vincent B, Naslund J. Estrogen reduces neuronal generation of Alzheimer β-amyloid peptides. Nature Medicine. 1998;**4**(4):447-451

[73] Dhandapani KM, Brann DW. Protective effects of estrogen and selective estrogen receptor modulators in the brain. Biology of Reproduction. 2002;**67**(5):1379-1385

[74] Garcia-Segura LM, Azcoitia I, DonCarlos LL. Neuroprotection by estradiol. Progress in Neurobiology. 2001;**63**(1):29-60

[75] Moosmann B, Behl C. The antioxidant neuroprotective effects of estrogens and phenolic compounds are independent from their estrogenic properties. Proceedings of the National Academy of Sciences of the United States of America. 1999;**96**(16):8867-8872

[76] Dimayuga FO, Reed JL, Carnero GA, et al. Estrogen and brain inflammation: Effects on microglial expression of MHC, costimulatory molecules and cytokines. Journal of Neuroimmunology. 2005;**161**(1):123-136

[77] Samantaray S, Sribnick EA, Das A, et al. Neuroprotective efficacy of estrogen in experimental spinal cord injury in rats. Annals of the New York Academy of Sciences. 2010;**1199**:90-94

[78] Kettenmann H, Hanisch U-K, Noda M, Verkhratsky A. Physiology of microglia. Physiological Reviews. 2011;**91**(2):461-553

[79] Hanisch U-K, Kettenmann H. Microglia: Active sensor and versatile effector cells in the normal and pathologic brain. Nature Neuroscience. 2007;**10**(11):1387-1394

[80] Block ML, Zecca L, Hong J-S. Microglia-mediated neurotoxicity: Uncovering the molecular mechanisms. Nature Reviews. Neuroscience. 2007;**8**(1):57-69

[81] Yenari MA, Kauppinen TM, Swanson RA. Microglial activation in stroke: Therapeutic targets. Neurotherapeutics. 2010;**7**(4):378-391

[82] Tambuyzer BR, Ponsaerts P, Nouwen EJ. Microglia: Gatekeepers of central nervous system immunology. Journal of Leukocyte Biology. 2009;**85**(3):352-370

[83] Neniskyte U, Brown GC. Lactadherin/MFG-E8 is essential for microglia-mediated neuronal loss and phagoptosis induced by amyloid β. Journal of Neurochemistry. 2013; **126**(3):312-317

[84] García-Ovejero D, Veiga S, García-Segura LM, Doncarlos LL. Glial expression of estrogen and androgen receptors after rat brain injury. Journal of Comparative Neurology. 2002;**450**(3):256-271

[85] Cheepsunthorn P, Mairaue N, Nasee K. Estrogen enhances the inhibitory effect of iron on microglial nitric oxide production. Journal of the Medical Association of Thailand. 2006;**89**(6):840

[86] Vegeto E, Pollio G, Ciana P, Maggi A. Estrogen blocks inducible nitric oxide synthase accumulation in LPS-activated microglia cells. Experimental Gerontology. 2000;**35**(9): 1309-1316

[87] Brettschneider J, Libon DJ, Toledo JB, et al. Microglial activation and TDP-43 pathology correlate with executive dysfunction in amyotrophic lateral sclerosis. Acta Neuropathologica. 2012;**123**(3):395-407

[88] Chinta SJ, Ganesan A, Reis-Rodrigues P, Lithgow GJ, Andersen JK. Anti-inflammatory role of the isoflavone diadzein in lipopolysaccharide-stimulated microglia: Implications for Parkinson's disease. Neurotoxicity Research. 2013;**23**(2):145-153

[89] Cameron B, Landreth GE. Inflammation, microglia, and Alzheimer's disease. Neurobiology of Disease. 2010;**37**(3):503-509

[90] Cutolo M, Sulli A, Seriolo B, Accardo S, Masi AT. Estrogens, the immune response and autoimmunity. Clinical and Experimental Rheumatology. 1995;**13**(2):217-226

[91] Dodel RC, Du Y, Bales KR, Gao F, Paul SM. Sodium salicylate and 17beta-estradiol attenuate nuclear transcription factor NF-kappaB translocation in cultured rat astroglial cultures following exposure to amyloid A beta(1-40) and lipopolysaccharides. Journal of Neurochemistry. 1999;**73**(4):1453-1460

[92] Segal AW. The function of the NADPH oxidase of phagocytes and its relationship to other NOXs in plants, invertebrates, & mammals. International Journal of Biochemistry & Cell Biology. 2008;**40**(4):604-618

[93] Qin L, Liu Y, Wang T, et al. NADPH oxidase mediates lipopolysaccharide-induced neurotoxicity and proinflammatory gene expression in activated microglia. The Journal of Biological Chemistry. 2004;**279**(2):1415-1421

[94] Bruce-Keller AJ, Keeling JL, Keller JN, et al. Antiinflammatory effects of estrogen on microglial activation. Endocrinology. 2000;**141**(10):3646-3656

[95] Bruce-Keller AJ. Microglial-neuronal interactions in synaptic damage and recovery. Journal of Neuroscience Research. 1999;**58**(1):191-201

[96] Brown CM, Choi E, Xu Q, Vitek MP, Colton CA. The APOE4 genotype alters the response of microglia and macrophages to 17beta-estradiol. Neurobiology of Aging. 2008;**29**(12):1783-1794

[97] Vegeto E, Belcredito S, Etteri S, et al. Estrogen receptor-alpha mediates the brain anti-inflammatory activity of estradiol. Proceedings of the National Academy of Sciences of the United States of America. 2003;**100**(16):9614-9619

[98] Dubal DB, Zhu H, Yu J, et al. Estrogen receptor alpha, not beta, is a critical link in estradiol-mediated protection against brain injury. Proceedings of the National Academy of Sciences of the United States of America. 2001;**98**(4):1952-1957

[99] Garidou L, Laffont S, Douin-Echinard V, et al. Estrogen receptor alpha signaling in inflammatory leukocytes is dispensable for 17beta-estradiol-mediated inhibition of experimental autoimmune encephalomyelitis. Journal of Immunology. 2004;**173**(4):2435-2442

[100] Polanczyk MJ, Carson BD, Subramanian S, et al. Cutting edge: Estrogen drives expansion of the CD4+CD25+ regulatory T cell compartment. Journal of Immunology. 2004; **173**(4):2227-2230

[101] Ghisletti S, Meda C, Maggi A, Vegeto E. 17beta-estradiol inhibits inflammatory gene expression by controlling NF-kappaB intracellular localization. Molecular and Cellular Biology. 2005;**25**(8):2957-2968

[102] Colton CA, Brown CM, Vitek MP. Sex steroids, APOE genotype and the innate immune system. Neurobiology of Aging. 2005;**26**(3):363-372

[103] Drew PD, Chavis JA. Female sex steroids: Effects upon microglial cell activation. Journal of Neuroimmunology. 2000;**111**(1-2):77-85

[104] Zemlyak I, Brooke S, Sapolsky R. Estrogenic protection against gp120 neurotoxicity: Role of microglia. Brain Research. 2005;**1046**(1-2):130-136

[105] Suzuki S, Brown CM, Dela Cruz CD, et al. Timing of estrogen therapy after ovariectomy dictates the efficacy of its neuroprotective and antiinflammatory actions. P Natl Acad Sci USA. 2007;**104**(14):6013-6018

[106] Liu SF, Adcock IM, Old RW, Barnes PJ, Evans TW. Differential regulation of the constitutive and inducible nitric oxide synthase mRNA by lipopolysacchride treatment in vivo in the rat. Critical Care Medicine. 1996;**24**(7):1219-1225

[107] Bruckdorfer R. The basics about nitric oxide. Molecular Aspects of Medicine. 2005;**26**(1): 3-31

[108] Saito S, Aras RS, Lou H, Ramwell PW, Foegh ML. Effects of estrogen on nitric oxide synthase expression in rat aorta allograft and smooth muscle cells. The Journal of Heart and Lung Transplantation. 1999;**18**(10):937-945

[109] Dang J, Mitkari B, Kipp M, Beyer C. Gonadal steroids prevent cell damage and stimulate behavioral recovery after transient middle cerebral artery occlusion in male and female rats. Brain, Behavior, and Immunity. 2011;**25**(4):715-726

[110] Smith JA, Das A, Butler JT, Ray SK, Banik NL. Estrogen or estrogen receptor agonist inhibits lipopolysaccharide induced microglial activation and death. Neurochemical Research. 2011;**36**(9):1587-1593

[111] Kipp M, Karakaya S, Johann S, et al. Oestrogen and progesterone reduce lipopolysaccharide-induced expression of tumour necrosis factor-α and interleukin-18 in midbrain astrocytes. Journal of Neuroendocrinology. 2007;**19**(10):819-822

[112] Giraud SN, Caron CM, Pham-Dinh D, Kitabgi P, Nicot AB. Estradiol inhibits ongoing autoimmune neuroinflammation and NFκB-dependent CCL2 expression in reactive astrocytes. Proceedings of the National Academy of Sciences of the United States of America. 2010;**107**(18):8416-8421

[113] Brown CM, Mulcahey TA, Filipek NC, Wise PM. Production of proinflammatory cytokines and chemokines during neuroinflammation: Novel roles for estrogen receptors α and β. Endocrinology. 2010;**151**(10):4916-4925

[114] Manning G, Whyte DB, Martinez R, Hunter T, Sudarsanam S. The protein kinase complement of the human genome. Science. 2002;**298**(5600):1912-1934

[115] Pearson G, Robinson F, Beers Gibson T, et al. Mitogen-activated protein (MAP) kinase pathways: Regulation and physiological functions. Endocrine Reviews. 2001;**22**(2): 153-183

[116] Merchenthaler I, Lane MV, Numan S, Dellovade TL. Distribution of estrogen receptor alpha and beta in the mouse central nervous system: In vivo autoradiographic and immunocytochemical analyses. Journal of Comparative Neurology. 2004;**473**(2):270-291

[117] Singh M, Setalo G Jr, Guan X, Warren M, Toran-Allerand CD. Estrogen-induced activation of mitogen-activated protein kinase in cerebral cortical explants: Convergence of estrogen and neurotrophin signaling pathways. The Journal of Neuroscience. 1999; **19**(4):1179-1188

[118] Reed JL, Dimayuga FO, Davies LM, Keller JN, Bruce-Keller AJ. Estrogen increases proteasome activity in murine microglial cells. Neuroscience Letters. 2004;**367**(1):60-65

[119] Vosler P, Brennan C, Chen J. Calpain-mediated signaling mechanisms in neuronal injury and neurodegeneration. Molecular Neurobiology. 2008;**38**(1):78-100

[120] Ray SK, Banik NL. Calpain and its involvement in the pathophysiology of CNS injuries and diseases: Therapeutic potential of calpain inhibitors for prevention of neurodegeneration. Current Drug Targets. CNS and Neurological Disorders. 2003;**2**(3):173-189

[121] Pike BR, Zhao X, Newcomb JK, et al. Regional calpain and caspase-3 proteolysis of spectrin after traumatic brain injury. Neuroreport. 1998;**9**(11):2437-2442

[122] Blomgren K, Zhu C, Wang X, et al. Synergistic activation of caspase-3 by m-calpain after neonatal hypoxia-ischemia: A mechanism of "pathological apoptosis"? The Journal of Biological Chemistry. 2001;**276**(13):10191-10198

[123] Levesque S, Wilson B, Gregoria V, et al. Reactive microgliosis: Extracellular μ-calpain and microglia-mediated dopaminergic neurotoxicity. Brain. 2010;**133**(3):808-821

[124] Sribnick EA, Del Re AM, Ray SK, Woodward JJ, Banik NL. Estrogen attenuates glutamate-induced cell death by inhibiting Ca^{2+} influx through L-type voltage-gated Ca^{2+} channels. Brain Research. 2009;**1276**:159-170

[125] Sribnick EA, Ray SK, Nowak MW, Li L, Banik NL. 17β-estradiol attenuates glutamate-induced apoptosis and preserves electrophysiologic function in primary cortical neurons. Journal of Neuroscience Research. 2004;**76**(5):688-696

[126] Hwang-Levine J, Stanczyk FZ, Hodis HN. The role of progestogens in regulating matrix metalloproteinase activity in macrophages and microglial cells. Neurochemical Research. 2011;**36**(10):1870-1875

[127] Nakanishi H. Microglial functions and proteases. Molecular Neurobiology. 2003;**27**(2): 163-176

[128] Gold S, Sasidhar M, Morales L, Du S, Sicotte N, Tiwari-Woodruff S, Voskuhl R. Estrogen treatment decreases matrix metalloproteinase (MMP)-9 in autoimmune demyelinating disease through estrogen receptor alpha (ERα). Laboratory Investigation. 2009;**89**(10): 1076-1083. DOI: 10.1038/labinvest. 2009.79

[129] Thomas M, Alegre-Abarrategui J, Wade-Martins R. RNA dysfunction and aggrephagy at the centre of an amyotrophic lateral sclerosis/frontotemporal dementia disease continuum. Brain. 2013;**136**:1345-1360

[130] Irwin DJ, Trojanowski JQ, Grossman M. Cerebrospinal fluid biomarkers for differentiation of frontotemporal lobar degeneration from Alzheimer's Disease. Frontiers in Aging Neuroscience. 2013;**5**(6):1-11

[131] Ahmed R, Latheef S, Bartley L, Irish M, Halliday G, Kiernan M. Eating behavior in frontotemporal dementia. Peripheral hormones vs hypothalamic pathology. Neurology. 2015;**85**(15):1310-1317

[132] Ikeda M, Brown J, Holland A, Fukuhara R, Hodges J. Changes in appetite, food preference, and eating habits in frontotemporal dementia and Alzheimer's disease. Journal of Neurology, Neurosurgery, and Psychiatry. 2002;**73**(4):371-376

[133] Piguet O, Hornberger M, Mioshi E, Hodges JR. Behavioural-variant frontotemporal dementia: Diagnosis, clinical staging, and management. Lancet Neurology. 2011;**10**: 162-172

[134] Asarian L, Geary N. Modulation of appetite by gonadal steroid hormones. Philosophical Transactions of the Royal Society B: Biological Sciences. 2006;**361**(1471):1251-1263

[135] Sotonyi P, Gao Q, Bechmann I, Horvath TL. Estrogen promotes parvalbumin expression in arcuate nucleus POMC neurons. Reproductive Sciences. 2010;**17**(12):1077-1080

[136] Gooley JJ, Schomer A, Saper CB. The dorsomedial hypothalamic nucleus is critical for the expression of food-entrainable circadian rhythms. Nature Neuroscience. 2006;**9**: 398-407

[137] Yang L, Scott KA, Hyun J, et al. Role of dorsomedial hypothalamic neuropeptide Y in modulating food intake and energy balance. The Journal of Neuroscience. 2009;**29**: 179-190

[138] Sinchack K, Wagner E. Estradiol signaling in the regulation of reproduction and energy balance. Frontiers in Neuroendocrinology. 2012;**33**(4):342-363

[139] Lanuta S, Miller B. The behavioural variant frontotemporal dementia (bvFTD) syndromein psychiatry. Neuropsychiatry. 2016;**87**(5):501-511. DOI: 10.1136/jnnp-2015-310697

[140] Bush G, Luu P, Posner MI. Cognitive and emotional influences in anterior cingulate cortex. Trends in Cognitive Sciences. 2000;**4**(6):215-222

[141] Weitzner M, Kanfer S, Booth-Jones M. Apathy and pituitary disease: It has nothing to do with depression. Journal of Neuropsychiatry & Clinical Neurosciences. 2005;**17**:159-166

[142] Haber SN, Knutson B. The reward circuit: linking primate anatomy and human imaging. Neuropsychopharmacology. 2010;**35**:4-26

[143] Leger G, Banks S, Cummings J. Clinical trials in frontotemporal lobar degeneration. In: Miller B, Cummings J, editors. The Human Frontal Lobes. 3rd ed. NY: Guilford Press. p. 563

[144] Gajjar TM, Anderson LI, Dluzen DE. Acute effects of estrogen upon methamphetamine induced neurotoxicity of the nigrostriatal dopaminergic system. Journal of Neural Transmission. 2003;**110**:1215-1224

[145] Garnier M, Di Lorenzo D, Albertini A, Maggi A. Identification of estrogenresponsive genes in neuroblastoma SK-ER3 cells. The Journal of Neuroscience. 1997;**17**:4591-4599

[146] Morissette M, Di Paolo T. Effect of chronic estradiol and progesterone treatments of ovariectomized rats on brain dopamine uptake sites. Journal of Neurochemistry. 1993; **60**:1876-1883

[147] Sarvari M, Kallo I, Hrabovszky E, Solymosi N, Toth K, Liko I, Molnar B, et al. Estradiol replacement alters expression of genes related to neurotransmission and immune Surveillance in the frontal cortex of middle aged, ovariectomized rats. Endocrinology. 2010;**151**:3847-3862

[148] Knickmeyer R. Turner syndrome: Advances in understanding altered cognition, brain structure and function. Current Opinion in Neurology. 2012;**25**(2):144

[149] Christopoulos P, Deligeoroglou E, Laggari V, Christogiorgos S, Creatsas G. Psychological and behavioural aspects of patients with Turner syndrome from childhood to adulthood: A review of the clinical literature. Journal of Psychosomatic Obstetrics and Gynecology. 2008;**29**(1):45-51

[150] Flaherty-Craig C, Brothers A, McFalls A, Yang C, Simmons ZVALUES. A national multicenter study of regional and gender differences in frontotemporal disease in amyotrophic lateral sclerosis. Neurodegenerative Disease Management. 2012;**2**(3):325-336

[151] Diehl J, Kurtz A. Frontotemporal dementia: Patient characteristics, cognition, and behavior. International Journal of Geriatric Psychiatry. 2002;**17**:914-918

[152] Gustafson L. Clinical picture of frontal lobe degeneration of non-Alzheimer type. Dementia. 1993;**4**:143-148

[153] Alberici A, Boccio L, Geroldi C, Zanardini R, Bomomini C, Bugari G, et al. Serum leptin levels are higher in females affected by frontotemporal lobar degeneration than Alzheimer's disease. Journal of Neurology, Neurosurgery, and Psychiatry. 2008;**79**: 712-715. DOI: 10.1136/jnnp.2007.137026

5

Neuroprotection in Perimenopausal Women

Manuela Cristina Russu and
Alexandra Cristina Antonescu

Abstract

Endocrine and neural senescence overlap in time, by intertwined complex feedback loops. Womens' brain is genetically more prone to suffer during life, and perimenopause is a "critical period" in neuroaging, when the degenerative processes begin. Many hypotheses on the multifactorial nature of women's brain aging are elaborated, and tested in high-tech research centers. The most analyzed Alzheimer's disease (AD) is characterized not only by Aβ oligomers and fibrils accumulation, but also by metabolic and inflammatory changes, with the onset during menopausal transition and early years of menopause. Deep analysis of endocrine, neural, and metabolic pathways are giving new insights to the sequential view of Aβ-centric in AD pathogenesis, prevention, and treatment from perimenopause, for maintaining women's neurological health.

Keywords: neuroaging, perimenopause, critical period

1. Introduction: sex differences in contemporary neurodegenerative disorders

Ovarian aging is very well-known in contemporary women's life, and the jeopardizing menopausal effects of sex steroid hormones deficiency are clinically evident in late-life mental disorders. Endocrine and neural senescence overlap in time, and are mechanistically intertwined in complex feedback loops.

In the past century, both life expectancy and the average age of onset of menopause for women in many countries from Western Europe and North America were slightly over 50 years, whereas currently, women can expect to live until the age of 80 years, although the average age of menopause remains in the early 50s. Given the importance of the brain as a target organ for sex steroids, it is not surprising that many of the complaints that prompt women to seek treatment related to menopause are neurological in origin.

Dementia with its most severe entities, such as the Alzheimer's disease (AD), Parkinson's disease (PD), multiple sclerosis (MS), and amyotrophic lateral sclerosis (ALS), are the most frequent contemporary neurodegenerative disorders, connected in majority by neural cell loss and neuroinflammation.

There are sex/gender differences in cognitive trajectories in clinically normal older adults [1], and women are known to have a higher propensity to develop AD versus men [2, 3], a higher risk of mild cognitive impairment and a lower risk, but poorer outcomes after stroke [4]. Women's risk for AD is considered to be through their organizational effects during developmental sexual differentiation of the fetal brain [5].

The AD is the most prevalent form of old-life mental failure in worldwide humans, being a progressive neurodegenerative disorder, for which a number of genetic, environmental, and lifestyle risk factors have been identified. The estimated prevalence of all-cause of dementia varies from 4.7% in Central Europe to 8.7% in North Africa/Middle East, with North America falling at 6.4%. Currently, over 46 million individuals live with dementia worldwide and the number is projected to increase to 131.5 million by 2050 [6]. The AD is familial with early-onset and sporadic with late-onset, and the present chapter will discuss the sporadic AD with late-onset in women, the most common form of AD representing more than 95% of the current human AD population [7].

In this very moment, the geroscience research is imperative with aims to forward a better and full understanding of neurodegeneration/neuroprotection of "the sexome" [8], and to prevent or delay by every tool the deleterious effects of brain aging [9]. Estrogen deficiency or estrogen disrupters are associated from menopause transition with episodic memory troubles, a cognitive domain in which impairments are associated with the increased risk of AD, being less known the onset of the other neurodegenerative disorders [10].

AD has an insidious onset and a gradual progression over several years—from 1.5 to 8 or up to 10 years, or a preclinical stage with a subtle loss of cognitive functioning—as verbal memory on new information, that precede several years the AD diagnostic, period considered as a transition period from normal aging brain to AD [11]. During this period, there are discovered several subtypes of mild cognitive impairment (MCI), 10–15% with the risk to future evolution to AD per year [12], or a 12% conversion rate from MIC to dementia yearly [13]. The characteristic deposits of β-amyloid and tau proteins depicted by neuroimaging or at autopsy located in the hippocampus, medial temporal regions, parietal, and frontal cortical regions [14] may be prevented from extension, as other structural degenerative diseases. It is imperious to prevent the intracellular appearance of the amyloid peptide, which induces by its toxicity neuronal apoptosis and cell death, events that can be prevented by sex steroid hormones [15].

The clinical symptoms/signs of MCI are considered by neuroscientists as prodrome to AD [16], and their algorithms for diagnosis may permit to initiate the hormone/estrogen therapy (HT/ET), because their onset moment is coincidental to perimenopause, as considering the North American clinicians [17]. The "timing" theory regarding the reproductive stage and role of time since menopause at initiation of HT/ET may work in preventing the mental deterioration due to aging [17], and perimenopause can be the "critical window" for opportunity in neuroprotection with steroids. The perimenopausal transition might also represent a "window of opportunity" to prevent age-related neurological diseases [10, 18, 19].

2. Hormonal and genetic data on perimenopausal neuroaging

The data of this chapter are regarding brain aging in perimenopause—a part in woman's reproductive life, systematized in the stages of reproductive aging (STRAW) [20].

Menopausal transition starts with the variation of cycles duration and ends with the last period (recognized only after 12 months of amenorrhea), natural menopause at the average age 51 years, premature menopause [premature ovarian failure (POF)] before 40 years, and early menopause between 40 and 45 years [21, 22]. Women with POF have been reported to have more anxiety, depression, somatization, sensitivity, hostility, and psychological distress than women with normal ovaries [23]. Perimenopause or "near menopause" starts from the stage −2 of menopausal transition and ends at 12 months after last menstruation, may be of 10–15 years. During this period, there are important variations of sex steroids, summarized by low ovarian inhibin [24], which in turn reduces the restraint on both the hypothalamus and pituitary gland, and results in elevated pituitary gonadotropin FSH, increased also by the hypothalamic gonadotropin-releasing hormone (GnRH). During the late menopause transition and a part of perimenopause, despite occasional episodes of normal cycling, women are exposed to periods of estrogen withdrawal, fewer ovulatory cycles, and prolonged hypogonadism, ultimately leading to the last menstrual period, after which is an elevated level of gonadotrophin secretion (only tonic, not phasic) [25]. During this phase, besides the low ovarian E2 and progesterone, there are productions of androgens and growth factors, which will decline in future years of postmenopause [26]. The ovaries are stimulated during menopausal transition and early postmenopausal years by gonadotropins, but the pulsatile GnRH pattern is different in different species before reproductive failure. It is a decrease of GnRH gene expression in many middle-aged rats [27], and an increase in perimenopausal rhesus monkeys [28].

Premature menopause/early menopause can be spontaneous or induced; after medical interventions such as chemotherapy/radiotherapy or surgery. The most common cause of premature/early menopause is bilateral oophorectomy with/without hysterectomy. Primary ovarian failure (POF) may be a cause of early/premature menopause, for ischemic stroke [29], as for all cardiovascular diseases risks [30], and these conditions were first described as a cause of neurological disturbances in different European, North American, and Japanese populations [21, 31–33].

Bilateral oophorectomy at premenopausal ages is inducing drops of E2 and testosterone levels, by 40–50%, and an abruptly rise in FSH levels, the levels of androgen being lower than in natural menopause at ages of 65 years, when women in normal or in premature/early menopause continue to have some levels of androgens [34]. As it is shown in the **Table 1**, the hazard ratios reached statistical significance in cases with bilateral oophorectomy: at the

Adjusted odd ratio for dementia after unilateral oophorectomy			
Age at surgery (years)	Hazard ratio	CI 95%	P value
<43	1.74	0.97–3.14	0.06
43–48	1.68	1.06–2.66	0.03
>48	1.09	0.74–1.61	0.66
Adjusted odd ratio for dementia after bilateral oophorectomy			
<34	4.61	2.52–8.43	<0.0001
34–41	1.23	0.67–2.26	0.51
>41	1.50	1.05–2.13	0.03
Adjusted odd ratio for PD after bilateral oophorectomy			
<38	2.85	1.28–6.35	0.001
38–45	1.38	1.28–6.35	0.42
>45	1.38	0.92–3.03	0.09

Cases of cognitive impairment/dementia and Parkinson disease (PD) in women with unilateral (813) and bilateral (676) oophorectomy: For a nonmalignant disease, in Olmsted County, Minnesota (USA) during 1950–1987, followed up the death or the finish of study at 2001–2006 (Rocca et al. [32]).

Table 1. Utero-ovarian surgery and neurological disturbances in premenopause.

age < 34 years for dementia and <38 years for PD. Perimenopause is a "fragile" period in woman's life, comparable to the fragility of the adolescence, if we speak about "hormonal storms," but the hormonal pyramid is upside down, and more than these, the North American neurologists are considering perimenopause as a neurological transition state [35], because the characteristic symptoms regarding thermoregulation, sleep, circadian rhythms, and sensory processing are of neurological nature, besides the changes of cognitive function [36].

The central and peripheral hormonal changes in menopausal transition and perimenopause were assessed in many research centers from Western Europe [37], Australia [24, 38], North America [25], and besides these, the rat models on gene expression analyses demonstrated that there are two distinct aging programs: chronological and endocrine, regarding bioenergetic gene expression involved in brain metabolism and synaptic plasticity [39].

The endocrine transition marked by changing from regular to irregular menstrual cycles is characterized by the impairment of the energy metabolism, glucose hypometabolism, and chronic oxidative stress, which were demonstrated by gene expression in brain metabolism, mitochondrial function, and long-term potentiation. Rat model analysis on brain energetic metabolism in menopausal transition demonstrated that insulin/insulin-like growth factor 1 and adenosine monophosphate-activated protein kinase/peroxisome proliferator-activated receptor gamma coactivator-1-alpha (AMPK/PGC1α) signaling pathways are upstream regulators [39], and these pathways suggest the critical role of E2 in neuronal survival. E2 stimulates the mitochondrial sequestration of Ca^{2+} and protects neurons against adverse consequences of excess cytoplasmic Ca^{2+} and subsequent dysregulation of Ca^{2+} homeostasis, with concomitant preservation of mitochondrial respiratory capacity [40].

Genetic analyses demonstrated that the menstrual cycles acyclicity is accompanied by a rise in genes required for fatty acid metabolism, a decline of genes required for mitochondrial function, β-amyloid degradation, and neuroinflammation including increased number in microglia population in aging hippocampus [41], plus the shift of microglia activation with predominant production of inflammatory cytokines [42], and a higher basal level of complement cascade genes and interleukin 1 receptor-like 1 in women versus men [43].

There are neuroimmune modulation differences in normal memory processes and memory dysregulation, in the roles of cytokines, astrocytes, and microglia in females and males [44]. These differences are from early development and differentiation of the brain [5], making women's brain inherently vulnerable to neurodegenerative diseases, to a higher risk of mild cognitive impairment and AD in advanced ages [45] (though not all studies are in agreement on this point, [1]), and non-neurodegenerative cognitive impairments fact that drive to the deleterious/beneficial consequences for estrogen therapy. The metabolic and neuroinflammatory changes are connected *via* redox regulation during normal brain aging, and may be predictive for later-life vulnerability to hypometabolic conditions of AD [46].

There are new animal studies on female neuroaging, regarding the microglia involvement in neurogenesis [47], to innate immune system [48], being revealed the microglia sensome by direct RNA sequencing [49]. Molecular studies on mice aging [50] revealed a central role of gender in the transcriptomic response in hippocampal and cortex aging, demonstrating sexually divergent changes of neuroinflammation, mainly an increase of microglia-specific genes, and C1q protein expression of the complement system, in the activation of astrocytes, and in cytokine release and function in aging. C1qa induction is a driver of synapse loss with greater C1qa induction associated with poorer cognitive performance. It is considered that the age-related changes in inflammatory hippocampal genes amplified in women after estrogen failure may contribute to sex differences in age-related neurological diseases. There are classes of genes in which inductions and reductions in gene expression are acting synergistically in female aging hippocampus [50].

The rise of microglia-specific genes in aging females is interrelated to a significant decrease in the activation of two pro-neurogenesis pathways evident in aging hippocampus: Notch1 and Presenilin 1 and 2 (PSEN1 and PSEN2) regulated genes [51]: Notch1 is necessary for neural stem cell maintenance [52], the PSEN1 expression regulates neuroprogenitor cell differentiation [53], and the defects in PSEN1 expression are associated with the manifestation of AD in old age [54]. Another change of neuroinflammatory genes in aging women is that of Tyrobp known as TREM2, as a causal regulator in microglia-associated changes in AD [55], and its proper mechanism in AD etiology is still being determined [56].

3. Hypothesis on brain aging and neurodegeneration during perimenopause

The months/years of perimenopause represent an important moment during women's aging, when steroids and their receptors decline is evident in the hippocampal and cortical neurons, after estrogen exposure during the reproductive years. The estrogens decline is associated/acts synergic to other factors as hypertension, diabetes, hypoxia/obstructive sleep apnea, obesity, vitamin B12/folate deficiency, depression, and traumatic brain injury to promote different pathological mechanisms involved in brain aging, memory impairment, and AD.

The Californian and Australian neuroscientists had shown that chronic cerebral hypoperfusion deprives the brain from its two paramount trophic substances, oxygen and glucose, and consequently, the brain suffers from synaptic dysfunction and neuronal degeneration/loss, leading to both gray and white matter atrophy. The magnetic resonance imaging of the head used in the North American studies from Kronos Early Estrogen Prevention Study (KEEPS) showed a brain volume decrease with an average of 0.30–0.35% per year, and an increase of 3.59–3.73% in the ventricular volumes in the first 18 months of menopause [57], with a regional reduction of volume, which is more important in the hippocampus [58].

There are two hypotheses regarding neurodegeneration in brain aging, connected to low energy fuel supply, glucose hypometabolism and its complications for normal functioning [59], and microglia activation with associated secondary effect. In these hypothetical conditions, there are sexually divergent differences in gene expression in aging brain with comparing the number of gene expression changes in both males and females, and separating gene expression profiles based on up or downregulation.

The first hypothesis regards to the deficiency in glucose availability and mitochondrial dysfunction well-known as hallmarks of brain aging, which are particularly accentuated in neurodegenerative disorders, and the shift from an aerobic glycolytic to a ketogenic phenotype of bioenergetic metabolism. The model on female rat brain aging revealed that bioenergetic decline is starting from perimenopausal transition, which is followed by the decrease of brain synaptic plasticity [39]. The mouse female transgenic model of familial AD revealed that ovariectomy induces a shift in fuel availability and metabolism in the hippocampus, with an increase of enzymes required for long-chain fatty acid and ketone body metabolism, to obtain brain energy [46, 60]. Glucose hypometabolism associated to cerebral hypoperfusion initiated with perimenopausal atherosclerosis [61], hypercholesterolemia, nitric oxide, and impairment of redox homeostasis is considered as the key pathophysiologic promoter of neurodegeneration [59], and the known differences in regional brain metabolism make some women prone to AD [62].

Posterior cingulated and prefrontal cortex, which closely resembles the hypometabolic profile of AD brains are the postmenopausal women's brain areas with reduced cerebral blood flow, with alteration of brain blood barrier glucose transport, and with significant decline in glucose metabolism [63].

It was demonstrated that brain aging is associated with a decrease of central insulin concentration [64–66], with an impairment of insulin receptor binding ability, resulting in an increase in deterioration of glucose homeostasis in the brain. Brain insulin resistance [67] is associated to peripheral insulin resistance–a typical feature of elder ages, associated to atherogenic dyslipidemia [68], and ET influences insulin resistance in medial prefrontal gyrus metabolism.

The second hypothesis is focusing on neuroinflammation specifically after low estrogen levels, connected to the shift of microglia activation, with the changing rate of microglia after activation M1 (classical) to M2 (alternative) type [68] or it is a maladaptive microglia activation [69], or a shift from neuroprotection to neurotoxicity, underlining chronic neuroinflammation and parainflammation, which is different in women and men [70, 71]. The shift is connected to proinflammatory cytokines and oxidative-nitrosative stress, which plus elevated levels of complement pathway components and other immune factors plays a key pathophysiological role in promoting cognitive dysfunction by enhancing endothelin, Amyloid-β deposition, cerebral amyloid angiopathy, aberrant synapse elimination in the hippocampus [72], and blood-brain barrier disruption.

AD is characterized by the loss of neurons and synapses from the cerebral cortex and certain subcortical regions of the temporal and parietal lobes, and parts of the frontal cortex and cingulated gyrus [73], and accumulation of plaque made up of small peptides called β-amiloid (also written as A-beta or Aβ). β-amyloid is a fragment from a larger protein called amyloid precursor protein (APP), a transmembrane protein that penetrates through the neuron's membrane. The Italian studies from Florence have demonstrated that estradiol is restoring in menopause the neuroprotective gene, seladin-1 (for SELective Alzheimer's Disease INdicator-1), or the gene DHCR24, which is downregulated in AD [74]. This gene inhibits the activation of caspase-3, a key modulator of apoptosis, and the gene encodes 3β-hydroxysterol, which catalyzes the conversion of desmosterol into cholesterol, and an appropriate amount of membrane cholesterol plays a pivotal role to protect nerve cells against Aβ toxicity and counteracts the synthesis of Aβ in AD [75, 76].

Microglia, a type of glial cell derived from myeloid precursors in the bone marrow that populate the CNS during development, as well as a brain resident innate immune cell, is the first line of defense in the CNS, as a monitor/sensor of neuronal activity in normal brain [77], protecting the local environment against invading pathogens, helping recovery from injury, and also in synapse pruning and neurodevelopment [78]. It is crucial in clearing debris, apoptotic/necrotic cells, or products from necrotic cells, infiltration of infectious agents, mediating the brain's inflammatory and repair response to traumatic injury, stroke, or neurodegeneration [79]. It was suggested that age-dependent and senescence-driven impairments of microglia functions and responses play essential roles during onset and progression of neurodegenerative diseases as AD and PD, in which molecular changes on microglia senescence are similar [80]. The unique nature and developmental origin of microglia causing microglial self-renewal and telomere shortening led to the hypothesis that these CNS-specific innate immune cells become senescent [81]. There are two important characteristics of human brain microglia: their heterogeneity observed in brain regions, and their different sensitivity to aging; the microglia from cortex, basal forebrain, and hippocampus are more sensible [81].

Microglia is activated from its normal state of a functionally "resting" resident immune cell of the CNS, and upon activation, microglia may proliferate and undergo a morphological transformation from a ramified to amoeboid appearance, and movement to sites of injury or stress can occur along with a release soluble immune mediators [82]. The activated microglia are functioning like a phagocyte or macrophage, having toll-like receptors (TLRs), that recognize specific molecular patterns as complement, mannose, scavenger, C-type lectin, nucleotide-binding oligomerization domain-like, and this specific action of microglia is called autophagy.

The autophagy is crucial for neuronal health and survival, the delivery of toxic molecules and organelles from neuronal apoptotic cells to microglia lysosomes may be acutely and/or chronically dysregulated by senescence, affecting phagocytosis and inflammation-innate immune functions in all age-associated neurodegenerative diseases [83]. There are two phenotypes of activated microglia: M1 (the cells become more cytotoxic by releasing additional pro-inflammatory cytokines- TNF, Il-1β, Il-6, and free radicals [84]), and M2, which becomes more anti-inflammatory, by secreting anti-inflammatory cytokines and neurotrophic factors and helps repair local damage [82]. The mouse model on AD is showing a distinct shift in activated microglia phenotypes, that occurs between the beginning of Aβ pathology (alternative phenotype), and advanced stages (classical phenotype), the latter may cause disease-associated neuron loss.

In this context, there are comments/discussions on microglia: if it is a scapegoat, a saboteur, or something else. A multicenter research group has discovered the presence of microglia amylin receptors mediating Aβ inflammation and neurodegeneration on primary cultures of fetal human and rats microglia [84], these receptors being common to neurons and microglia. It was proposed a model of microglia activation for AD, and neuronal death, involving these receptors, microglia, neurons, inflammation, amyloid precursor protein, and Aβ (**Figure 1**).

The amylin receptors are increasing as microglia responds to inflammatory triggers, such as lipopolysaccharide, resulting in microglia activation. The interaction of Aβ with amylin receptors of the activated microglia leads to increased production and release of cytokines, which act directly on neurons to produce cell death, with additionally increased production of Aβ *via* processing the amyloid precursor protein. The Aβ interacts with neurons and microglia amylin receptors to produce cell death [84].

The microglia activation is *via* the release of ATP, neurotransmitters, growth factors or cytokines, ion changes, special of Ca^{+2} in the CNS environment, or loss of inhibitor molecules displayed by healthy neurons, or when microglia cells encounter molecules not normally found in the healthy CNS, as blood clotting factors, intracellular constituents released by necrotic cells (hypomethylated mammalian DNA, RNA), externalized phosphatidylserine on apoptotic cells, immunoglobulin-antigen complexes, opsonizing complement, abnormally folded proteins or pathogen-related structures. When microglia activation occurs, the activation is correlated to the severity degree of the stressor, being recorded the disruptions of microglia functions causing synaptic dysfunction and excess synapse loss early in abnormalities of learning and memory [77].

Being a debate about the initiator from the two hypotheses: first, the bioenergetic hypothesis based on mitochondrial dysfunction, and the second on the microglia activation as the driving force for neuroinflammation, which is "a lesson learned from microglia depletion models" [85], there are multiple evidences that these abnormalities exacerbate each other, and these mechanistic diversities have cellular redox dysregulation as a common denominator and connector [86]. According to these, one may consider a metabolic inflammatory axis during brain aging and in neurodegenerative diseases [42]. In conditions of hypoglycemia, lactate can serve as an auxiliary fuel by metabolism of glycogen stores to generate glucose and subsequently lactate; some studies revealed that glial cells are likely to produce lactate in excess to its utilization by neurons [46].

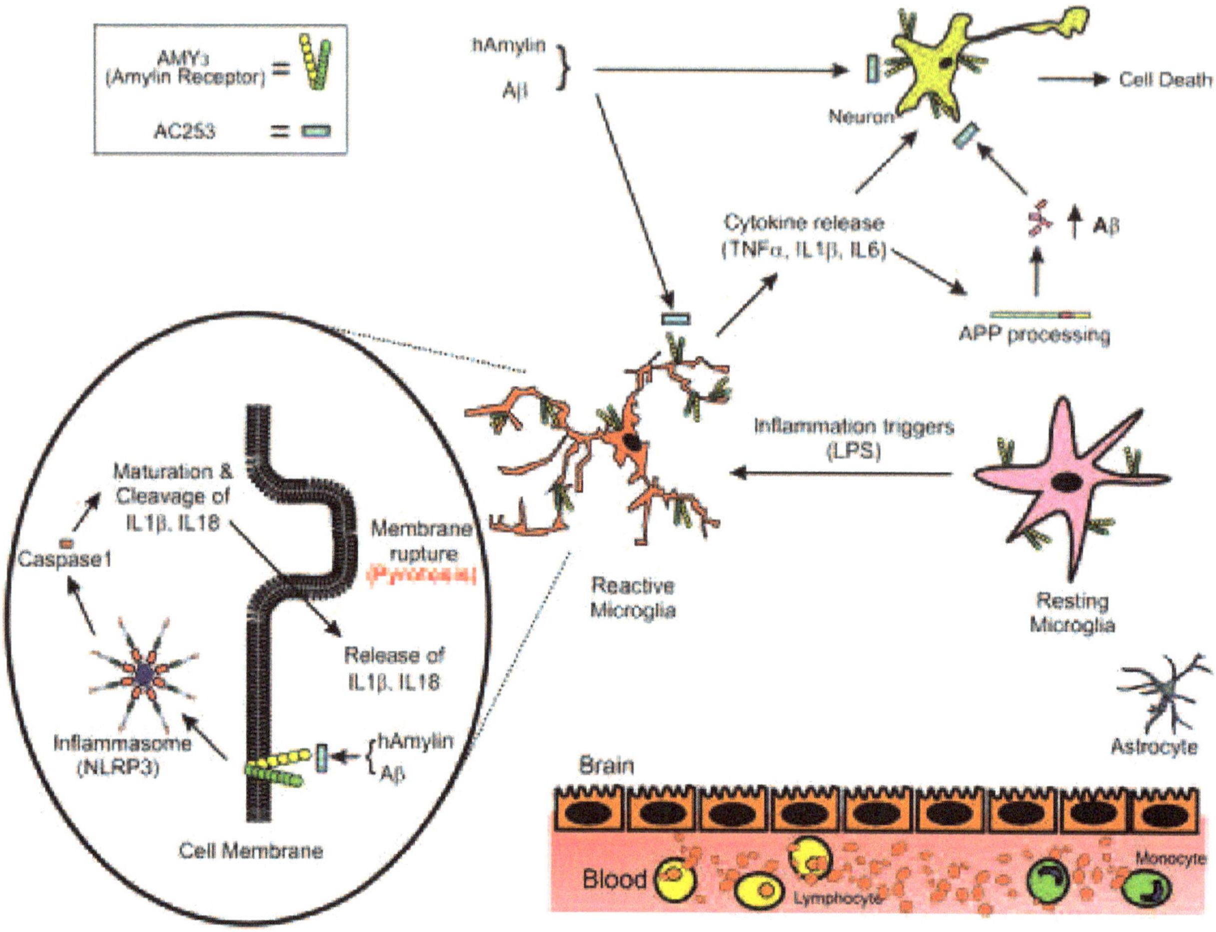

Figure 1. Model of neurodegeneration in AD proposed by Fu et al. [84]: Through the involvement microglia and neural amylin receptors in mediating the Aβ-induced neurodegeneration. *Legend:* The expression of amylin receptors of resting microglia, increased in response to inflammatory triggers like LPS, induces microglial cells activation. The interaction of Aβ with amylin receptors of the activated microglia leads to increased production and release of cytokines (TNF, Il-1β, and Il-6), which act directly on neurons to produce cell death and additionally augment the production of Aβ *via* processing of the amyloid precursor protein (APP). The Aβ, in turn, interacts with neuronal and microglial amylin receptors to produce cell death. Adapted from Fu et al. [84]. Open access to this article is distributed under the terms of the creative commons attribution 4.0 international license (http://creativecommons.org/licenses/by/4.0/), which permits unrestricted use, distribution, and reproduction in any medium, provided you give appropriate credit to the original author(s) and the source, provide a link to the creative commons license, and indicate if changes were made. The creative commons public domain dedication waiver (http://creativecommons.org/publicdomain/zero/1.0/) applies to the data made available in this article, unless otherwise stated.

Neurological symptoms that emerge during perimenopause are indicative of disruption in multiple estrogen-regulated systems, and affect multiple domains of cognitive and memory functions [87].

Estrogens (special E2) are appreciated as a master regulator of bioenergetic systems in the body and brain [88].

The hypothesis on estrogen action or "healthy-cell bias" hypothesis [87, 89] is similar to the understanding of the different cardiovascular protective/harmful effects of estrogens at different women ages—protective before 60 years and harmful after 65 years. The protective effect of E2 is altered in the presence of the APOE4 genotype, which alters the response of microglia and macrophages to 17β-E2 [90], and this fact may be an explanation of some studies showing better results with ET on memory recall in women aged around 70 and 20 years postmenopausal, if women have not demonstrated memory impairment [91].

It was demonstrated how during reproductive ages the estrogen-induced signaling pathways in hippocampal and cortical neurons converge upon the mitochondria to enhance aerobic glycolysis coupled to the citric acid cycle, mitochondrial respiration, and ATP generation, and in senescence when estrogens are missing, it is a chronic oxidative stress due to the shift from an aerobic glycolytic to a ketogenic profile/phenotype/ [35, 60], and this shift is preceded by the early, already mentioned decline in glucose transport and metabolism [46]. In mouse model, the mitochondrial bioenergetic deficit precedes AD [92]. The estrogen decline in perimenopause is associated to the decline in mitochondria bioenergetics and together with the shift to ketogenetic profile are steps to Aβ depositions in AD [93, 94]. Hexokinase, the first rate limiting step in glycolysis, interacts with mitochondria and prevents mitochondria-mediated apoptosis and through this mechanism, is promoting survival in neurons and other cell types [95], but AD patients exhibit declined hexokinase activity in the brain, cerebral microvessels, leukocytes, and fibroblasts.

Calcium dynamics play a pivotal and mandatory role in the estradiol-inducible cascade that leads to neurotrophic and neuroprotective benefit [89]. Dynamics of Ca^{2+} homeostasis are tightly regulated in healthy neurons and dysfunctional in degenerating neurons at elder ages.

The emergence of glucose hypometabolism, microglia activation, and impaired synaptic function in brain provide plausible mechanisms of neurological symptoms of perimenopause and can be predictive of later-life vulnerability to hypometabolic conditions such as AD. The alteration in the bioenergetic profile of the brain in the months/years of perimenopause may be an explanation for the controversies on estrogen therapy/hormone therapy divergent outcomes, beneficial [18, 19] or harmful (WHI Memory Study) effects on neural health, on memory and cognition [46].

Author details

Manuela Cristina Russu[1]* and Alexandra Cristina Antonescu[2]

*Address all correspondence to: manuela_russu@yahoo.com

1 "Dr. I. Cantacuzino" Clinic of Obstetrics and Gynecology, "Carol Davila" University of Medicine and Pharmacy, Bucharest, Romania

2 Intromed Laboratories, Bucharest, Romania

References

[1] McCarrey AC, An Y, Kitner-Triolo MH, Ferrucci L, Resnick SM. Sex differences in cognitive trajectories in clinically normal older adults. Psychology and Aging. 2016;**31**(2):166-175. DOI: 10.1037

[2] Vina J, Lloret A. Why women have more Alzheimer's disease than men: Gender and mitochondrial toxicity of amyloid-beta peptide. Journal of Alzheimer's Disease. 2010; **20**(Suppl 2):S527-S533. DOI: 10.3233

[3] Alzheimer's A. Alzheimer's disease facts and figures. Alzheimer's & Dementia. 2013; **9**(2):208-245. DOI:10.1016

[4] Appelros P, Stegmayr B, Terent A. Sex differences in stroke epidemiology: A systematic review. Stroke. 2009;**40**(4):1082-1090. DOI: 10.1161

[5] Pike CJ. Sex and the development of Alzheimer's disease. Journal of Neuroscience Research. 2017 Jan 2;**95**(1-2):671-680. DOI: 10.1002

[6] Prince M, Wimo A, Prina M, et al. Alzheimer's Disease International. World Alzheimer Report 2015: The Global Impact of Dementia: An Analysis of Prevalence, Incidence, Cost and Trend. https://www.alz.co.uk/research/world-report-2015

[7] Marin R, Guerra B, Diaz M, et al. Estrogen activates classical and alternative mechanisms to orchestrate neuroprotection. Current Neurovascular Research. 2005 Oct;**2**(4):287-301

[8] Arnold AP, Lusis AJ. Understanding the sexome: Measuring and reporting sex differences in gene systems. Endocrinology. 2012;**153**(6):2551-2555. DOI: 10.1210

[9] Baron AM, Pike CJ. Sex hormones, aging, and Alzheimer's disease. Frontiers in Bioscience. 2012;**4**:976-997

[10] Henderson VW. Cognition and cognitive aging. Climacteric. 2007 Oct;**10**(Suppl 2):88-91

[11] Blacker D, Lee H, Muzikansky A, et al. Neuropsychological measures in normal individuals that predict subsequent cognitive decline. Archives of Neurology. 2007;**64**(6): 862-871

[12] Levey J, Lah J, Goldstein F, Steenland K, Bliwise D. Mild cognitive impairment: An opportunity to identify patients at high risk for progression to Alzheimer's disease. Clinical Therapeutics. 2006;**28**(7):991-1001

[13] Gauthier S, Reisberg B, Zaudig M, Winblad B, et al. Mild cognitive impairment. Lancet 2006;**367**:1262-1270

[14] Yan Y, Cheng L, Chen X, Ai J, et al. Estrogen deficiency is associated with hippocampal morphological remodeling of early postmenopausal mice. Oncotarget. 2017 Mar 28;**8**(13):21892-21902. DOI: 10.18632

[15] Zhang Y, Champagne N, Beitel KL, Goodyer GC, Trifiro M, LeBlanc A. Estrogen and androgen protection of human neurons against intracellular amyloid toxicity through heat shock protein 70. The Journal of Neuroscience. 2004;**24**(23):5315-5321

[16] Kohannim O, Hua X, Hibar DP, et al. Boosting power for clinical trials using classifiers based on multiple biomarkers. Neurobiology of Aging. 2010;**31**(8):1429-1442

[17] Dye VR, Miller JK, Singer JE, Levine JA. Hormone replacement therapy and risk for neurodegenerative diseases. International Journal of Alzheimer's Disease. 2012:**18**. Jagannatha Rao KS, editor. Article ID 258454. DOI: doi.org/10.1155/2012/258454

[18] Maki PM et al. Perimenopausal use of hormone therapy is associated with enhanced memory and hippocampal function later in life. Brain Research. 2011;**1379**:232-243

[19] Maki PM. Minireview: Effects of different HT formulations on cognition. Endocrinology. 2012;**153**:3564-3570

[20] Soules MR, Sherman S, Parrott E, Rebar R, Santoro N, Utian W, et al. Executive summary: Stages of reproductive aging workshop (STRAW). Fertility and Sterility. 2001; **76**(5):874-878

[21] Shuster LT, Rhodes DJ, Rocca WA, et al. Premature menopause or early menopause: Long-term health consequences. Maturitas 2010;**65**:161-166

[22] North American Menopause Society Menopause Practice–A Clinician's Guide. 4. Cleveland, OH: North American menopause Society; 2010

[23] van der Stege JG, Groen H, van Kasteren YM, et al. Decreased androgen concentrations and diminished general and sexual well-being in women with premature ovarian failure. Menopause. 2008;**15**:23-31

[24] Burger HG, Dudley EC, Robertson DM, Dennerstein L. Hormonal changes in the menopause transition. Recent Progress in Hormone Research. 2002;**57**:257-275

[25] Butler L, Santoro N. The reproductive endocrinology of the menopausal transition. Steroids. 2011 Jun;**76**(7):627-635. DOI: 10.1016

[26] Davison SL, Bell R, Davis SR, et al. Androgen levels in adult females: Changes with age, menopause, and oophorectomy. The Journal of Clinical Endocrinology and Metabolism. 2005;**90**:3847-3853

[27] Gore AC, Oung T, Woller MJ, et al. Neuroendocrine mechanisms for reproductive senescence in the female rat: Gonadotropin-releasing hormone neurons. Endocrine. 2000;**13**:315-323

[28] Gore AC, Windsor-Engnell BM, Terasawa E. Menopausal increases in pulsatile gonadotropin-releasing hormone (GnRH) release in a non-human primate (*Macaca mulatta*). Endocrinology. 2004;**145**:4653-4659

[29] Rocca AW, Miller MV, Brown DR, et al. Premature menopause or early menopause and risk of ischemic stroke. Menopause. 2012 Mar;**19**(3):271-277. DOI: 10.1097

[30] Rivera CM, Grossardt BR, Rhodes DJ, et al. Increased cardiovascular mortality after early bilateral oophorectomy. Menopause. 2009;**16**:15-23

[31] Nappi ER, Sinforiani E, Nappi G, et al. Memory functioning at menopause: Impact of age in ovariectomized women. Gynecologic and Obstetric Investigation 1999;**47**:29-36

[32] Rocca WA, Grossardt BR, Melton LJ 3rd, et al. Survival patterns after oophorectomy in premenopausal women: A population-based cohort study. The Lancet Oncology. 2006; **7**:821-828

[33] Baba Y, Ishikawa S, Kajii E, et al. Premature menopause is associated with increased risk of cerebral infarction in Japanese women. Menopause 2010;**17**:506-510

[34] De Vos M, Devroey P, Fauser BC. Primary ovarian insufficiency. Lancet. 2010;**376**:911-921

[35] Brinton DR, Yao J, Cadenas E, et al. Perimenopause as a neurological transition state. Nature Reviews Endocrinology. 2015;**11**:393-405. DOI:10.1038

[36] Weber MT, Rubin LH, Maki PM. Cognition in perimenopause: The effect of transition stage. Menopause 2013;**20**:511-517

[37] Genazzani AR, Bernardi F, Luisi M, et al. Endocrinology of menopausal transition and its brain implications. CNS Spectrums. 2005 Jun;**10**(6):449-457

[38] Burger HG et al. Nomenclature and endocrinology of menopause and perimenopause. Expert Review of Neurotherapeutics. 2007;**7**(11 Suppl):S35-S43

[39] Yin F, Yao J, Sancheti H, Cadenas E, Brinton RD, et al. The perimenopausal aging transition in the female rat brain: Decline in bioenergetic systems and synaptic plasticity. Neurobiology of Aging. 2015 Jul;**36**(7):2282-2295. DOI: 10.1016

[40] Nilsen J, Irwin RW, Brinton RD, et al. Estradiol *in vivo* regulation of brain mitochondrial proteome. The Journal of Neuroscience. 2007 Dec 19;**27**(51):14069-14077. DOI: 10.1523

[41] Mouton PR, Long JM, Ingram DK, et al. Age and gender effects on microglia and astrocyte numbers in brains of mice. Brain Research. 2002;**956**(1):30-35. DOI: 10.1016

[42] Yin F, Sancheti H, Patil I, Cadenas E. Energy metabolism and inflammation in brain aging and Alzheimer's disease. Free Radical Biology and Medicine. 2016 Nov;**100**:108-122. DOI: 10.1016

[43] Trabzuni D, Ramasamy A, Ryten M, et al. North American Brain Expression C Widespread sex differences in gene expression and splicing in the adult human brain. Nature Communications. 2013;**4**:2771. DOI: 10.1038

[44] Tronson NC, Collette KM. (Putative) sex differences in neuroimmune modulation of memory. Journal of Neuroscience Research. 2017 Jan 2;**95**(1-2):472-486. DOI: 10.1002

[45] Zhang Z. Gender differentials in cognitive impairment and decline of the oldest old in China. Journals of Gerontology. Series B, Psychological Sciences and Social Sciences. 2006;**61**(2):S107-S115. DOI: 10.1093

[46] Ding F, Yao J, Brinton RD, et al. Early decline in glucose transport and metabolism precedes shift to ketogenic system in female aging and Alzheimer's mouse brain: Implication for bioenergetic intervention. PLoS One. 2013 Nov 11;**8**(11):e79977. DOI: 10.1371

[47] Holtman IR, Raj DD, Kamphuis W, et al. Induction of a common microglia gene expression signature by aging and neurodegenerative conditions: A co-expression meta-analysis. Acta Neuropathologica Communications. 2015;**3**:31. DOI: 10.1186

[48] Ziv Y, Ron N, Schwartz M, et al. Immune cells contribute to the maintenance of neurogenesis and spatial learning abilities in adulthood. Nature Neuroscience. 2006;**9**(2):268-275. DOI: 10.1038

[49] Hickman SE, Kingery ND, El Khoury J, et al. The microglial sensome revealed by direct RNA sequencing. Nature Neuroscience. 2013;**16**(12):1896-1905. DOI: 10.1038

[50] Mangold AC, Wronowski B, Freeman MW, et al. Sexually divergent induction of microglial-associated neuroinflammation with hippocampal aging. Journal of Neuroinflammation. 2017;**14**:141. DOI: 10.1186

[51] Gebara E, Sultan S, Kocher-Braissant J, Toni N. Adult hippocampal neurogenesis inversely correlates with microglia in conditions of voluntary running and aging. Frontiers in Neuroscience 2013;**7**:145. DOI: 10.3389

[52] Ables JL, Decarolis NA, Eisch AJ, et al. Notch1 is required for maintenance of the reservoir of adult hippocampal stem cells. The Journal of Neuroscience 2010;**30**(31): 10484-10492. DOI: 10.1523

[53] Gadadhar A, Marr R, Lazarov O. Presenilin-1 regulates neural progenitor cell differentiation in the adult brain. The Journal of Neuroscience. 2011;**31**(7):2615-2623. DOI: 10.1523

[54] Bekris LM, Yu CE, Bird TD, Tsuang DW. Genetics of Alzheimer disease. Journal of Geriatric Psychiatry and Neurology . 2010;**23**(4):213-227. DOI: 10.1177

[55] Zhang B, Gaiteri C, Bodea LG, Dobrin R, et al. Integrated systems approach identifies genetic nodes and networks in late-onset Alzheimer's disease. Cell. 2013;**153**(3):707-720. DOI: 10.1016

[56] Ma J, Jiang T, Tan L, Yu JT. TYROBP in Alzheimer's disease. Molecular Neurobiology. 2015;**51**(2):820-826. DOI: 10.1007

[57] Kantarci K, Miller VM, Jack Jr CR, et al. Brain Volume Changes in Recently Menopausal Women in a Hormone Replacement Trial.: International Menopause Society Meeting. May 21, 2008. Madrid, Spain

[58] Raz N, Lindenberger U, Acker JD, et al. Regional brain changes in aging healthy adults: General trends, individual differences and modifiers. Cereberal Cortex. 2005;**15**(11):1676-1689. DOI: 10.1093

[59] Daulatzai MA. Cerebral hypoperfusion and glucose hypometabolism: Key pathophysiological modulators promote neurodegeneration, cognitive impairment, and Alzheimer's disease. Journal of Neuroscience Research. 2017 Apr;**95**(4):943-972. DOI: 10.1002

[60] Yao J, Hamilton RT, Cadenas E, Brinton RD. Decline in mitochondrial bioenergetics and shift to ketogenic profile in brain during reproductive senescence. Biochimica et Biophysica Acta. 2010 Oct;**1800**(10):1121-1126. DOI: 10.1016

[61] Lerner DJ, Kannel WB. Patterns of coronary heart disease morbidity and mortality in the sexes. A 26-year follow up of the Framingham population. American Heart Journal. 1986;**111**:383-390

[62] Silverman DHS, Geist CL, Kenna HA, et al. Differences in regional brain metabolism associated with specific formulations of hormone therapy in postmenopausal women at risk for AD. Psychoneuroendocrinology. 2010;**36**:502-513

[63] Zhao L, Mao Z, Woody SK, Brinton RD. Sex differences in metabolic aging of the brain: Insights into female susceptibility to Alzheimer's disease. Neurobiology of Aging. 2016; **42**:69-79. DOI: 10.1016

[64] Rasgon NL, et al. Insulin resistance and hippocampal volume in women at risk for Alzheimer's disease. Neurobiology of Aging. 2011;**32**:1942-1948

[65] Rasgon NL, et al. Insulin resistance and medial prefrontal gyrus metabolism in women receiving hormone therapy. Psychiatry Research. 2014;**223**:28-36

[66] Baranowska – Bik A, Bik W. Insulin and brain aging. Przeglad Menopauzalny. 2017 Jun;**16**(2): 44-46. DOI: 10.5114

[67] Kullmann S, Heni M, Haring HU, et al. Brain insulin resistance at the crossroads of metabolic and cognitive disorders in humans. Physiological Reviews. 2016 Oct;**96**(4):1169-1209. DOI: 10.1152

[68] Nikodemova M, Small AL, Kimyon RS, Watters JJ. Age-dependent differences in microglial responses to systemic inflammation are evident as early as middle age. Physiological Genomics. 2016;**48**(5):336-344. DOI: 10.1152/physiolgenomics.00129.2015

[69] Hume DA. The many alternative faces of macrophage activation. Frontiers in Immunology. 2015;**6**:370. DOI: 10.3389/fimmu.2015.00370

[70] Mirza MA, Ritzel R, Liu F, et al. Sexually dimorphic outcomes and inflammatory responses in hypoxic-ischemic encephalopathy. Journal of Neuroinflammation. 2015;**12**:32. DOI: 10.1186/s12974-015-0251-6

[71] Lenz KM, McCarthy MM. A starring role for microglia in brain sex differences. The Neuroscientist. 2015;**21**(3):306-321. DOI: 10.1177/1073858414536468

[72] Hong S, Beja-Glasser VF, Nfonoyim BM, Barres BA, et al. Complement and microglia mediate early synapse loss in Alzheimer mouse models. Science 2016;**352**(6286):712-716. DOI: 10.1126/science.aad8373

[73] Wenk GL. Neuropathologic changes in Alzheimer's disease. The Journal of Clinical Psychiatry. 2003;**64**(Suppl 9):7-10

[74] Luciani P, Deledda C, Peri A, et al. Seladin-1 is a fundamental mediator of the neuroprotective effects of estrogen in human neuroblast long-term cell cultures. Endocrinology 2008 Sep;**149**(9):4256-4266. DOI: 10.1210/en.2007-1795

[75] Peri A, Benvenuti S, Cellai I, et al. Membrane cholesterol as a mediator of the neuroprotective effects of estrogens. Neuroscience. 2011;**191**:107-117. DOI: 10.1016

[76] Peri A. Neuroprotective effects of estrogens: The role of cholesterol. Journal of Endocrinological Investigation. 2016 Jan;**39**(1):11-18. DOI: 10.1007/s40618-015-0332-5

[77] Morris GP, Clark IA, Zinn R, Vissel B. Microglia: A new frontier for synaptic plasticity, learning and memory, and neurodegenerative disease research. Neurobiology of Learning and Memory. 2013 Oct;**105**:40-53. DOI: 10.1016/j.nlm.2013.07.002

[78] Conde JR, Streit WJ. Microglia in the aging brain. Journal of Neuropathology and Experimental Neurology. 2006;**65**(3):199-203. DOI: 10.1097/01.jnen.0000202887.22082.63

[79] Lucin KM, Wyss-Coray T. Immune activation in brain aging and neurodegeneration: Too much or too little? Neuron. 2009 Oct 15;**64**(1):110-122. DOI: 10.1016

[80] Spittau B. Aging microglia-phenotypes, functions and implications for age-related neurodegenerative diseases. Frontiers in Aging Neuroscience. 2017 Jun 14;**9**:194. DOI: 10.3389/fnagi.2017.00194

[81] Grabert K, Michoel T, Karavolos MH, McColl BW, et al. Microglial brain region-dependent diversity and selective regional sensitivities to aging. Nature Neuroscience 2016;**19**(3):504-516. DOI: 10.1038/nn.4222

[82] Ekdahl CT. Microglial activation—Tuning and pruning adult neurogenesis. Frontiers in Pharmacology. 2012;**3**:41. DOI: 10.3389/fphar.2012.00041

[83] Plaza-Zabala A, Sirra-Torre V, Sierra A. Autophagy and microglia: Novel partners in neurodegeneration and aging. International Journal of Molecular Sciences. 2017 Mar 9;**18**(3). pii: E598. DOI: 10.3390/ijms18030598

[84] Fu W, Vukojevic V, Patel A, Jhamandas J, et al. Role of microglial amylin receptors in mediating beta amyloid (Aβ)-induced inflammation. Journal of Neuroinflammation, 2017 Oct 6;**14**(1):199. DOI: 10.1186/s12974-017-0972-9

[85] Spangenberg EE, Green KN. Inflammation in Alzheimer's disease: Lessons learned from microglia-depletion models. Brain, Behavior, and Immunity 2017 Mar;**61**:1-11. DOI: 10.1016/j.bbi.2016.07.003

[86] Uchoa MF, Moser VA, Pike CJ. Interactions between inflammation, sex steroids, and Alzheimer's disease risk factors. Frontiers in Neuroendocrinology. 2016 Oct;**43**:60-82. DOI: 10.1016/j.yfrne.2016.09.001

[87] Brinton RD. Investigative models for determining hormone therapy-induced outcomes in brain: Evidence in support of a healthy cell bias of estrogen action. Annals of the New York Academy of Sciences. 2005;**1052**:57-74

[88] Rettberg JR, Yao J, Brinton RD. Estrogen: A master regulator of bioenergetic systems in the brain and body. Frontiers in Neuroendocrinology. 2014 Jan;**35**(1):8-30. DOI: 10.1016

[89] Chen S, Nilsen J, Brinton RD. Dose and temporal pattern of estrogen exposure determines neuroprotective outcome in hippocampal neurons: Therapeutic implications. Endocrinology. 2006;**147**(11):5303-5313. DOI: 10.1210/en.2006-049

[90] Brown CM, Colton CA, et al. The APOE4 genotype alters the response of microglia and macrophages to 17β-estradiol. Neurobiology of Aging. 2008;**29**(12):1783-1794

[91] Dumas J, Hancur-Bucci C, Newhouse P, et al. Estradiol interacts with the cholinergic system to affect verbal memory in postmenopausal women: Evidence for the critical period hypothesis. Hormones and Behavior. 2008;**53**(1):159-169

[92] Yao J, Irwin RW, Brinton RD, et al. Mitochondrial bioenergetic deficit precedes Alzheimer's pathology in female mouse model of Alzheimer's disease. Proceedings of National Academy of Sciences of United States of America. 2009;**106**:14670-14675

[93] Yao J, Rettberg JR, Brinton RD, et al. Shift in brain metabolism in late onset Alzheimer's disease: Implications for biomarkers and therapeutic interventions. Molecular Aspects of Medicine. 2011;**32**:247-257

[94] Yao J, Irwin R, Brinton RD, et al. Ovarian hormone loss induces bioenergetic deficits and mitochondrial beta-amyloid. Neurobiology of Aging. 2012;**33**:1507-1521

[95] Gimenez-Cassina A, Lim F, Diaz-Nido J, et al. Mitochondrial hexokinase II promotes neuronal survival and acts downstream of glycogen synthase kinase-3. The Journal of Biological Chemistry. 2009;**284**:3001-3011

6

Sex Hormones and Alzheimer's Disease

Wafik Said Bahnasy, Yasser A. El-Heneedy and Ehab A. El-Seidy

Abstract

Alzheimer's disease (AD) is the most common type of dementia and the most common neurodegenerative disorder of elderly. It is not an accelerated form of aging but it is characterized by distinct temporospatial brain pathological changes, including amyloid plaques accumulation, neurofibrillary tangles deposition, synaptic loss and neuronal death with gross brain atrophy. These changes result in persistent progressive memory and cognitive decline interfering with the usual daily activities. AD is a multifactorial disorder results from the interaction of genetic, epigenetic, environmental and lifestyle factors. Estrogen, progesterone and androgen effects are important building stones in AD pathogenesis, and their effect in brain modulation and development results in different gender susceptibility to the disease. These sex hormones whether gonadal or neurosteroids (synthesized locally in the brain) play important neuroprotective roles influencing the individual's vulnerability to AD development, rate of mild cognitive impairment (MCI)/AD conversion and speed of AD progression. Despite the little therapeutic implications of hormonal replacement therapy in AD treatment, yet this topic still represents a challenging hopeful way to construct a strategy for the development of personalized, gender-specific AD management.

Keywords: Alzheimer's disease, sex hormones, neurosteroids, estrogens, progesterone, androgens

1. Introduction

Alzheimer's disease (AD) is the most common type of dementia and a key determinant of healthcare costs. It is an age-related neurodegenerative disorder, and due to increased people life expectancy, AD becomes one of the most burdensome threats to public health and a grand international research challenges. It is a system-specific brain disease affecting discrete neurons in a nearly consistent temporospatial pattern and is characterized by progressive memory decline and persistent cognitive impairment enough to interfere with the person's performance of the usual daily activities.

1.1. History

The gender difference in the cognitive and neurobehavioral performance had been noticed since ancient time which may be the origin of the popular legend (men are from Mars, women are from Venus and had met here in Earth) [1]. The concept of age-related cognitive decline was well known since antiquity, which progressed through the ages till reached the term dementia. The link between female sex and dementia had also noticed since a very long period and this made Jean Etienne Esquirol put menstrual disorders and sequelae of delivery as direct causes of dementia in his book Des Maladies Mentales [2, 3]. In 25 November 1901, the German neurologist, Dr. Alois Alzheimer admitted a patient presented by recent cognitive decline to the public mental asylum in Frankfurt. Surprisingly, this first description was on a 51-year-old lady named Auguste Deter, who experienced marked memory decline, fear of people and became jealous of her husband in the last year preceded her admission in Frankfurt asylum by Dr. Alois Alzheimer and Dr. Hermann P. Nitsche. Later, the patient developed severe behavioral abnormalities, delusions, disorientation of time and place, hallucinations and severe language difficulties. In 1906, Auguste died and her autopsy revealed gross brain atrophy and microscopically increased silver staining by using Bielschowsky method, which later named amyloid plaques and neurofibrillary tangles (NFTs) [4].

1.2. Epidemiology

Dementia affects about 47 million people worldwide, and this number is expected to double every 20 years due to increased life expectancy. AD is the leading cause of dementia accounting for about 30% of early onset cases before the age of 50 years and 60–80% of late onset ones either as pure or mixed form [5]. It is one of the commonest causes of prolonged disability in old age, the sixth cause of death in USA globally and the fifth cause for seniors above the age of 65. Old age is the most important AD risk with estimated prevalence of 3% in people aged 65–74 years, 17% between 75 and 84 years and 32% in those >85 years [6, 7].

AD disproportionately affects both sexes, with females have 2–3 times higher incidence of AD than males of the same age. The age-specific risk of developing AD is almost twofold greater in women than men, 17.2% vs. 9.1% at 65 years and 28.5% vs. 10.2% at 75 years. The incidence of amnestic mild cognitive impairment (MCI) is equal both in male and female, denoting that females take shorter MCI/AD transitional state with rapid conversion to manifest AD [5, 8, 9].

1.3. Pathology

AD is not an accelerated form of aging but it is characterized by distinct cellular and molecular pathological changes, including amyloid plaque deposition, NFTs accumulations, synaptic loss and neuronal death with gross brain atrophy.

1.3.1. *The amyloid hypothesis*

The amyloid cascade theory with the resultant extracellular amyloid plaque aggregation is the leading one for AD pathogenesis. Amyloid plaques are aggregates of amyloid beta (Aβ) peptide derived mainly from the cleavage of a transmembrane protein named amyloid precursor protein (APP) by the sequential action of two aspartyl protease enzymes, β- and γ-secretases (amyloidogenic pathway) in which the APP is firstly cleaved by β-secretase to soluble APP and residual C-terminal segment that is further digested by the γ-secretase to Aβ-40/42 segments. The insoluble Aβ aggregates start to appear 15–25 years prior to the onset of cognitive decline or tau pathology, and their formation is triggered by enhancement of the amyloidogenic pathway with increasing the pool of soluble Aβ production, which in turn aggregate to form monomeric, oligomeric, protofibrils and finally mature insoluble Aβ [10]. Under normal circumstances, the ratio of Aβ-42: Aβ-40 is 1:9 and increase in this ratio due to either aberrant production (increased γ-secretase activity) or clearance (abnormal microglial activities) is the cause of Aβ accumulation as the former has a high tendency to aggregate. The amyloid aggregates spark a sequence of events that lead to AD development including neuronal injury and synaptic loss. It is generally accepted that brain β-amyloid deposition is relatively diffuse, and there is non-linear correlation between the density of mature Aβ aggregate and severity of AD, which denotes that soluble Aβ oligomers per se are neurotoxic and cause synaptic dysfunction even in the absence of insoluble aggregate [11, 12].

1.3.2. *Neurofibrillary tangles*

Tau pathology, including NFTs, neuritic plaques and neuropil threads intraneural deposition is assumed to be the consequence of amyloid accumulation. NFTs are intraneural misfolded twisted paired helical filaments, which accumulate to form intracellular deposits composed of hyperphosphorylated tau protein that concentrates in the inner side of the cell membrane, but when the neurons die, NFT may migrate to other healthy or less affected neurons or may be found extracellular. Tau is essential for NMDA-dependent long-term potentiation and AMPA-dependent long-term depression and acts as autophagy regulator by inhibiting histone deacetylase-6 enzyme. Thus, tauopathies result in marked synaptic disturbances and impaired selective autophagic clearance. Tau has more than 25 serine, threonine and tyrosine residue sites, which can be phosphorylated by specific protein kinases and phosphatases [13]. Genetic or acquired

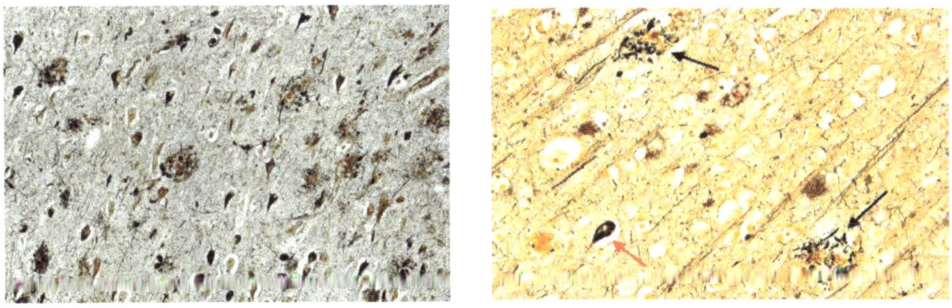

Figure 1. Photomicrography of Alzheimer's disease pathology using Bielschowsky stain demonstrating neurofibrillary tangles and amyloid plaques.

induced dysfunctions result in tau hyperphosphorylation, misfolding and fibrillar formation ending in NFTs deposition. On the other hand, tau dephosphorylation is regulated by protein phosphatase 2A enzyme, which activity is impaired in AD. NFTs accumulation starts several years after Aβ deposition but still before AD clinical manifestations and its accumulation dense and distribution is directly proportional with the severity of AD cognitive decline. NFTs deposition usually follows a stepwise progression typically starting in the transentorhinal cortex, the entorhinal cortex, hippocampus, medial temporal cortex and lastly other areas of the neocortex [14, 15] (**Figure 1**).

1.3.3. Microglia and neuroinflammation

It is well known that the density of β-amyloid deposition is not proportional with the severity of AD cognitive decline making the amyloid hypothesis alone is not sufficient to explain the whole AD pathological cascade and in turn the possible role of additional pathogenetic factors, including neuroinflammation and vascular amyloidosis. The neuroinflammatory theory was supposed after identification of activated microglia within the vicinity of the amyloid plaques, which number was proportional with the size of the plaques. At the same time, several microglial expressed genes were associated with AD predisposition, including TREM2, CD33, CR1, CLU, CD2AP, EPHA1, ABCA7 and INPP5D. Under normal circumstances, microglial activities are modulated by several neuroimmune regulatory proteins, including insulin-like growth factor-1, brain-derived neurotrophic factor, transforming growth factor-b and nerve growth factor, which help in slowdown and resolving the inflammatory process [16].

Microglia have no role in Aβ production; however, they act as Aβ scavengers as they play major roles in its clearance either directly through phagocytosis or indirectly via the secretion of several enzymes, including insulin degrading enzyme, neprilysin, matrix metalloproteinase-9 and plasminogen. At the same time, microglia regulate synaptic network remodeling (synaptic pruning) and neural circuit maintenance [17].

In AD, chronic reactivation and excessive proliferation of microglia result in the production of inflammatory mediators, including reactive oxygen species, interleukin-1, interferon-γ and tumor necrosis factor-alpha. This imbalanced microglial function results in aberrant synaptic pruning, pathological synaptic stripping, neuronal loss, enhancing the endothelial response to hypoxia with impaired blood-brain barrier (BBB) stability, disturbed Aβ clearance, increased levels of phosphorylated tau protein, promoting NFTs accumulation and, consequently, cognitive decline. Microglia also transport amyloid and tau from one brain area to another; thus, they play a major role in spatial AD progression. Microglia are candidate for the action of sex hormones, and they express abundant sex hormone receptors. These receptors modulate microglial activities producing potent anti-inflammatory actions that resist AD development and progression [18, 19].

1.3.4. Vascular theory

Diabetes, hypertension, smoking and heart diseases are associated with increased risk of AD. This concept resulted in the emergence of the AD vascular theory, which can explain why aging is the major risk of AD as vascular dysfunction is considered as a universal feature of aging and why AD progression increases after cerebral ischemic events like stroke and transient ischemic attacks. Cerebral amyloid angiopathy (CAA) is present in more than 75% of autopsy confirmed AD brains especially in mixed AD/vascular dementia where the vascular risk factors predominate. Cerebral microvascular compromise is more common among subjects having the APOE4 allele making them at increased risk of AD development. CAA represents imbalanced Aβ production and clearance with consequent deposition within the basement membrane of the leptomeningeal vessels, intracerebral arteries and arterioles, and less frequently in capillaries and veins [20].

Amyloid deposition in and around the blood vessel wall impairs its endothelial integrity and disturbs the BBB leading to Aβ trapping in the CSF and its diminished clearance to the venous circulation. At the same time, CAA disrupts the microvascular homeostasis leading to chronic cerebral parenchymal hypoperfusion with focal ischemia, microinfarcts, release of inflammatory mediators, oxygen-free radicals, loss of nitric oxide bioavailability and mitochondrial dysfunction. The net result is neurotoxicity, reduced neural plasticity, neural apoptosis and synaptic loss [21]. Sex hormone receptors are heavily expressed in the cerebral blood vessels and exert very important actions to keep the vascular integrity and prevent chronic ischemic hypoperfusion through promoting endothelial relaxation by increasing the production/activity of nitric oxide and prostacyclin and at the same time prevent vascular smooth muscle contraction by inhibiting intracellular Ca^{2+} influx and antagonize the actions of protein kinases [22].

1.3.5. Monoaminergic and cholinergic abnormalities

Synaptic failure is an important factor in the cognitive manifestations of AD before manifest neuronal loss takes place. The neurochemical changes in AD include extensive serotonergic denervation in the hippocampus and neocortex, depletion of the cholinergic neurons in the basal forebrain, loss of >70% of noradrenergic locus coeruleus neurons, reduction of dopamine, dopamine metabolites and dopamine receptors, histaminergic tuberomammillary nucleus degeneration and impaired melatonin secretion and action in the pineal body and suprachiasmatic hypothalamic nucleus, respectively [23].

Glutamate is a non-essential amino acid but it is one of the most important excitatory synaptic neurotransmitter as most of the CNS myelinated axons are glutamatergic. AD patients show aberrant increase in extracellular glutamate, which enhances tau pathology and enhances glutamate receptors expressed oligodendroglia to transport tau from one brain area to another leading to AD spatial progression. At the same time, there is a reciprocal relationship between glutamate and Aβ as soluble amyloid oligomers as well as insoluble Aβ deposits increases the extracellular glutamate concentration resulting in AMPA (α-amino-3-hydroxy-5-methyl-4-isoxazolepropionate) and NMDA (N-methyl-D-aspartate) receptors dysfunction, disturbed synaptic pruning and impaired synaptic plasticity with promotion of long-term synaptic depression and inhibition of long-term synaptic potentiation leading to cognitive decline especially memory domain. At the same time, NMDA receptor inhibition promotes amyloidogenic γ-secretase activities and inhibits non-amyloidogenic α-secretase with the resultant increase in Aβ production and accumulation and vice versa. Many studies revealed protective effects of sex hormones against glutamate-induced neurotoxicity through inhibition of glutamate release by reducing the activities of lactate dehydrogenase, inhibiting intracellular Ca^{2+} influx, exerting antioxidant action and enhancing mitogen-activated protein kinase action [24, 25].

1.4. Genetics and epigenetics of AD

Genetic predisposition to AD is very complex although positive family history is a common patients' finding. The rare early onset AD constitutes less than 1% of cases and often transmitted as autosomal dominant and fully penetrant inheritance. Common affected genes include APP (genes encoding γ-secretase complex), presenelin-1 (PSNL1) and presenelin-2 (PSNL2) gene mutation in chromosomes 21, 14 and 1, respectively. Overexpression of these genes results in increased production of the highly hydrophobic fibrillogenic longer Aβ-42 and on the expense of the relatively shorter Aβ-40 [23].

In late onset AD, apolipoprotein E series, especially APOE4, is the major genetic risk as >60% of AD patients harbor at least one APOE4 allele. APOE is a lipid-binding cholesterol transporter protein essential for maintenance of myelin and neuronal membranes, synaptogenesis and dendritic reorganization. Three APOE isoforms exist in humans: APOE2, APOE3 and APOE4. Heterozygous and homozygous APOE4 are at increased risk of significantly lower age of AD onset and higher rate of AD development by about 4 and 15 folds than other allele types. At the same time, males with APOE4 are more liable to develop MCI than others. APOE4 allele expression interacts with the sex hormones leading to increased risk of AD in women than men of the same age. APOE4 expression results in decreased soluble APPα/Aβ ratio, reduced Sirtuin T1 expression (NAD+-dependent deacetylases that attenuate amyloidogenic), triggered tau phosphorylation and induced neuronal apoptosis [26].

Many studies revealed that people with a rare missense mutation (rs75932628-T) in the gene encoding TREM2 (Triggering Receptor Expressed on Myeloid Cells 2) are at increased risk of developing AD 2–3 folds than others possibly due to reduced clearing abilities of their microglia to Aβ and apoptotic cells [10]. At the same time, other studies suggested a possible role of epigenetic changes and aberrantly expressed micro-RNAs (miRNAs) in the pathogenesis of AD through disturbing neurogenesis, synaptic plasticity, synaptogenesis and neuronal network preservation as well as enhancing Aβ production and neuroinflammation [27]. Both epigenetics and miRNAs are influenced by sex hormone receptor activation, and they are potentially versatile and adaptive, which gives a challenging hope for novel therapeutic approaches in AD management. The epigenetics represents alterations in genetic functions without changing DNA sequence and constitutes an interface of genetic/environmental factors interplay, e.g. DNA methylation, histone modifications, non-coding RNAs regulation and higher order chromatin remodeling [28]. MiRNAs are 18–22 nucleotide long, non-coding RNAs that are involved in post-transcriptional suppression of gene expression [29].

1.5. Clinical signs and symptoms

Dementia of Alzheimer's type typically presents by episodic memory impairment, which gradually progresses to interfere with the activities of daily living. Memory impairment is usually followed by other cognitive domains declines which vary according to the pattern of cortical progression, including apathy, loss of interest in hobbies, sleep disturbances, impaired spatial and temporal navigations, inability to solve problems due to executive dysfunction, behavioral changes, difficulty in using common instruments due to apraxia, language difficulties, incontinence and high dependency on others [7, 11].

The AD cognitive decline is usually preceded by a period of mild cognitive impairment (MCI) in which the individual retains his usual daily activities but has subnormal performance in cognitive neuropsychological testing. Many researchers reported a prodromal stage of subjective cognitive decline in which the person experiences worsening in his memory and/or cognitive performance despite the normal objective performance in standardized cognitive neuropsychological tests [30]. Atypical AD types start by non-amnestic manifestations but have the same pathological hallmarks include logopenic aphasia type, dysexecutive type, parietal dominant and frontal dominant atrophy subtypes [31, 32].

1.6. Investigations and biomarkers

It is generally accepted that AD pathological changes begin decades before the appearance of dementia symptoms and this leads to the introduction of the term preclinical AD, which is defined as biomarker evidences of AD pathological changes in a cognitively healthy individual. The current challenge is to develop reliable biomarkers for early pre-dementia AD diagnosis to maintain longer patients' independence and prepare the floor for the discovery of disease modifying agents including hormonal replacement therapy before irreversible neural damage takes place [11].

The ADNI-2 (Alzheimer Disease Neuroimaging Initiative-2) established CSF biomarkers include reduced CSF Aβ-42 and elevated total and phosphorylated tau-181, which are very accurate in prediction of MCI/AD conversion with 85% sensitivity and 90% specificity. Novel but still non-approved CSF biomarkers include high Aβ oligomers and neurogranin levels [33].

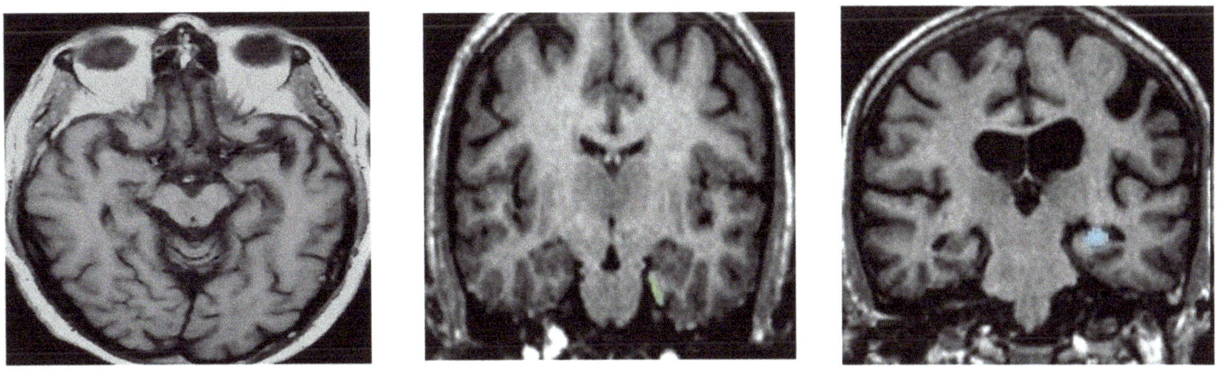

Figure 2. Brain MRI of a 56 years old female with early Alzheimer Disease showing medial temporal atrophy in T1 axial section (left), decreased right entorhinal cortex volume (middle) and right hippocampus volume (right) in coronal 3D spoiled gradient magnetic resonance images.

Blood biomarkers include high plasma homocysteine, high serum angiotensin converting enzyme activities and low plasma levels of the obesity-related hormone leptin [20]. Other ongoing research biomarkers include prostate-specific antigen complexed to α1-antichymotrypsin, pancreatic prohormone, clusterin and fetuin B [34].

The imaging biomarkers that can predict MCI/AD conversion are usually directed to measure the neural and synaptic densities in the commonly affected cortical areas. In volumetric MRI, manual and/or automated techniques can detect hippocampus and entorhinal cortex atrophy with concomitant dilatation of the temporal horns of the lateral ventricle. Other early neuroimaging biomarkers include task-free functional MRI (measures network failure quotient), diffusion tensor imaging (DTI) MRI, SPECT, FDG-PET, amyloid PET and tau PET [35] (**Figure 2**).

2. Sex hormones in normal cognition

Better keep progestogen as it is a wider term than progesterone and this is clarified in the section of progesterone are synthesized from cholesterol by the action of aromatase enzyme, and they play important roles in shaping the neural functions and behavior throughout all stages of human life. The sex steroid hormones are potent regulators of neuronal survival and function in multiple CNS regions during normal development, aging and in some neurodegenerative disorders including AD. In aging individuals, low levels of gonadal sex hormones are associated with decline in neurogenesis especially in the hippocampus with the resultant age-dependent memory decline and executive function difficulties [36].

2.1. Gender cognitive variability

Over a long time, obvious sexual dimorphism in adult human brain was observed with females harbor larger frontal and medial paralimbic cortices, while males exhibit bigger medial frontal cortex, amygdala and hypothalamic volumes. This gender difference is mainly due to variability in sex chromosome and sex hormone neuronal action. Genetic studies revealed that X-chromosome carry genes which expressions enhance visuospatial, executive and/or social cognitive tasks, whereas genes on Y-chromosome are more responsible for behavioral sexual differentiation [37].

At the same time, there is different gender cognitive performance starting during the early neonatal period and persists throughout human survival. This sex difference may be the base of the striking variable susceptibilities to various cognitive disorders in men and women [38]. Under normal circumstances, there is non-significant sex difference in global cognitive performance, but generally, males are better in mathematics and 3D spatial tests, while females are superior in autobiographic, episodic memory and verbal tests. Regarding spatial navigation, males perform better in allocentric strategy (world-centered object-to-object spatial relations) but females excel in egocentric navigation (self-centered subject-to-object spatial relations). This different cognitive performance is universal and evident in humans and animals which weaken the suggestion that environmental factors or gendered socialization are the causes of these gender variations [39, 40].

2.2. Estrogen actions in normal cognition

Estrogen is the primary female sex hormone, which regulates fundamental physiological processes in both reproductive and nonreproductive organs, including the CNS. The brain can synthesize estrogens (neuroestrogens) either by the aromatization of androgens or via a series of enzymatic steps from the precursor of all steroids, cholesterol. This neuroestrogen plays major roles in sexual differentiation of brain in both male and female. Four natural types of estrogens exist: estrone (E1; a weak estrogen and the main postmenopausal type), estradiol (E2; the most potent endogenous estrogen and the main type during the reproductive age), estriol (E3; very weak estrogen and hardly detected in non-pregnant females) and estetrol (E4; secreted only during pregnancy) [41].

Estrogens can cross the cell membrane lipid bilayer to bind to the estrogen receptors (ER), which are of two types: nuclear and membrane ER. The nuclear ER are either ERα or ERβ, which are responsible for the estrogen genomic action through regulation of various transcriptional gene expression mechanisms. The brain contains both types of nuclear ER, which are abundant in the hippocampus, pyramidal cells and glial tissue [42]. The membrane estrogen receptors (mERs) are G protein-coupled and ligand-gated ion channels, including GPER1 (previously known as GPR30), ER-X and Gq-mER, which are responsible for the rapid non-genomic actions of estrogen that is initiated within minutes after estrogen administration (estrogen neurotransmitter actions) due to recruitment and activation of kinase-dependent signaling pathways. Membrane ER are abundant in the neocortex and their activation results in increased activity of nitric oxide synthase and Ca^{2+} influx to the cells through N-methyl-D-aspartate (NMDA) receptor-mediated mechanism [43, 44].

The cellular mechanisms underlying estrogen CNS actions are still uncertain due to the different estrogen expression in both sexes and in different brain areas, but it is generally accepted that estrogens usually promote neurogenesis, exert neuroprotective actions and support neuronal survival by antiapoptotic action, stimulating nerve growth factor and brain-derived neurotrophic factor [45]. Estrogens also improve neuronal plasticity especially in the hippocampus, increase cerebral blood flow by enhancing endothelial derived nitric oxide and prostacyclin pathways, regulate neural mitochondrial functions (both types of ER are expressed in the mitochondria) especially in stressful conditions by stimulating anti-apoptotic proteins and decrease free radical production. At the same time, estrogen exerts anti-inflammatory actions by reducing the expression of astrocyte to chemokines, promoting the maturation of oligodendrocyte precursor cells and improve their ability for CNS repair, which enhances the growth and differentiation of axons and dendrites and prevents axonal loss and demyelination [46].

Estrogens also have well-documented direct cognitive and behavioral actions, and their postmenopausal depletion been associated with cognitive decline and increased risk of AD. The rapid estrogen non-genomic actions are important for hippocampal memory consolidation and hippocampal-dependent spatial navigation memory and improve learning performance, novel objects recognition and object placement tasks when administered before the cognitive tests. At the same time, estrogens improve choline acetyltransferase activity, promote serotonergic neuronal function and stimulate dopamine release in the caudate, prefrontal cortex, nucleus accumbens and dorsal raphe nucleus, which in turn enhance age-related learning and memory declines [36, 47].

2.3. Progesterone actions in normal cognition

Progesterone is a steroid hormone and it is most active natural progestogen, synthesized in the gonads, placenta, adrenal glands and CNS (neurosteroids). It has many reproductive and non-reproductive functions, including regulation of a wide range of brain functions [48]. Progesterone has a lipophilic structure, which can cross the cell membrane to interact with its specific intracellular progesterone receptors (PRs) expressed throughout the brain without sex difference with special higher expression in the hypothalamus, hippocampus, frontal cortex, medial amygdaloid nucleus, norepinephrine neurons of the nucleus tractus solitaries and cerebellum. Progesterone exerts its CNS actions through regulation of gene expression, modulation of neurotransmitter systems and epigenetic actions as well as enhancing estrogen actions [49].

PRs are either nuclear type (PR-A and PR-B), transmembrane PR (7TMPRβ) or membrane-associated 25-Dx PR (PGRMC1). Nuclear PRs are ligand inducible transcription factors that regulate target genes expression and play important roles in sexual brain differentiation, reproductive behavior, neuroprotection, neurogenesis, Schwan cell activities and their myelination programs, proliferation of neural progenitor cells and the release of the brain-derived neurotrophic factor important for cell differentiation and survival. Progesterone also has anti-inflammatory actions through regulation of the activities of astrocytes, microglia and oligodendrocytes [50, 51].

Transmembrane PRs are G protein-coupled receptors responsible for the rapid action of progesterone, and when activated, they block the activity of adenylyl cyclase, including enhancement of mitochondrial functions and regulation of cell viability. At the same time, progesterone alters dopaminergic and GABAergic system activities in many brain regions mainly the hippocampus, amygdala and fusiform gyrus enhancing the memory and learning performances [52, 53].

2.4. Androgen actions in normal cognition

Androgens are very important sex steroids that exert cognitive functions in both males and females as they not only regulate the CNS development but also help to maintain its proper function from infancy to adulthood [54]. It is generally accepted that androgens play a pivotal role in cognitive performance and their depletion or signaling inhibition (in normal aging or anti-androgen hormonal therapy in cancer prostate) results in dysfunction in androgen-responsive tissues, including the brain and consequently deleterious cognitive impairment. At the same time, discontinuation of anti-androgen in cancer therapy restores cognitive performance especially verbal memory [55].

The CNS action of androgens is mediated either directly through stimulation of androgen receptors (ARs) (nuclear receptors regulating target genes expression at transcriptional level) or indirectly after conversion to estrogen by the action of aromatase enzyme. ARs are highly expressed in the septum pellucidum, stria terminalis, preoptic area, ventromedial hypothalamus and cerebellum where they regulate the sexual reproductive behaviors [56, 57]. Neuroandrogens production had detected in the hippocampus where they modulate the hippocampal structure specifically CA1 and CA3 areas. In the medial amygdala and prefrontal cortex, androgens exert important roles in cognitive function regulation through promoting neuroprotection (anti-glutamate action) and neurogenesis, improving neuronal survival and anti-apoptotic effect (regulating mitochondrial genome activities and suppressing reactive oxygen species), modulating hippocampal synaptic plasticity, enhancing remyelination and exerting anti-inflammatory action by regulating astrocytic and oligodendrocytic activities [58]. Beside the delayed genomic effects of androgens, non-genomic rapid actions are mediated by trans-membrane G-protein-coupled ARs, which stimulations increase the intracellular Ca^{2+} influx and result in improved inhibitory avoidance task, spatial learning and memory performance [59, 60].

Androgens especially anabolic androgen steroids (AAS) are not always neurobehaviorally beneficial, and their short-term use results in aggressive and manic behaviors, whereas their long-term use is associated with impairment of decision making, behavioral flexibility, cognitive control and spatial memory [61, 62].

3. Brain responses variability to sex hormones

The neurocognitive actions of sex hormones are not simple but several factors may interact to control their beneficial effects including the inter-balance between their levels as well as the age and sex of the individual. In pregnancy, simultaneous increase in progesterone and estrogens results in impaired mood and decreased memory [63]. At the same time, sex hormones seem to play their major neuromodulatory action in early person's prepubertal life with subsequent decrease in the neuronal sensitivity to their actions with advancement of age. Some studies revealed that prepubertal sex hormones have permanent effects in individual's behaviors and cognition including spatial abilities. Early pubertal testosterone administration to gonadectomized male Syrian hamsters resulted in their attaining adult mating behaviors while administration in late puberty did not give the same results denoting that neurons are highly sensitive to the organizational effect of sex hormones at certain age with decreased sensitivity later after passage of this time [64–66]. On the other hand, brain estrogen expression was reduced in adult female mice previously exposed to stress in adolescence but not in early adulthood which concludes that adolescent stresses suppress estrogen activities and interfere with its organizational actions to attain adult mating behavior. From these results, we can conclude that the individual's susceptibility to many neurodegenerative disorders including AD may be attained since early life and we may not be able to reverse it easily later [67, 68].

4. Sex hormones in MCI and Alzheimer's disease

Alzheimer's disease is a heterogenous disorder with multiple variants and wide variety of manifestations, which result from the interactions between multiple etiological factors, including genetic, epigenetic, environmental and lifestyle factors. Neuronal action of sex hormones represents one of the well-defined AD pathogenetic factors and may represent a hope to understand the biology of sex-dependent variability in AD predisposition and in turn leads to the development of personalized, gender-specific AD management.

4.1. Sex hormones and MCI

The concept of MCI had received much attention nowadays for early detection of those candidates to AD conversion which open a gate for future disease modifying agents including hormonal therapy before irreversible neuronal damages take place. MCI is a clinical condition lies between normal aging and dementia in which the cognitive dysfunctions are greater than expected for age but is not severe enough to significantly interfere with the daily life or warrant the diagnosis of dementia [8, 69]. MCI is classified to amnestic (am-MCI) and non-amnestic (nam-MCI) types. In the former, memory impairment is the dominating manifestation, and in the latter, non-memory cognitive domain is the affected one (language, attention, executive function, visual-spatial). Amnestic MCI is termed multiple domain if another cognitive domain is affected, whereas nam-MCI becomes multiple domain if more than one cognitive non-memory domain is affected. People with am-MCI are more liable to develop AD [11, 70].

The prevalence of am-MCI is about 8.5–25.9 per 1000 of general population and 10–20% of those above the age of 60 years; 10–15% of am-MCI persons will develop AD compared to 1–2% of nam-MCI people. Several clinical and biochemical markers had been studied to be used as predictors of MCI/AD progression. In general, women have a higher prevalence of nam-MCI but most metanalytic studies showed non-significant gender difference in the prevalence of am-MCI, which means that women take shorter time to convert from am-MCI to manifest AD [71, 72].

4.2. Sex hormones and Alzheimer's disease

One of the most common observations associated with AD onset is decreased levels of sex hormones, including estrogens, progesterone and androgens, pointing the potential role of these hormones in AD pathogenesis and the possible benefits of their targeting in AD management strategies.

4.2.1. Estrogens and Alzheimer's disease

Estrogen neuroprotective actions in AD are well documented by decades of researches showing that women used estrogen supplements or those with late menopause are at significantly decreased risk of AD development. On the other hand, early menopause because of increased sex hormone-binding globulin is associated with higher risk of AD in later life [73]. Estrogens exert anti-AD actions through different mechanisms including inhibition of tau deposition and Aβ accumulation. The former action is exerted through inhibition of tau hyperphosphorylation and promotion of tau dephosphorylation in an estrogen receptor-dependent mode through inhibition of protein kinases and promotion of protein phosphatase 2A enzyme activities, respectively [13, 74]. Estrogens inhibit Aβ accumulation by several mechanisms, one of which is decreasing Aβ production by enhancement of non-amyloidogenic APP pathway through activation of α-secretase enzyme that cleaves APP to soluble APP-α peptides and shorter membrane-attached C-terminal segment. The latter is further digested by γ-secretase to non-toxic P3 and C59 segments. Other estrogen actions include inhibition of β-secretase (amyloidogenic pathway) and stimulation of APP-containing vesicle budding by trans-Golgi network [75]. Estrogens also promote Aβ clearance by stimulation of microglial Aβ phagocytosis and enzymes involved in Aβ degradation, including metalloproteases-2 and -9, insulin-degrading enzyme and neprilysin [76].

At the same time, estrogens exert anti-AD actions by increasing dendritic spine densities, promoting synaptogenesis, inhibiting the neurotoxic effects of oxidized low-density lipoproteins and glutamate, improving mitochondrial functions and enhancing the hippocampal cholinergic neurotransmitter system. Estrogens also regulate the epigenetic DNA methylation and miRNAs biogenesis especially in the hippocampus and thus master the genes expressions both transcriptionally and post-transcriptionally, which in turn play pivotal roles in enhancement of neuroprotection and prevention of neurodegeneration. Estrogen actions seem to be age dependent with obvious dysregulation in old-aged people. At the same time, estrogens have neuroprotective actions through increasing the expression of antiapoptotic Bcl-xL and Bcl-w and suppressing the expression of proapoptotic Bim, which lead to prevention of neuronal loss from Aβ toxicity [77–80].

Women are at increased risk of AD due to age-related sharp decline in sex steroid hormones and spending a large proportion of their life in the postmenopausal period because of increased their life longevity with the resultant prolonged hypoestrogenic state and its negative neurological consequences. Studies showed that postmenopausal women with AD had lower estradiol (E2) and estrone (E1) levels in both blood and CSF compared to normal controls. Moreover, female CSF-E2 level is positively correlated with CSF-Aβ level and cerebral glucose metabolism in the left hippocampus PET scan, which denotes that they are at increased risk to develop AD. In short-term studies, transdermal estrogen administration is associated with increased attention, verbal and visual memories; however, long-term studies failed to slow down AD progression or adding benefits to rivastigmine therapy in postmenopausal women [47, 81].

The neuroprotective effect of estrogen is not the same in both sexes as brain E1 and E2 levels have no relations with Aβ accumulation in males pointing to different gender expression of sex steroid hormones. At the same time, estrogen administration in male to female cross sex subjects results in significant decreases in the hippocampal volume despite producing neurogenesis, which means that the estrogen AD risk prevention in males is negligible [82, 83] (**Figure 3**).

4.2.2. Progesterone and Alzheimer's disease

Studies in progesterone neuroprotective actions against AD predisposition are not so plenty like those on estrogens but despite this, it is generally accepted that progesterone has a direct neuroprotective action while its indirect actions against AD development by regulating the neuroestrogen effects are matter of controversy as in some studies, progesterone enhances estradiol neuroprotective actions and in others antagonizes them beside reducing the cerebral blood flow [84].

The direct progesterone protecting actions against AD development and/or progression include regulation of β-amyloid metabolism by reducing Aβ production and decreasing the pool of soluble Aβ by enhancement of the non-amyloidogenic α-secretase pathway, decreasing Aβ accumulation through modulation of γ-secretases activities and increasing Aβ

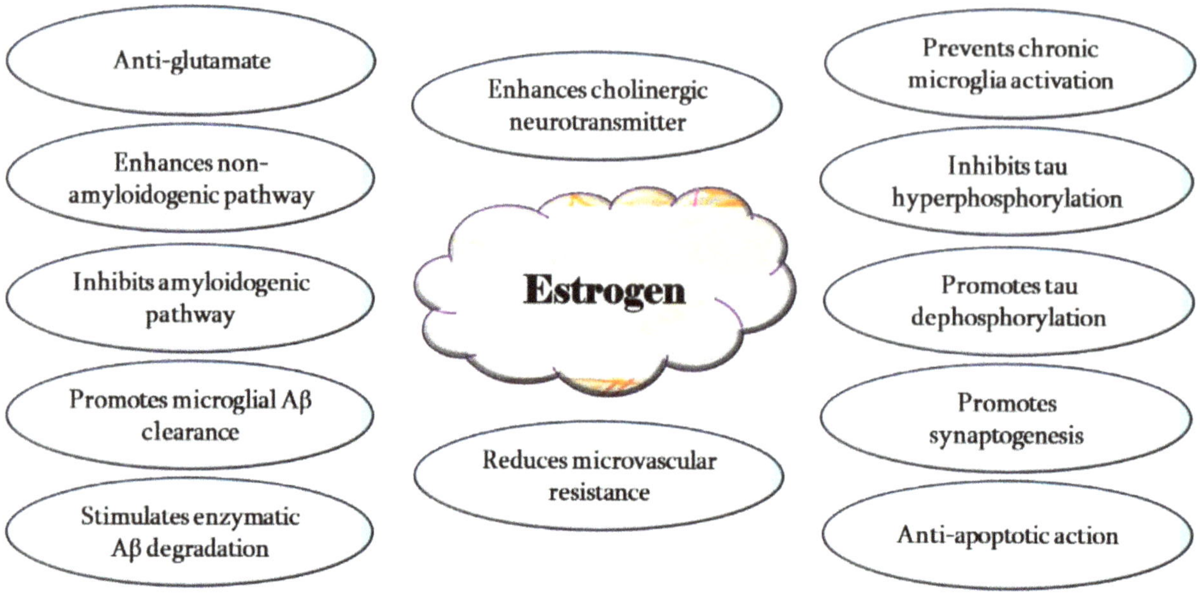

Figure 3. Estrogen anti-Alzheimer's neuroprotective actions.

clearance by enhancing insulin-degrading enzyme expression and downregulation of β-secretase gene expression [85, 86]. At the same time, progesterone reduces tau hyperphosphorylation and the serum level of endogenous progesterone is inversely correlated with tau accumulation, and at the same time, progesterone administration in transgenic AD mice improved cognitive performance in object recognition and T-maze task [87].

4.2.3. Androgens and Alzheimer's disease

Androgens have neuroprotective effects against AD in both males and females. Many studies had detected lower testosterone level in men with AD relative to normal age-matched control both in the blood and CSF. At the same time, APOE4 allele, which is a major risk of late onset AD, is associated with significantly lower level of circulating testosterone [88]. In accordance with these results, the Baltimore Longitudinal Study on Aging had detected significantly lower testosterone level 5–10 years in healthy men prior to their development of clinically manifest AD compared to those who did not develop AD [89].

Short-term testosterone administration improves cognitive functions in MCI and AD patients possibly through non-genomic transmembrane ARs activation [90, 91]. The long-term direct genomic action of androgens results in reduction of Aβ accumulation through enhancement of non-amyloidogenic APP pathway and promoting Aβ clearance by stimulation of Aβ-degrading enzyme action. Postmortem studies had shown that brain levels of testosterone were inversely correlated with cerebral soluble Aβ, which precedes insoluble fibrillar Aβ accumulation. These androgenic anti-amyloid actions are exerted in both sexes [92, 93]. Androgens can also indirectly reduce Aβ accumulation either through enhancing the estrogen pathway or through hypothalamo-hypophyseal-gonadal axis where they inhibit the release of gonadotropin luteinizing hormone secretion by the negative feedback, and it is well known that the latter hormone increases Aβ production by enhancement of APP/β-secretase initiated amyloidogenic pathway [94].

Males are subjected to andropause due to age-dependent high level of sex hormone-binding globulin with subsequent decrease in androgen levels and effects. Sex hormone-binding globulin is significantly higher in AD patients than age- and sex-matched control resulting in functional impairments of androgen-responsive tissues including the brain with consequent increase in AD risk [73]. Male andropause occurs very slowly over a long period of time where total androgen level starts to decline in thirties in a rate of 0.2–1% per year, while free testosterone decreases in a higher rate (2–3% yearly). This slowly gradual andropause relative to the rapid menopause may be one of the explanations of decreased male gender AD risk, delayed male MCI/AD conversion and slower AD cognitive deterioration [78, 95].

5. Sex hormone therapy trials for Alzheimer's disease

Based on the abundant data supporting the numerous neuroprotective actions of sex hormones in ameliorating many pathological processes occurring in AD, hormonal replacement therapy (HRT) seems to be theoretically beneficial but the translation of this hypothesis to practice met a lot of difficulties which made the use of HRT in AD management still a matter of skepticism [36, 94]. The values of female estrogens and progesterone replacement therapies carry controversial results, which are mainly dependent on the timing, dose and duration of their application to the AD predisposed individual. Promising results were only attained on early HRT initiation at a close menopause temporal proximity and any delayed administration may even give counterproductive bad consequence. This time limit of proper HRT initiation resulted in introduction of the term the critical window of intervention or the window of opportunity which describes the time after which HRT become worthless. HRT has not the same effect in all genotypes but it is found to be more beneficial in people with APOE2 and APOE3 genotypes than APOE4 [96–100]. At the same time, some studies revealed that the protective effect of HRT against AD is only achieved in long-term users (>10 years), while short-term therapy had no AD preventive actions pointing to the need of long-term HRT use to gain significantly beneficial AD protection [101, 102]. The need for long-term use of conventional HRT opens a new obstacle due to the high cardiovascular risks which in some instances may overwhelm the anti-AD cognitive benefits. This makes AD patients in ultimate need for future introduction of new hormonal drugs with little side effects [103, 104]. At the androgenic level and despite their numerous anti-AD neuroprotective actions, the long-term androgens use carries many neurological and extra-neurological risks including decreased dendritic reorganization and spine density in the limbic regions after initial increase due to increased glutamate turnover and neurotoxicity in amygdala structures with functional impaired connectivity with areas involved in cognitive functions [105, 106].

6. Conclusions and future prospect

Alzheimer's disease is a complex multifactorial neurodegenerative disorder resulted from dysregulation of many biological processes at multiple levels in a specific neuronal temporo-spatial pattern. Sex hormones, including estrogens, progesterone and androgens, play crucial

CNS modulatory functions and their disturbances result in impairment of neuroprotection, neurogenesis, synaptogenesis, synaptic plasticity and myelination as well as abnormal glial cell activities. The sharp decrease of neurosteroids influences in menopause relative to the slow andropause makes females sex at increased risk of AD development, rapid MCI/AD conversion and rapid course of cognitive deterioration. Trials used sex hormones as a disease modifying neuroprotective anti-AD agents revealed that their possible beneficial effect can be achieved only by early HRT before the beginning of critical window of intervention and the therapy must continue for long time which may put the treated individuals at increased risk of cardiovascular complications.

So, what is nowadays considered normal menopausal or andropausal sex hormones' declines may be sufficient triggers irreversible neuropathological changes which latter on progress to AD in susceptible individuals, and it is the time to use these changes as early AD biomarkers in high risk persons and in turn correct them before the onset of the window of opportunity by safe and effective HRT for long-term use and sufficient to produce significant AD prophylaxis.

Author details

Wafik Said Bahnasy*, Yasser A. El-Heneedy and Ehab A. El-Seidy

*Address all correspondence to: wafikbahnasy@gmail.com

Department of Neurology, Faculty of Medicine, Tanta University, Tanta, Egypt

References

[1] Li R, Singh M. Sex differences in cognitive impairment and Alzheimer's disease. Frontiers in Neuroendocrinology. 2014;**35**:385-403. DOI: 10.1016/j.yfrne.2014.01.002

[2] Esquirol J. Des maladies mentales. Paris: Baillie're; 1838

[3] Boller F, Forbes MM. History of dementia and dementia in history: An overview. Journal of the Neurological Sciences. 1998;**158**:125-133

[4] Cipriani G, Dolciotti C, Picchi L, Bonuccelli U. Alzheimer and his disease: A brief his tory. Neurological Sciences. 2011;**32**:275-279. DOI: 10.1007/s10072-010-0454-7

[5] Alzheimer's Association. Alzheimer's Association Report 2017 Alzheimer's disease facts and figures. Alzheimer's & Dementia. 2017;**13**:325-373. DOI: 10.1016/j.jalz.2017.02.001

[6] Scheltens P, Blennow K, Breteler MB, de Strooper B, Frisoni GB, Salloway S, Van der Flier WM. Alzheimer's disease. Lancet. 2016;**388**:505-517. DOI: 10.1016/S0140-6736(15)01124-1

[7] Ulrich JD, Ulland TK, Colonna M, Holtzman DM. Elucidating the role of TREM2 in Alzheimer's disease. Neuron. 2017;**94**:237-248. DOI: 10.1016/j.neuron.2017.02.042

[8] Au B, Dale-McGrath S, Tierney MC. Sex differences in the prevalence and incidence of mild cognitive impairment: A meta-analysis. Ageing Research Reviews. 2017;**35**:176-199. DOI: 10.1016/j.arr.2016.09.005

[9] Phung KTT, Chaaya M, Prince M, Atweh S, El Asmar K, Karam G, Khoury RM, Ghandour L, Nielsen TR, Waldemar G. Dementia prevalence, care arrangement, and access to care in Lebanon: A pilot study. Alzheimer's & Dementia. 2017;**13**(12):1317-1326. DOI: 10.1016/j.jalz.2017.04.007

[10] Roher AE, Kokjohn TA, Clarke SG, Sierks MR, Maarouf CL, Serrano GE, Sabbagh MS, Beach TG. APP/Aβ structural diversity and Alzheimer's disease pathogenesis. Neurochemistry International. 2017;**110**:1-13. DOI: https://doi.org/10.1016/j.neuint.2017.08.007

[11] Peterson R, Graff-Radford J. Alzheimer disease and other dementias. In: Daroff RB, Jankovic J, Mazziotta JC, Pomeroy SL, editors. Bradley's Neurology in Clinical Practice. 7th ed. Vol. 95. Elsevier; 2016. pp. 1380-1421

[12] Mohamed T, Shaker A, Rao PPN. Amyloid cascade in Alzheimer's disease: Recent advances in medicinal chemistry. European Journal of Medicinal Chemistry. 2016;**113**: 258-272. DOI: 10.1016/ j.ejmech.2016.02.049

[13] Arendt T, Stieler JT, Holzer M. Tau and tauopathies. Brain Research Bulletin. 2016;**126**:238-292. DOI: 10.1016/j.brainresbull.2016.08.018

[14] Mishra S, Gordon BA, Su Y, Christensen J, Friedrichsen K, Jackson K, Hornbeck R, Balota DA, Cairns NJ, Morris JC, Ances BM, Benzinger TLS. AV-1451 PET imaging of tau pathology in preclinical Alzheimer disease: Defining a summary measure. NeuroImage. 2017;**161**:171-178. DOI: 10.1016/j.neuroimage.2017.07.050

[15] Theendakara V, Bredesen DE, Rao RV. Downregulation of protein phosphatase 2A by apolipoprotein E: Implications for Alzheimer's disease. Molecular and Cellular Neuroscience. 2017;**83**:83-91. DOI: 10.1016/j.mcn.2017.07.002

[16] Carlsen EM, Rasmussen R. Protein networks in Alzheimer's disease. Cell Systems. 2017; **4**:153-155. DOI: 10.1016/j.cels.2017.02.006

[17] El Ali A, Rivest S. Microglia in Alzheimer's disease: A multifaceted relationship. Brain, Behavior, and Immunity. 2016;**55**:138-150. DOI: 10.1016/j.bbi.2015.07.021

[18] Piirainen S, Youssef A, Song C, Kalueff AV, Landreth GE, Malm T, Tian L. Psychosocial stress on neuroinflammation and cognitive dysfunctions in Alzheimer's disease: The emerging role for microglia? Neuroscience and Biobehavioral Reviews. 2017;**77**:148-164. DOI: 10.1016/j.neubiorev.2017.01.046

[19] Spangenberg EE, Green KN. Inflammation in Alzheimer's disease: Lessons learned from microglia-depletion models. Brain, Behavior, and Immunity. 2017;**61**:1-11. DOI: 10.1016/j.bbi.2016.07.003

[20] Chakraborty A, de Wit NM, van der Flier WM, de Vries HE. The blood brain barrier in Alzheimer's disease. Vascular Pharmacology. 2017;**89**:12-18. DOI: 10.1016 /j.vph.2016.11.008

[21] Kapasi A, Schneider JA. Vascular contributions to cognitive impairment, clinical Alzheimer's disease, and dementia in older persons. Biochimica et Biophysica Acta. 2016; **1862**:878-886. DOI: 10.1016/j.bbadis.2015.12.023

[22] do Nascimento GRA, Barros YVR, Wells AK, Khalil RA. Research into specific modulators of vascular sex hormone receptors in the management of postmenopausal cardiovascular disease. Current Hypertension Reviews. 2009;**5**(4):283-306. DOI: 10.2174/157340209789587717

[23] Šimic G, Leko MB, Wray S, Harrington CR, Delalle I, Jovanov-Miloševic N, Bažadona D, Buée L, de Silva R, Giovanni GD, Wischik CM, Hof PR. Monoaminergic neuropathology in Alzheimer's disease. Progress in Neurobiology. 2017;**151**:101-138. DOI: 10.1016/j.pneurobio.2016.04.001

[24] Hu NW, Ondrejcak T, Rowan MJ. Glutamate receptors in preclinical research on Alzheimer's disease: Update on recent advances. Pharmacology, Biochemistry and Behavior. 2012;**100**:855-862. DOI: 10.1016/j.pbb.2011.04.013

[25] Kilian JG, Hsu HW, Mata K, Wolf FW, Kitazawa M. Astrocyte transport of glutamate and neuronal activity reciprocally modulate tau pathology in drosophila. Neuroscience. 2017;**348**:191-200. DOI: 10.1016/j.neuroscience.2017.02.011

[26] Theendakara V, Peters-Libeu CA, Spilman P, Poksay KS, Bredesen DE, Rao RV. Direct transcriptional effects of apolipoprotein E. Journal of Neuroscience. 2016;**36**(3):685-700. DOI: 10.1523/JNEUROSCI.3562-15.2016

[27] Wang J, JT Y, Tan MS, Jiang T, Tan L. Epigenetic mechanisms in Alzheimer's disease: Implications for pathogenesis and therapy. Ageing Research Reviews. 2013;**12**:1024-1041. DOI: 10.1016/j.arr.2013.05.003

[28] Shamsi MB, Firoz AS, Imam SN, Alzaman N, Samman MA. Epigenetics of human diseases and scope in future therapeutics. Journal of Taibah University Medical Sciences. 2017;**12**(3):205-211. DOI: 10.1016/j.jtumed.2017.04.003

[29] Van den Hove DL, Kompotis K, Lardenoije R, Kenis G, Mill J, Steinbusch HW, Lesch KP, Fitzsimons CP, De Strooper B, Rutten BPF. Epigenetically regulated microRNAs in Alzheimer's disease. Neurobiology of Aging. 2014;**35**:731-745. DOI: 10.1016/j.neurobiolaging.2013.10.082

[30] Buckley RF, Maruff P, Ames D, Bourgeat P, Martins RN, Masters CL, et al. Subjective memory decline predicts greater rates of clinical progression in preclinical Alzheimer's disease. Alzheimer's & Dementia. 2016;**12**(7):796-804. DOI: 10.1016/j.jalz.2015.12.013

[31] Kenawy WS, Bahnasy WS, Aboelsafa AA, Ramadan ES. Sleep disorders in Alzheimer's and vascular dementia [master thesis]. Tanta (Egypt): Tanta University; 2016. 108-120 p 10.13140/RG.2.2.23574.24649

[32] Leyton CE, Hodges JR, Piguet O, Ballard KJ. Common and divergent neural correlates of anomia in amnestic and logopenic presentations of Alzheimer's disease. Cortex. 2017;**86**:45-54. DOI: 10.1016/j.cortex.2016.10.019

[33] Mattsson N, Lönneborg A, Boccardi M, Blennow K, Hansson O. Clinical validity of cerebrospinal fluid Aß-42, tau, and phospho-tau as biomarkers for Alzheimer's disease in the context of a structured 5-phase development framework. Neurobiology of Aging. 2017;**52**:196-213. DOI: 10.1016/j.neurobiolaging.2016.02.034

[34] Sattlecker M, Kiddle SJ, Newhouse S, Proitsi P, Nelson S, Williams S, Johnston C, Killick R, Simmons A, Westman E, Hodges A, Soininen H, Kłoszewska I, Mecocci P, Tsolaki M, Vellas B, Lovestone S. Alzheimer's disease biomarker discovery using SOMA scan multiplexed protein technology. Alzheimer's & Dementia. 2014;**10**(6):724-734. DOI: 10.1016/j.jalz.2013.09.016

[35] Beheshti I, Demirel H, Matsuda H. Classification of Alzheimer's disease and predic tion of mild cognitive impairment-to-Alzheimer's conversion from structural magnetic resource imaging using feature ranking and a genetic algorithm. Computers in Biology and Medicine. 2017;**83**:109-119. DOI: 10.1016/j.compbiomed.2017.02.011

[36] Engler-Chiurazzi EB, Brown CM, Povroznik JM, Simpkins JW. Estrogens as neuropro tectants: Estrogenic actions in the context of cognitive aging and brain injury. Progress in Neurobiology. 2017;**157**:188-211. DOI: 10.1016/j.pneurobio. 2015.12.008

[37] Hong DS, Reiss AL. Cognitive and neurological aspects of sex chromosome aneuploidies. Lancet Neurology. 2014;**13**:306-318. DOI: 10.1016/S1474-4422(13)70302-8

[38] Hyde JS. Sex and cognition: Gender and cognitive functions. Current Opinion in Neurobiology. 2016;**38**:53-56. DOI: 10.1016/j.conb.2016.02.007

[39] Shah DS, Prados J, Gamble J, De Lillo C, Gibson CL. Sex differences in spatial memory using serial and search tasks. Behavioural Brain Research. 2013;**257**:90-99. DOI: 10.1016/j.bbr.2013.09.027

[40] Sommer W, Hildebrandt A, Kunina-Habenicht O, Schacht A, Wilhelm O. Sex differences in face cognition. Acta Psychologica. 2013;**142**:62-73. DOI: 10.1016/j.actpsy. 2012.11.001

[41] Cornil CA, Ball GF, Balthazart J. The dual action of estrogen hypothesis. Trends in Neurosciences. 2015;**38**(7):408-416. DOI: 10.1016/j.tins.2015.05.004

[42] Alexander A, Irving AJ, Harvey J. Emerging roles for the novel estrogen-sensing receptor GPER1 in the CNS. Neuropharmacology. 2017;**113**:652-660. DOI: 10.1016/j.neuropharm.2016.07.003

[43] Hamilton KJ, Hewitt SC, Arao Y, Korach KS. Estrogen Hormone Biology. In: Wassarman PM, editor. Current Topics in Developmental Biology. 1st ed. Elsevier; 2017;**125**(4); 110-146. DOI: http://dx.doi.org/10.1016/bs.ctdb.2016.12.005

[44] Warner M, Huang B, Gustafsson J. Estrogen receptor β as a pharmaceutical target. Trends in Pharmacological Sciences. 2017;**38**(1):92-99. DOI: 10.1016/j.tips.2016.10.006

[45] Mennenga SE, Baxter LC, Grunfeld IS, Brewer GA, Aiken LS, Engler-Chiurazzi EB, Camp BW, Acosta JI, Braden BB, Schaefer KR, Gerson JE, Lavery CN, Tsang CW, Hewitt LT, Kingston ML, Koebele SV, Patten KJ, Ball BH, McBeath MK, Bimonte-Nelson HA. Navigating to new frontiers in behavioral neuroscience: Traditional neuropsychological tests predict human performance on a rodent-inspired radial-arm maze. Frontiers in Behavioral Neuroscience. 2014;**8**:294. DOI: 10.3389/fnbeh.2014.00294

[46] Koebele SV, Bimonte-Nelson HA. The endocrine-brain-aging triad where many paths meet: Female reproductive hormone changes at midlife and their influence on circuits

important for learning and memory. Experimental Gerontology. 2017;**94**:14-23. DOI: 10.1016/j.exger.2016.12.011

[47] Kim J, Frick KM. Distinct effects of estrogen receptor antagonism on object recognition and spatial memory consolidation in ovariectomized mice. Psychoneuroendocrinology. 2017;**85**:110-114. DOI: 10.1016/j.psyneuen.2017.08.013

[48] Mani SK, Blaustein JD. Neural progestin receptors and female sexual behavior. Neuroendocrinology. 2012;**96**(2):152-161. DOI: 10.1159/000338668

[49] Camacho-Arroyo I, Hansberg-Pastor V, Vázquez-Martínez ER, Cerbón, M. Mechanism of Progesterone Action in the Brain. In: Pfaff DW, Joëls M, editors. Hormones, Brain, and Behavior. 3rd ed. Oxford: Academic Press; 2017;**3**:181-214. DOI: 10.1016/B978-0-12-803592-4.00053-5

[50] Gagnidze K, Weil ZM, Faustino LC, Schaafsma SM, Pfaff DW. Early histone modifications in the ventromedial hypothalamus and preoptic area following estradiol administration. Journal of Neuroendocrinology. 2013;**25**(10):939-955. DOI: 10.1111/jne.12085

[51] Guennoun R, Labombarda F, Gonzalez Deniselle MC, Liere P, De Nicola AF, Schumacher M. Progesterone and allopregnanolone in the central nervous system: Response to injury and implication for neuroprotection. Journal of Steroid Biochemistry and Molecular Biology. 2015;**146**:48-61. DOI: 10.1016/j.jsbmb.2014.09.001

[52] Su C, Cunningham RL, Rybalchenko N, Singh M. Progesterone increases the release of brain-derived neurotrophic factor from glia via progesterone receptor membrane component 1 (Pgrmc1)-dependent ERK5 signaling. Endocrinology. 2012;**153**(9):4389-4400. DOI: 10.1210/en.2011-2177

[53] Berent-Spillson A, Briceno E, Pinsky A, Simmen A, Persad CC, Zubieta JK, Smith YR. Distinct cognitive effects of estrogen and progesterone in menopausal women. Psychoneuroendocrinology. 2015;**59**:25-36. DOI: 10.1016/j.psyneuen.2015.04.020

[54] Moghadami S, Jahanshahi M, Sepehri H, Amini H. Gonadectomy reduces the density of androgen receptor-immunoreactive neurons in male rat's hippocampus: testosterone replacement compensates it. Behavioral and Brain Functions. 2016;**12**:5-14. DOI: https://doi.org/10.1186/ s12993-016-0089-9

[55] Carcaillon L, Brailly-Tabard S, Ancelin ML, Tzourio C, Foubert-Samier A, Dartigues JF, Guiochon-Mantel A, Scarabin PY. Low testosterone and the risk of dementia in elderly men: Impact of age and education. Alzheimer's & Dementia. 2014;**10**:S306-S314. DOI: 10.1016/j.jalz.2013.06.006

[56] Zup SL, Edwards NS, Mccarthy MM. Sex- and age-dependent effects of androgens on glutamate-induced cell death and intracellular calcium regulation in the developing hippocampus. Neuroscience. 2014;**281**:77-87. DOI: http://dx.doi.org/10.1016/j.neuroscience.2014.09.040

[57] Perez-Pouchoulen M, Toledo R, Garcia LI, Perez-Estudillo CA, Coria-Avila GA, Hernandez ME, Carrillo P, Manzo J. Androgen receptors in Purkinje neurons are modulated by systemic testosterone and sexual training in a region-specific manner in the male rat. Physiology & Behavior. 2016;**156**:191-198. DOI: 10.1016/j.physbeh.2016.01.027

[58] Bielecki B, Mattern C, Abdel G, Javaid S, Smietanka K, Abi Ghanem C, Mhaouty-Kodja S, Ghandour MS, Baulieu EE, Franklin RJ, Schumacher M, Traiffort E. The spontaneous regeneration of myelin: an unexpected central role of the androgen receptor. Proceedings of the National Academy of Sciences of the United States of America. 2016;**113**:14,829-14,834. DOI: 10.1073/pnas.1614826113

[59] Christou MA, Christou PA, Markozannes G, Tsatsoulis A, Mastorakos G, Tigas S. Effects of anabolic androgenic steroids on the reproductive system of athletes and recreational users: A systematic review and meta-analysis. Sports Med. 2017;**47**(9):1869-1883. DOI: 10.1007/s40279-017-0709-z

[60] Klores M, Moon JT, Duncan KA. Expression of glial CBP in steroid mediated neuroprotection in male and female zebra finches. Journal of Chemical Neuroanatomy. 2017;**79**:32-37. DOI: 10.1016/j.jchemneu.2016.11.002

[61] Westlye LT, Kaufmann T, Alnæs D, Hullstein IR, Bjørnebekk A. Brain connectivity aberrations in anabolic-androgenic steroid users. NeuroImage: Clinical. 2017;**13**:62-69. DOI: 10.1016/j.nicl.2016.11.014

[62] Bjørnebekk A, Walhovd KB, Jørstad ML, Due-Tønnessen P, Hullstein IR, Fjell AM. Structural brain imaging of long-term anabolic-androgenic steroid users and non-using weightlifters. Biological Psychiatry. 2017;**82**:294-302. DOI: 10.1016/j.biopsych.2016.06.017

[63] Keiser AA, Tronson NC. Molecular mechanisms of memory in males and females. In: Shansky RM, editor. Sex Differences in the Central Nervous System. Elsevier; 2016;**2**: 27-51. DOI: 10.1016/B978-0-12-802114-9.00002-0

[64] Berenbaum SA, Bryk KLK, Beltz AM. Early androgen effects on spatial and mechanical abilities: Evidence from congenital adrenal hyperplasia. Behavioral Neuroscience. 2012;**126**:86-96. DOI: 10.1037/a0026652

[65] Beltz AM, Berenbaum SA. Cognitive effects of variations in pubertal timing: Is puberty a period of brain organization for human sex-typed cognition? Hormones and Behavior. 2013;**63**:823-828. DOI: 10.1016/j.yhbeh.2013.04.002

[66] Nelson LH, Warden S, Lenz KM. Sex differences in microglial phagocytosis in the neonatal hippocampus. Brain, Behavior, and Immunity. 2017;**64**:11-22. DOI: 10.1016/j.bbi.2017.03.010

[67] Mahmoud R, Wainwright SR, Galea LAM. Sex hormones and adult hippocampal neurogenesis: Regulation, implications, and potential mechanisms. Frontiers in Neuroendocrinology. 2016;**41**:129-152. DOI: 10.1016/j.yfrne.2016.03.002

[68] Heberden C. Sex steroids and neurogenesis. Biochemical Pharmacology. 2017;**141**:56-62. DOI: 10.1016/j.bcp.2017.05.019

[69] Petersen RC, Roberts RO, Knopman DS, Boeve BF, Geda YE, Ivnik RJ, Smith GE, Jack CR. Mild cognitive impairment: Ten years later. Archives of neurology. 2009;**66**(12):1447-1455. DOI: 10.1001/archneurol. 2009.266

[70] Lee LK, Shahar S, Chin AV, Yusoff NAM, Rajab NF, Abdul Aziz S. Prevalence of gender disparities and predictors affecting the occurrence of mild cognitive impairment. Archives of Gerontology and Geriatrics. 2012;**54**:185-191. DOI: 10.1016/j.archger.2011.03.015

[71] Ward A, Arrighi HM, Michels S, Cedarbaum JM. Mild cognitive impairment: Disparity of incidence and prevalence estimates. Alzheimer's & Dementia. 2012;**8**:14-21. DOI: 10.1016/j.jalz.2011.01.002

[72] Roberts RO, Knopman DS, Mielke MM, Cha RH, Pankratz VS, Christianson TJ, Geda YE, Boeve BF, Ivnik RJ, Tangalos EG, Rocca WA, Petersen RC. Higher risk of progression to dementia in mild cognitive impairment cases who revert to normal. Neurology. 2014;**82**(4):317-325. DOI: 10.1212/WNL.0000000000000055

[73] Muller M, Schupf N, Manly JJ, Mayeux R, Luchsinger JA. Sex hormone binding globulin and incident Alzheimer's disease in elderly men and women. Neurobiology of Aging. 2010;**31**:1758-1765. DOI: 10.1016/j.neurobiolaging.2008.10.001

[74] Zhang HZ, Simpkins JW. Okadaic acid induces tau phosphorylation in SH-SY5Y cells in an estrogen-preventable manner. Brain Research. 2010;**1345**:176-181. DOI: 10.1016/j.brainres. 2010.04.074

[75] Merlo S, Spampinato SF, Sortino MA. Estrogen and Alzheimer's disease: Still an attractive topic despite disappointment from early clinical results. European Journal of Pharmacology. 2017;**817**:51-58. DOI: 10.1016/j.ejphar.2017.05.059

[76] Barratt HE, Budnick HC, Parra R, Lolley RJ, Perry CN, Nesic O. Tamoxifen promotes differentiation of oligodendrocyte progenitors in vitro. Neuroscience. 2016;**319**:146-154. DOI: 10.1016/j.neuroscience.2016.01.026

[77] Jung JI, Ladd TB, Kukar T, Price AR, Moore BD, Koo EH, Golde TE, Felsenstein KM. Steroids as γ-secretase modulators. FASEB Journal. 2013;**27**(9):3775-3785. DOI: 10.1096/fj.12-225,649

[78] Vest RS, Pike CJ. Gender, sex steroid hormones, and Alzheimer's disease. Hormones and Behavior. 2013;**63**:301-307. DOI: 10.1016/j.yhbeh.2012.04.006

[79] Fortress AM, Frick KM. Epigenetic regulation of estrogen-dependent memory. Frontiers in Neuroendocrinology. 2014;**35**(4):530-549. DOI: 10.1016/j.yfrne.2014.05.001

[80] Rao YS, Shult CL, Pinceti E, Pak TR. Prolonged ovarian hormone deprivation alters the effects of 17beta-estradiol on microRNA expression in the aged female rat hypothalamus. Oncotarget. 2015;**6**:36965-36983. DOI: 10.18632/oncotarget.5433

[81] Tschiffely AE, Schuh RA, Prokai-Tatrai K, Prokai L, Ottinger MA. A comparative evaluation of treatments with 17β-estradiol and its brain-selective prodrug in a double-transgenic mouse model of Alzheimer's disease. Hormones and Behavior. 2016;**83**:39-44. DOI: 10.1016 /j.yhbeh.2016.05.009

[82] Rosario ER, Chang L, Head EH, Stanczyk FZ, Pike CJ. Brain levels of sex steroid hormones in men and women during normal aging and in Alzheimer's disease. Neurobiology of Aging. 2011;**32**(4):604-613. DOI: 10.1016/j.neurobiolaging.2009.04.008

[83] Seiger R, Hahn A, Hummer A, Kranz GS, Ganger S, Woletz M, Kraus C, Sladky R, Kautzky A, Kasper S, Windischberger C, Lanzenberger R. Subcortical gray matter

changes in transgender subjects after long-term cross-sex hormone administration. Psychoneuroendocrinology. 2016;**74**:371-379. DOI: 10.1016/j.psyneuen.2016.09.028

[84] Garcia-Segura LM, Jacques Balthazart J. Steroids and neuroprotection: New advances. Frontiers in Neuroendocrinology. 2009;**30**:v-ix. DOI: 10.1016/j.yfrne.2009.04.006

[85] Carroll JC, Rosario ER, Villamagna A, Pike CJ. Continuous and cyclic progesterone differentially interact with estradiol in the regulation of Alzheimer-like pathology in female 3xTransgenic-Alzheimer's disease mice. Endocrinology. 2010;**151**:2713-2722. DOI: 10.1210/en.2009-1487

[86] Jayaraman A, Carroll JC, Morgan TE, Lin S, Zhao L, Arimoto JM, Murphy MP, Murphy MP, Beckett TL, Finch CE, Brinton RD, Pike CJ. 17 beta-estradiol and progesterone regulate expression of beta-amyloid clearance factors in primary neuron cultures and female rat brain. Endocrinology. 2012;**153**:5467-5479. DOI: 10.1210/en.2012-1464

[87] Zhao L, Morgan TE, Mao Z, Lin S, Cadenas E, Finch CE, Pike CJ, Mack WJ, Brinton RD. Continuous versus cyclic progesterone exposure differentially regulates hippocampal gene expression and functional profiles. PLoS ONE. 2012;**7**:e31267. DOI: 10.1371/journal.pone.0031267

[88] Raber J. AR, apoE, and cognitive function. Hormones and Behavior. 2008;**53**:706-715. DOI: 10.1016/j.yhbeh.2008.02.012

[89] Moffat SD, Zonderman AB, Metter EJ, Kawas C, Blackman MR, Harman SM, Resnick SM. Free testosterone and risk for Alzheimer disease in older men. Neurology. 2004; **62**:188-193 PMID: 14745052

[90] Cherrier MM, Matsumoto AM, Amory JK, Asthana S, Bremner W, Peskind ER, Raskind MA, Craft S. Testosterone improves spatial memory in men with Alzheimer disease and mild cognitive impairment. Neurology. 2005;**64**:2063-2068. DOI. DOI: 10.1212/01.WNL.0000165995.98986.F1

[91] Filová B, Ostatníková D, Celec P, Hodosy J. The effect of testosterone on the formation of brain structures. Cells Tissues Organs. 2013;**197**(3):169-177. DOI: 10.1159/000345567

[92] Butchart J, Birch B, Bassily R, Wolfe L, Holmes C. Male sex hormones and systemic inflammation in Alzheimer disease. Alzheimer Disease and Associated Disorders. 2013; **27**:153-156. DOI: 10.1097/WAD.0b013e 318,258 cd63

[93] Lee JH, Byun MS, Yi D, Choe MC, Choi HJ, Baek H, Sohn BK, Lee JY, Kim HJ, Kim JW, Lee Y, Kim YK, Sohn CH, Woo JI, Lee DY. Sex-specific association of sex hormones and gonadotropins, with brain amyloid and hippocampal neurodegeneration. Neurobiology of Aging. 2017;**58**:34-40. DOI: 10.1016/j.neurobiolaging.2017.06.005

[94] Burnham VL, Thornton JE. Luteinizing hormone as a key player in the cognitive decline of Alzheimer's disease. Hormones and Behavior. 2015;**76**:48-56. DOI: 10.1016/j yhbeh.2015.05.010

[95] Wang S, Wang R, Chen L, Bennett DA, Dickson DW, Wang DS. Expression and functional profiling of neprilysin, insulin-degrading enzyme, and endothelin-convert-

ing enzyme in prospectively studied elderly and Alzheimer's brain. J Neurochem. 2010;**115**(1):47-57. DOI: 10.1111/j.1471-4159.2010. 06899.x

[96] Maki PM, Henderson VW. Hormone therapy, dementia, and cognition: The women's health initiative 10 years on. Climacteric. 2012;**15**(3):256-262. DOI: 10.3109/13697137. 2012.660613

[97] Maki P. Is timing everything? New insights into why the effect of estrogen therapy on memory might be age dependent. Endocrinology. 2013;**154**(8):2570-2572. DOI: 10.1210/ en.2013-1598

[98] Xu L, Freeman G, Cowling BJ, Schooling CM. Testosterone therapy and cardiovascular events among men: A systematic review and meta-analysis of placebo-controlled randomized trials. BMC Medicine. 2013;**11**(1):108. DOI: 10.1186/1741-7015-11-108

[99] Riedel BC, Thompson PM, Brinton RD. Age, APOE and sex: Triad of risk of Alzheimer's disease. Journal of Steroid Biochemistry & Molecular Biology. 2016;**160**:134-147. DOI: 10.1016/j.jsbmb.2016.03.012

[100] Wroolie TE, Kenna HA, Williams KE, Rasgon NL. Cognitive effects of hormone therapy continuation or discontinuation in a sample of women at risk for Alzheimer disease. American Journal of Geriatric Psychiatry. 2015;**23**(11):1117-1126. DOI: 10.1016/j. jagp.2015.05.009

[101] Shao H, Breitner JC, Whitmer RA, Wang Hayden K, Wengreen H, Corcoran C, Tschanz J, Norton M, Munger R, Welsh-Bohmer K, Zandi PP. Cache county investigators, hormone therapy and Alzheimer disease dementia: New findings from the cache county study. Neurology. 2012;**79**:1846-1852. DOI: 10.1212/WNL.0b013e318271f823

[102] Imtiaz B, Taipale H, Tanskanen A, Tiihonen M, Kivipelto M, Heikkinen AM, Tolppanen AM. Risk of Alzheimer's disease among users of postmenopausal hormone therapy: A nationwide case–control study. Maturitas. 2017;**98**:7-13. DOI: 10.1016/j.maturitas.2017.01.002

[103] O'Brien J, Jackson JW, Grodstein F, Blacker D, Weuve J. Postmenopausal hormone therapy is not associated with risk of all-cause dementia and Alzheimer's disease. Epidemiologic Reviews. 2014;**36**(1):83-103. DOI: 10.1093/epirev/mxt008

[104] Depypere H, Vierin A, Weyers S, Sieben A. Alzheimer's disease, apolipoprotein E and hormone replacement therapy. Maturitas. 2016;**94**:98-105. DOI: 10.1016/j.maturitas. 2016.09.009

[105] Maggio M, DeVita F, Fisichella A, Colizzi E, Provenzano S, Lauretani F, Luci M, Ceresini G, Dall'Aglio E, Caffarra P, Valenti G, Ceda GP. DHEA and cognitive function in the elderly. Journal of Steroid Biochemistry & Molecular Biology. 2015;**145**:281-292. DOI: 10.1016/j.jsbmb.2014.03.014

[106] Seitz J, Lyall AE, Kanayama G, Makris N, Hudson JI, Kubicki M, Pope HG, Kaufman MJ. White matter abnormalities in long-term anabolic-androgenic steroid users: A pilot study. Psychiatry Research: Neuroimaging. 2017;**260**:1-5. DOI: 10.1016/j. pscychresns.2016.12.003

7

Sex Hormones: Role in Neurodegenerative Diseases and Addiction

Jonathan Martínez Pinto, Rodrigo L. Castillo and Ramón Sotomayor-Zárate

Abstract

The brain is a complex organ in charge of regulating the homeostasis of our body and behaviors such as motivation, reward, memory, and movement control, between others. These behaviors are regulated by dopaminergic neurons, which can be modulated by several stimuli throughout the life of an individual. For example, early exposure to sex hormones or endocrine disruptors during critical period of neuronal development affects dopaminergic pathways permanently, producing some disorders such as drug addiction. On the other hand, current knowledge regarding neurodegeneration in Parkinson and Alzheimer diseases pointed out the neuroprotection that estradiol can exert, but contradictory information can also be found in the literature. To know the underlying mechanisms that are related to the above mentioned diseases will help to improve health policies and treatments development.

Keywords: sex hormones, neonatal programming, dopaminergic circuit, neuroprotection, drug addiction, Alzheimer, Parkinson disease

1. Introduction

In the current world, humans are exposed to different compounds that can exert deleterious modifications in their bodies, taking special attention of the short- and long-term effects of endocrine disruptor chemicals, which mimic or block hormonal activity. Endocrine disruptor chemicals are natural or synthetic molecules that can alter the endocrine homeostasis, especially if exposure to these molecules is during critical developmental windows [1]. These compounds are used in plastic industries, chemical, and pharmaceutical industries, and for different events that are bioavailable in the environment affecting animals and humans. Endocrine disruptors exert their action through different pathways that converge on the molecular targets such as hormone receptors, enzymatic pathways involved in biosynthesis and metabolism of endobiotics in endocrine, reproductive, and nervous system. In this sense, different brain areas are sensible to the action of endocrine disruptors and sex hormones due to the presence of its receptors that can modulate the synaptic transmission and neuronal survival. In this regard, nuclear receptors for sex hormones are ligand-activated transcriptional factors that regulate different neural process such as neurodevelopment and behaviors. Alterations in hormonal homeostasis (e.g., aging) or signaling (e.g., exposure to agonists or antagonists of sex hormone receptors) may induce the onset of diseases before mentioned, affecting lifespan, quality of life, and high medical costs.

Worldwide, drug abuse has increased dramatically, especially in susceptible populations such as youth. However, human and animal studies show that not all drug consumers become addicts. In addition, it has determined sex differences in behaviors related to motivation, reward, and cognition, among others. Clinical observation has shown that children who have developed precocious puberty show an increase in risky behaviors such as drugs abuse, sexual risk, and anti-social behaviors in adolescence.

Also, when Parkinson (PD) and Alzheimer disease (AD) is analyzed, it observed a sex difference in terms of prevalence, which draws the attention to the possible role of sex hormones in the onset of these pathologies. In this term, meta-analysis has shown that males have augmented prevalence of PD than women, overall in the age range of 50–59 years (134 per 100,000) compared to women (41 per 100,000) [2]. However, the prevalence of AD is greater in women compared to men, considering different age range and ethnicity [3, 4].

In this chapter, we will discuss about the exposure to abnormal levels of sex hormones, due to metabolic alterations or endocrine disruptor chemicals, during critical period of neurodevelopment; and based on clinical evidence and current scientific knowledge, we will discuss the mechanisms involved in the development of drug addiction, Alzheimer and Parkinson disease, and the sex differences observed between patients.

2. Programming: early exposure to sex hormones

Programming concept was defined by Lucas as the physiological redirection of a tissue or organ by a deleterious stimulus in a sensitive period of development produces adverse functional changes in adulthood [5]. Currently, research in programming has been focused in the study of stimuli that affects sensitive periods of development such as prenatal and neonatal stages.

In that sense, experiments are carried out in female rats, where precocious puberty is induced by neonatal exposure to estradiol valerate, is accompanied by increased catecholamine content in the adrenal gland, noradrenaline content in the ovary and reproductive alterations in the adulthood [6]. Using the same model of neonatal administration of estradiol valerate [7], it observed an increase in dopamine (DA) and noradrenaline content in dopaminergic neurons of tuberoinfundibular [8], nigrostriatal, and mesolimbic pathways [9] of the adult. Indeed, neonatal administration of estradiol valerate and testosterone propionate increases DA content and tyrosine hydroxylase (TH), (rate limiting enzyme of dopamine synthesis) expression in substantia nigra (SN), and ventral tegmental area (VTA) of adult male rats [10]. Others works have shown that neonatal administration of testosterone reduces spatial memory and TH positive terminals in prefrontal cortex in an animal model of attention deficit disorder with hyperactivity [11].

In recent years, it has been shown that environmental pollutants (being most of them chemical disruptors) produce a myriad of effects in the brain [12]. For example, in rats, neonatal and postnatal administration of bisphenol A produce an increase of spontaneous locomotion behavior associated with the decreased immunoreactivity for TH in SN and decreased expression of dopamine transporter (DAT) in midbrain nuclei [13].

Sex hormone levels affect cortical and subcortical brain areas, especially in sensitive periods of development in childhood and adolescence [14]. In this regard, dopaminergic brain areas such as SN, VTA, and hypothalamus are sensitive to the effects of sex hormones because they express estrogens and androgens receptors [7, 15, 16].

It has been demonstrated that exposure to a single dose of sex hormones during the neonatal period can change the profile expression of DA [8]; in fact, when female rats are exposed to a single dose of estradiol during the neonatal period, DA levels are increased in the ventromedial hypothalamus–arcuate nucleus, but not the exposure to testosterone, during adult life [8]. In addition, when male rats are exposed to estradiol or testosterone, DA levels and TH expression are increased in substantia nigra-ventral tegmental in addition to increased dopamine release in nucleus accumbens. This effect is not seen when rats are exposed to a nonaromatizable androgen, dihydrotestosterone, suggesting an estrogenic mechanism involving increased TH expression, either by direct estrogenic action or by aromatization of testosterone to estradiol in substantia nigra-ventral tegmental area [10].

2.1. Long-term epigenetic programming of the dopaminergic circuit

The programming is exerted through epigenetic modifications, which comprised DNA methylation and post-translational histone modifications, interacting with regulatory proteins and noncoding RNA to reorganize the chromatin in active or inactive domains (euchromatin or heterochromatin), being possible to be inherited from one generation to another without subsequent exposure to the endocrine disruptor [17]. The normal development of mammals involves the activity of DNA methyl transferase (DNMTs) to determine the *de novo* methylation, where DNMT3A and DNMT3B are involved, and to maintain the methylation pattern in the genome, where DNMT1 is involved. The expression levels of these enzymes are highly regulated during specific stages of life [18], and therefore, the impact of the exposure to endocrine disruptors and the consequences over the offspring are alarming.

In this view, in humans the social alcohol drinking during periconceptional or pregnancy period may induce changes in the promoter methylation of DAT in mothers and their babies. Specifically, using peripheral blood from mothers or cord blood from newborns, they found that alcohol intake decreases the methylation level of the locus-specific DAT promoter region of the parents and newborns [19]. However, these findings are controversial, since also found a decrease of DAT mRNA expression in drug addicts (to opioid drugs) compared to control subjects, but not in the methylation pattern of DAT promoter [20]. One of the methodological factors that could determine this difference is from where the samples are obtained, in the case of the peripheral blood, it is not a direct measurement of DAT expression in brain.

3. Sex hormones, dopaminergic neurotransmission, and addiction

Worldwide, drugs of abuse have increased dramatically, especially in susceptible populations such as youth. However, human and animal studies show that not all drug consumers become addicts [21, 22]. Lately, it has been determined differences in behaviors related to motivation reward and cognition between women and men (for review see 23). Accordingly, sex hormone levels affect cortical and subcortical brain areas, especially in sensitive periods of development in childhood and adolescence [14]. In this regard, dopaminergic brain areas such as SN, VTA, and hypothalamus are sensitive to the effects of sex hormones because they express estrogens and androgens receptors [7, 15, 16]. Interestingly, sex hormones induce opposite effects between female and males. While estrogens increase the expression of tyrosine hydroxylase in SN and VTA of adult female rats [24], androgens such as testosterone and dihydrotestosterone reduce TH expression in the same brain areas in adult male rats [25]. However, in adolescent male rats, androgens increase TH expression in SN [26].

In humans, it has been observed that an excess of testosterone levels during prenatal stage is related with the development and maintenance of alcohol dependence during adolescence and adulthood [27, 28]. Children who have developed precocious puberty (an early activation of the reproductive axis leading to the onset of puberty closer to 8, 9 years in girls and boys, respectively) shows an increase in risky behaviors such as drugs abuse, sexual risk, and anti-social behaviors in adolescence [29]. Many of these behaviors and the neuroendocrine pathways that regulate them are sexually dimorphic. These sex dimorphisms reflect adaptive differences for behavioral strategies in coping as a result of sexual selection. Disruptions in these behaviors may lead to reduced social adaptation and impaired responsiveness to environmental demands [30]. On the other hand, the exposure to several environmental pollutants, with neuroendocrine activity, has been associated with behavioral effects. For example, genistein (a phytoestrogen produced by legumes and present in soy bean-based food) increases locomotor activity in males, ethinylestradiol (a synthetic estrogen used as contraceptive) affects response to reward in females and bisphenol A, an endocrine disruptor, increases anxiety and sexual behavior in males (for review see [12]). In summary, our brain is modulated by sex hormones (or exogenous compounds) and depending on the stage of development, this interaction could affect the organization and activation of neural systems (for review see [31–33]). The alteration of sexually-dimorphic behaviors may be relevant for concerns regarding the increased developmental, cognitive, and/or emotional disabilities reported over the past 30 years [34].

Some studies of enrichment and deprivation of sensory inputs to the brain have provided information regarding the role of experience on the development of the brain. These studies suggest widespread effects of experience on the complexity and function of the developing system, while the deprivation studies document the capacity for neural reorganization within particular sensory systems [35]. These studies suggest that plasticity in developing neural systems can modulate the capacity to develop fundamentally different patterns of organization and function in response to injury. Therefore, the neurochemical interaction and environmental aspects can modulate the pathophysiological processes that determine the development of neurodegenerative events [36] (**Figure 1**).

The mesocorticolimbic system comprises the midbrain dopaminergic projection from the VTA to the nucleus accumbens (NAcc) [23, 37] and prefrontal and orbitofrontal cortexes [38]. One of the most important neurotransmitters in mesocorticolimbic system is DA, which is released in response to natural rewarding stimuli as food [39] or sex [40]. Drugs of abuse produce an increase in DA release in NAcc and striatum [41]; however, the magnitude and duration of this effect are much greater than with natural reinforces [42]. This acute supraphysiological DA release induced by drugs of abuse in the NAcc exherte its actions through the activation of the DA receptor type 1 (D_1 receptor), leading to early gene products induction (e.g., cFos) [43]. *In situ* hybridization studies have demonstrated the expression of estrogen receptors (ESR1, ESR2) and androgen receptors in SN-VTA [16, 44]. Using immunohistochemistry, it has been shown that ESR2 is expressed in high proportion in TH positive neurons of the VTA, whereas

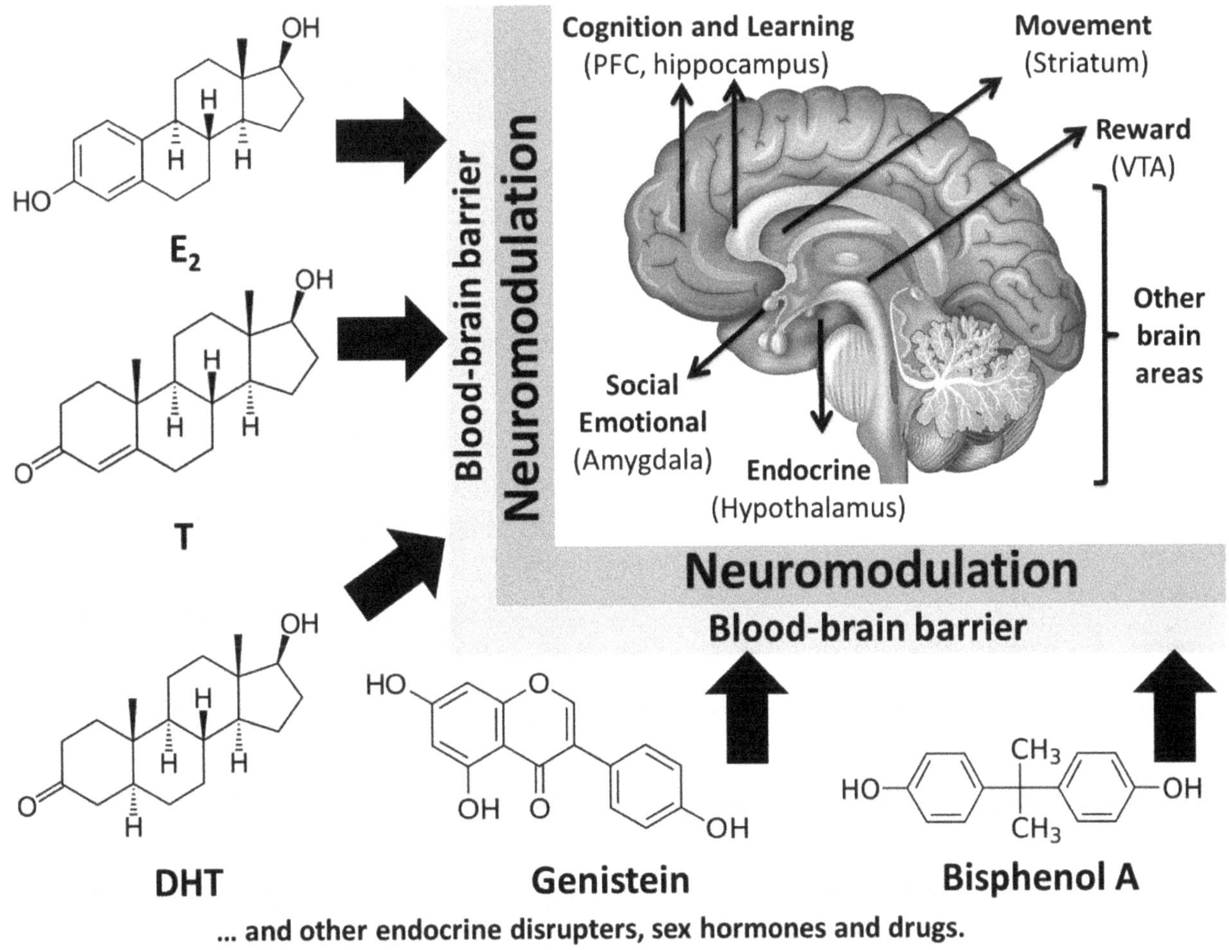

Figure 1. Schematic representation of the influence of neuroactive compounds like estradiol, testosterone, DHT, genistein, and bisphenol A on brain areas. These compounds can cross the blood–brain barrier, reaching brain areas that are related to cognition and learning (prefrontal cortex and hippocampus), movement (striatum), reward (VTA), social emotional (amygdala), the endocrine system (hypothalamus). Abbreviations: E_2, estradiol; T, testosterone; DHT, dihydrotestosterone; PFC, prefrontal cortex; VTA, ventral tegmental area.

androgen receptor is expressed in high proportion in TH positive neurons of NAcc [15]. Thus, sex hormones can regulate the expression of Tyrosine hydroxylase; specifically, estrogens can increase the expression of TH in SN and VTA of adult female rats [24], while androgens reduce TH expression in the same brain areas in adult male rats [25]. Noteworthy, in adolescent male rats, androgens increase TH expression in SN [26], suggesting a mechanism that depends on the physiological/hormonal context. The effects of sex hormones are mediated by the activation of specific receptors expressed in cell bodies of midbrain dopaminergic neurons and its limbic projections. The dopamine transporter, DAT, is a protein that mediates the active reuptake of dopamine from the synapse and is a principal regulator of dopaminergic neurotransmission, dopamine receptor 1 and 2 (D_1 and D_2, respectively) are modulated by 17β-estradiol and testosterone. Experiments using ovariectomized adult rats have shown a significant reduction of DAT levels in the NAcc and Striatum, which is restored to normal levels after E_2 replacement or the use of diarylpropionitrile (a selective ERβ agonist) and tamoxifen (selective estrogen receptor modulator) [45–48]. In the same model, levels of D_1 in mPOA are decreased after E_2 replacement [49]. Noteworthy, immunoreaction to D_2 is not affected by E_2 replacement, when is measured using immunohistochemistry. However, when western blot is used, levels of D_2 are apparently increased in mPOA and PLC [49]. In NAcc, D_2 levels are significantly increased in the NAcc and striatum of ovariectomized rats and E_2 replacement reduced D_2 receptors to lower levels than in controls rats [48].

It has been shown that circulating levels of female and male sex hormones modulate the mesocorticolimbic system, regulating the addictive behavior. Women in reproductive age who are users of drugs of abuse show greater rate of escalation of drug use than men [50], leading to the establishment of the addictive behavior quickly [51]. On the other hand, depending on circulating levels of sex hormones in menstrual cycle, the reward effects of psychostimulant drugs such as amphetamine are more potent in follicular phase when estradiol levels are higher than luteal phase, when progesterone levels are higher [52, 53].

Exposure to hormone disruptors has shown to produce effects on the behavior of animals. Thus, the prenatal administration of bisphenol A to pregnant mice and postnatal administration to offspring until postnatal day 15 produces anxiolytic behavior in elevated plus-maze and open field tests [54]. Interestingly, this behavior has been related to a significant decrease of DAT in striatum and NMDA receptor in frontal cortex [54]. Silverman and Koenig [55] showed the involvement of ESR2 in the reinforcement induced by low doses of amphetamine in female rats. In this work, ovariectomized female rats do not show conditional place preference to amphetamine compared with intact female rats. The replacement with estradiol or estradiol plus progesterone reestablishes the conditioned place preference induced by amphetamine in ovariectomized rats [55]. Interestingly, the authors found that conditioning with amphetamine was significant in the ovariectomized groups that were administered with estradiol or the ESR2-specific ligand DPN. These results provide new evidence of the specific requirement of ESR2 in response to drugs of abuse [55].

3.1. Attention-deficit/hyperactivity disorder (ADHD)

Regarding the behavioral effects produced by the administration of androgens, it has been observed that the neonatal administration of testosterone in spontaneously hypertensive rats

(SHR) (an animal model of attention-deficit hyperactivity disorder [ADHD]) decreases cognitive function and TH immunoreactivity in prefrontal cortex [11]. In this work, the authors implanted at postnatal day 1 pellets of testosterone in SHR rats, observing at postnatal day 45, through the Morris water maze test, an increased latency to find the platform. The authors conclude that the administration of androgens in neonatal period may predispose to ADHD-like behaviors in the adulthood.

With regard to pharmacological therapies of ADHD, animal studies and case reports have suggested that methylphenidate exerts adverse effects on gonadal hormones. In this case, methylphenidate could be altering testosterone levels in children with attention-deficit/hyperactivity disorder through the comparison of those with or without methylphenidate treatment [56].

Recently, prospective study conducted in Taiwan that included 203 ADHD patients with a mean age of 8.7 years (boys: 75.8%). After the initial recruitment, 137 received daily methylphenidate treatment and 66 were assessed through naturalistic observation (nonmedicated group). During the study period, salivary testosterone levels did not significantly change in the treated group (P = 0.389) or in the nontreated group (P = 0.488). After the correction for potential confounding effects of age and sex, salivary testosterone levels still remained unchanged in the treated and nontreated groups during the 4-week follow-up [57]. Findings suggest that the short-term treatment with methylphenidate at usual doses does not significantly alter salivary testosterone levels in attention-deficit/hyperactivity disorder patients. Future studies should clarify whether long-term methylphenidate treatment disrupts testosterone production as well as the function of the reproductive system.

In summary, these evidences indicate that sex hormones play an important role modulating the mesocorticolimbic system and behavioral, neurochemical, and neuroplastic effects of drugs of abuse.

4. Sex hormones and Alzheimer disease

During the menopause in women or andropause in men, there is a normal decrease in sexual hormones, due to the loss of ovarian sex hormones (estrone, estradiol, and progesterone) or to a decrease in testosterone levels, correspondingly. Noteworthy, postmortem analysis has shown lower brain levels of estrogens in women with AD, and lower levels of androgens in men with AD compared to nonAD patients. Specifically, studies performed in caucasic female subjects with neuropathological diagnosis of AD, according to Braak stages V–VI, with the absence of other neuropathologies (ranging in age from 61 to 90 years old) show a decrease of two times in estrone levels (midfrontal gyrus samples) when compared to controls, but not in estradiol, testosterone, or dihydrotestosterone (DHT) levels [58]. However, when male subjects with neuropathological diagnosis of AD, according to Braak stages V–VI, are analyzed (ranging in age from 50 to 97 years old) estradiol or estrone levels are not different between AD subjects and controls, but there is a decrease in androgen levels in AD patients, compared to controls [58]. Thus, it is proposed that the sex hormone decrease observed in brain samples from AD patients is not just related to the normal decrease in gonadal synthesis, but also to a decrease in local brain steroidogenesis [58, 59].

Supporting that, the premenopausal bilateral oophorectomy (surgical menopause), which induces early menopause through an abrupt decrease in circulating estrogen levels in young women, has shown lights about the role of sex hormones, its decline during the menopause and correct timing of hormonal replace therapy [60, 61]. Thus, in a study where 1884 women were followed longitudinally for upto 18 years (natural menopause n = 1277, surgical menopause n = 607) relating the onset of menopause (natural or surgical) to cognitive decline and AD. According to the study, surgical menopause at earlier age was associated with the decline in cognition (decline in episodic and semantic memory) as well as a greater level of Alzheimer disease in women who survived free of dementia to a mean age of 78 years [61]. Noteworthy, when the use of hormone therapy was considered in the study, a protective role was found when the treatment was administrated within 5-year perimenopausal period for at least 10 years: less decline in visuospatial ability, episodic, and semantic memory, but no influence over the onset of AD [61].

In women, it has been determined that the hormonal treatment with estradiol has more protective effects than the treatment with conjugated equine estrogen. Noteworthy, many studies have pointed out that the hormonal treatment needs to start during what is called a "window of opportunity", since the protective effects of estradiol treatment depend on when hormonal treatment is started. In particular, hormonal treatment needs to start during the perimenopause period (i.e., under age of 65 years). During this period is necessary to maintain a constant treatment (not withdraw), since doing so could decrease the memory improvement obtained by the hormonal treatment [62]. Verbal memory is enhanced with the treatment with E_2. Although there are many studies supporting the benefits of hormonal treatment, there are other studies that are against this statement. The window of efficient therapy depends on the capacity of the brain to respond to sexual hormones, and the presence of receptors in brain areas related to memory. This decrease is related to the normal decrease in sexual hormones due to aging, in man and woman. In that term, HT is focused on to keep the hormonal levels constant, so the brain cannot lose its responsiveness to hormones. Basic studies have shown that the role of estrogens or molecules like tamoxifen, a selective estrogen receptor modulator used as hormone therapy, may induce/modulate the dopamine system, inducing neuroprotection. In that term, the use of tamoxifen in murine AD model has shown an increment in dopamine content in striatum, and an improvement in memory tasks [63].

Recently, seven prospective cohort studies with a total of 5251 elderly men and 240 cases of Alzheimer's disease were included into the meta-analysis of AD follow-up. Meta-analysis using random effect model showed that low plasma testosterone level was significantly associated with an increased risk of Alzheimer's disease in elderly men (RR = 1.48, 95% CI 1.12-1.96, P = 0.006) [64]. This decrease is in direct relation with appearance of Aβ plaques in the brain, since androgen and estrogens can regulate the amount of Aβ through the modulation of signal transduction or enzymes related to the clearance of Aβ, like insulin-degrading enzyme, neprilysin, endothelin-converting enzymes 1 and 2, and angiotensin-converting enzyme. In that term, animal models of gonadectomy, to reduce the sexual hormones, have shown a direct relationship between the hormonal decrease and the increased amount of Aβ in the brain [65–67]. Also, in this type of models, the hormone therapy reduces the levels of Aβ and improves the memory. Thus, the formation of Aβ plaques can be induced by a reduction in sensitivity to estrogens or androgens due to long periods of low steroid hormones synthesis from gonads, modifying the mechanism of amyloid precursor protein elimination that is regulated by estradiol.

Clinical approach involved the estradiol and its role in maintaining brain architecture and metabolism, and chronically low levels of estradiol associated to anovulation may impair brain health. In women with functional hypothalamic amenorrhea, alterations in the thyroid axis impair neurogenesis and synaptic connectivity [68].

5. Sex hormones and Parkinson disease

Parkinson disease is a progressive neurodegenerative, multisystemic disorder characterized by a combination of motor symptoms like resting tremors, rigidity, bradykinesia, and postural abnormalities [69]. In addition, there are cognitive, neuropsychiatric, sleep, autonomic, and sensory disturbances associated to PD, which are related to the degeneration of serotoninergic neurons of the raphe nucleus, noradrenergic neurons of the locus coeruleus or cholinergic neurons of the nucleus basalis of Meynert [70]. PD is associated to degeneration of dopamine neurons in substantia nigra pars compacta, being PD the most common disease of dopamine dysfunction [71].

It has been reported that higher incidence rates of PD in men are compared to women [72, 73], and special interest has been put on sex hormones, due to its role on the regulation of dopamine synthesis, being estradiol the main regulator of this synthesis. In addition, studies performed to oophorectomized women, have revealed a higher risk of PD in this patients, suggesting that the abnormal decrease in estradiol prior to the menopause can be related to the onset of PD condition [74]. On other hand, increased exposure to endogenous estrogen can be associated with a late onset of PD and less sever motor impairment according to a study where 579 female patients were analyzed according to menarche age, menopause age, and PD onset age; also, delayed exposure to estrogens, through an increased age at menarche, is associated with older age at PD onset [75].

The synthesis of estrogen differs between reproductive and nonreproductive women, being the extragonadal tissues, like kidney, adipose tissue, skin, and brain, the main source of estrogen in nonreproductive women. In reproductive women, the main sources are ovaries, corpus luteum, and placenta. In men, the main source of testosterone is the testis.

As was mentioned for Alzheimer, sex hormones levels are crucial to maintain the proper functioning of brain circuits. Regarding to that, the normal decrease of estrogen levels in women, or testosterone in men, has been related to the onset of Parkinson. Many studies have shown that hormonal replacement therapy can reduce the risk of PD is applied during what is called a "window of opportunity", which is immediately after menopause. Using the same treatment after that period, the beneficial effects could be lost, due to a long-term hormone deprivation reviewed by [76] (**Figure 2**).

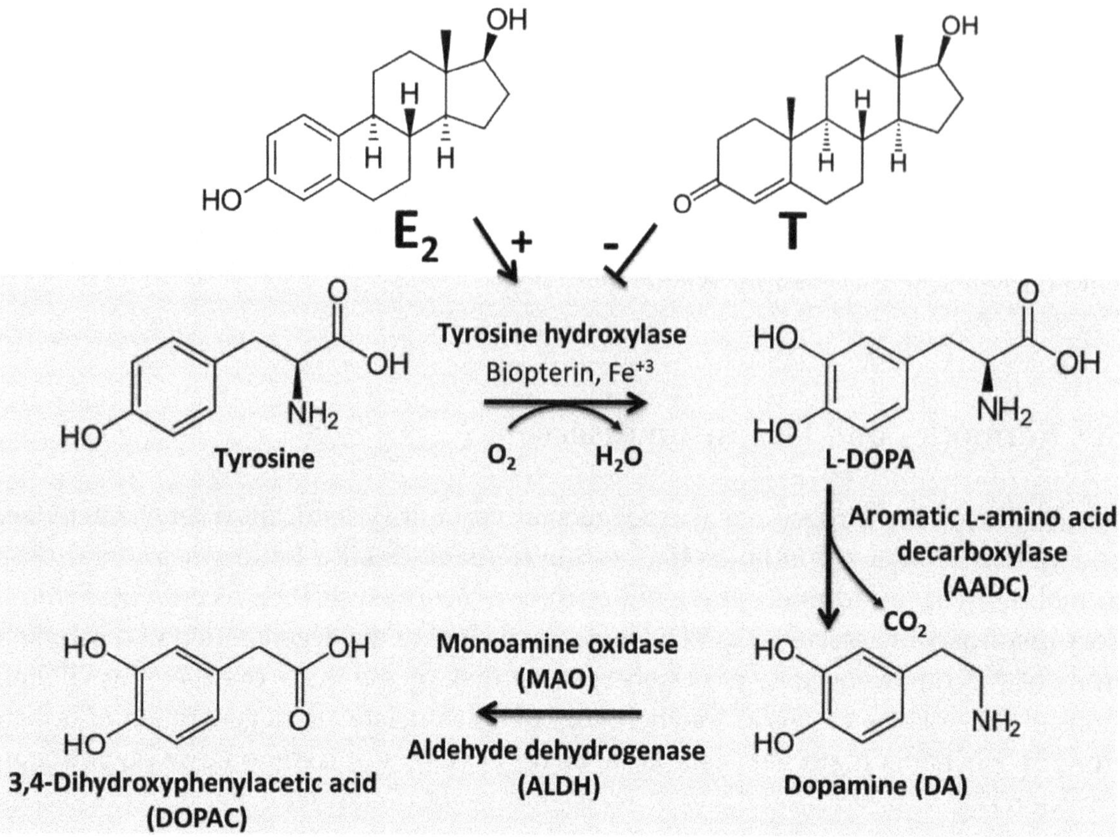

Figure 2. Effects of estradiol and testosterone on dopamine synthesis. Neonatal exposure to estradiol or testosterone increases TH expression in midbrain dopaminergic neurons. Abbreviations: E_2, estradiol; T, testosterone.

5.1. Clinical aspects in Parkinson disease

Male patients with Parkinson disease have less testosterone and estradiol than healthy males. In a recent study, it was determined if dopaminergic therapy using levodopa and dopamine agonist influenced testosterone levels. In this study, a cohort of 32 consecutive male patients from the INSPECT trial were used. INSPECT is a multi-center, prospective study that primarily examined the effects of short-term treatment with pramipexole or levodopa on cohort of PD patients [77]. There were statistically significant differences in the change in free testosterone level, increased in both the levodopa group and pramipexole group but decreased in the untreated group at 12-weeks post-treatment. These preliminary data support the premise that dopaminergic medications do not reduce testosterone levels in early PD patients. In a clinical study, where male subjects were analyzed (36 PD patients and 69 age-matched controls): prolactin levels were higher in PD subjects, compared to healthy ones. Also, concentrations of estradiol and testosterone in the control group were higher than those found in patients. In addition, the level of sex hormones was positively correlated with better mood and quality of life in patients affected with PD; prolactin levels correlated negatively with sex steroid concentrations [78, 79]. Therefore, it is extremely necessary to determine the level of hormones that may influence patients' cognition, mood, and quality of life of PD patients. The more important clinical trials that show the relationship between sex hormones and neurodegenerative disorders are shown in **Table 1**.

Pathology	Trial (N)	Primary end point	Treatment/Results (R)	Reference
ADHD	Phase III trial (n = 203)	Salivary testosterone levels	137 received daily methylphenidate treatment and 66 were assessed through naturalistic observation	[57]
Alzheimer disease	Phase II trial (n = 240)	Plasma testosterone	Meta-analysis using random effect model showed that low plasma testosterone level was significantly associated with an increased risk of Alzheimer's disease in elderly men	[64]
	Prospective brain imaging study (n = 54)	2-year prospective brain imaging study and randomized trial of HT continuation or discontinuation in a sample of middle-aged postmenopausal women (aged 49-69 years).	Continuation of HT use appears to protect cognition in women with heightened risk for AD when initiated close to menopause onset	[62]
Parkinson Disease	INSPECT trial–A multi-center Phase III trial (n = 32)	Testosterone levels and motor scores	There were statistically significant differences in the change in free testosterone level, increased in both the levodopa group and pramipexole group but decreased in the untreated group at 12-weeks post-treatment	[77]
	Phase II trial (n = 36)	The plasma levels of oestradiol, testosterone, prolactin and sex hormone-binding protein were examined in 36 patients affected with Parkinson's disease and in 69 age-matched control subjects, using chemiluminescent reactions.	The level of sex hormones was positively correlated with better mood and quality of life in patients affected with Parkinson's disease; prolactin levels correlated negatively with sex steroid concentrations.	[78]
Hormone decrease	Cognitive Impairment in postmenopausal women (n = 4532)		Participants received either one daily tablet of 0.625 mg of conjugated equine estrogen plus 2.5 mg of medroxyprogesterone acetate or a matching placebo. Results demonstrate that estrogen plus progestin therapy increases older women's risk for probable dementia, including Alzheimer	[80]
	Phase II trial Functional hypothalamic amenorrhea (n = 60)	Ovarian function (ovulating)	Randomized to Cognitive behavioral therapy or observation for 20 weeks	[68]

Table 1. More important clinical trials that show the relationship between sex hormones and neurodegenerative disorders.

6. Concluding remarks

Here, we review how sex hormones (i.e., neuroactive modulators) can differentially modulate neuronal neurodegeneration in animal and clinical models. Specifically, we provide an overview of the effects of sex hormones, stress hormones, and metabolic hormones on structural plasticity and some pharmacological targets. In addition, we also discuss how sex hormones such as estrogen and testosterone can be affected by variables such as duration and intensity of motor and cognitive impairment. Understanding the neurobiological mechanisms underlying the modulation of neuronal structural plasticity by intrinsic and extrinsic factors will impact the design of new therapeutic approaches aimed at restoring physiological state and determine some pharmacological therapies. This approach is very important for the design of phase III clinical trial (randomized clinical trial) in the clinical practical conditions.

Acknowledgements

This work was supported by FONDECYT Grant N° 116-0398 and DIUV-CI Grant 01/2006 to Ramón Sotomayor-Zárate.

Author details

Jonathan Martínez Pinto[1], Rodrigo L. Castillo[2] and Ramón Sotomayor-Zárate[1]*

*Address all correspondence to: ramon.sotomayor@uv.cl

1 Laboratory of Neurochemistry and Neuropharmacology, Center of Neurobiology and Brain plasticity, Institute of Physiology, Faculty of Sciences, Universidad de Valparaíso, Valparaíso, Chile

2 Program of Pathophysiology, Institute of Biomedical Sciences, Faculty of Medicine, Universidad de Chile, Santiago, Chile

References

[1] Diamanti-Kandarakis E, Bourguignon J-P, Giudice LC, Hauser R, Prins GS, Soto AM, et al. Endocrine-disrupting chemicals: An Endocrine Society scientific statement. Endocrine Reviews. 2009;**30**(4):293-342

[2] Pringsheim T, Jette N, Frolkis A, Steeves TD. The prevalence of Parkinson's disease: A systematic review and meta-analysis. Movement Disorders. 2014;**29**(13):1583-1590. Epub 01-07-2014

[3] Seshadri S, Wolf PA, Beiser A, Au R, McNulty K, White R, et al. Lifetime risk of dementia and Alzheimer's disease. The impact of mortality on risk estimates in the Framingham study. Neurology. 1997;**49**(6):1498-1504. Epub 31-12-1997

[4] Baum LW. Sex, hormones, and Alzheimer's disease. The Journals of Gerontology: Series A. 2005;**60**(6):736-743

[5] Lucas A. Programming by early nutrition in man. Ciba Foundation Symposium. 1991; **156**:38-50; discussion-5. Epub 01-01-1991

[6] Sotomayor-Zarate R, Dorfman M, Paredes A, Lara HE. Neonatal exposure to estradiol valerate programs ovarian sympathetic innervation and follicular development in the adult rat. Biology of Reproduction. 2008;**78**(4):673-680. Epub 14-12-2007

[7] Perez SE, Chen EY, Mufson EJ. Distribution of estrogen receptor alpha and beta immunoreactive profiles in the postnatal rat brain. Brain research. Developmental Brain Research. 2003;**145**(1):117-139

[8] Sotomayor-Zarate R, Tiszavari M, Cruz G, Lara HE. Neonatal exposure to single doses of estradiol or testosterone programs ovarian follicular development-modified hypothalamic neurotransmitters and causes polycystic ovary during adulthood in the rat. Fertility and Sterility. 2011;**96**(6):1490-1496

[9] Cruz G, Riquelme R, Espinosa P, Jara P, Dagnino-Subiabre A, Renard GM, et al. Neonatal exposure to estradiol valerate increases dopamine content in nigrostriatal pathway during adulthood in the rat. Hormone and Metabolic Research = Hormon- und Stoffwechselforschung = Hormones et metabolisme. 2014;**46**(5):322-327

[10] Espinosa P, Silva RA, Sanguinetti NK, Venegas FC, Riquelme R, Gonzalez LF, et al. Programming of dopaminergic neurons by neonatal sex hormone exposure: Effects on dopamine content and tyrosine hydroxylase expression in adult male rats. Neural Plasticity. 2016;**2016**:4569785

[11] King JA, Barkley RA, Delville Y, Ferris CF. Early androgen treatment decreases cognitive function and catecholamine innervation in an animal model of ADHD. Behavioural Brain Research. 2000;**107**(1–2):35-43. Epub 11-01-2000

[12] Frye CA, Bo E, Calamandrei G, Calza L, Dessi-Fulgheri F, Fernandez M, et al. Endocrine disrupters: A review of some sources, effects, and mechanisms of actions on behaviour and neuroendocrine systems. Journal of Neuroendocrinology. 2012;**24**(1):144-159

[13] Ishido M, Yonemoto J, Morita M. Mesencephalic neurodegeneration in the orally administered bisphenol A-caused hyperactive rats. Toxicology Letters. 2007;**173**(1):66-72. Epub 11-08-2007

[14] Crone EA, Dahl RE. Understanding adolescence as a period of social-affective engagement and goal flexibility. Nature Reviews. Neuroscience. 2012;**13**(9):636-650

[15] Creutz LM, Kritzer MF. Mesostriatal and mesolimbic projections of midbrain neurons immunoreactive for estrogen receptor beta or androgen receptors in rats. The Journal of Comparative Neurology. 2004;**476**(4):348-362. Epub 30-07-2004

[16] Simerly RB, Chang C, Muramatsu M, Swanson LW. Distribution of androgen and estrogen receptor mRNA-containing cells in the rat brain: An in situ hybridization study. The Journal of Comparative Neurology. 1990;**294**(1):76-95

[17] Geneviève PD, Mojgan R, James RD. Epigenetic control. Journal of Cellular Physiology. 2009;**219**(2):243-250

[18] Schaefer CB, Ooi SK, Bestor TH, Bourc'his D. Epigenetic decisions in mammalian germ cells. Science. 2007;**316**(5823):398-399. Epub 21-04-2007

[19] Lee BY, Park SY, Ryu HM, Shin CY, Ko KN, Han JY, et al. Changes in the methylation status of DAT, SERT, and MeCP2 gene promoters in the blood cell in families exposed to alcohol during the periconceptional period. Alcoholism, Clinical and Experimental Research. 2015; **39**(2):239-250. Epub 07-02-2015

[20] Kordi-Tamandani DM, Tajoddini S, Salimi F. Promoter methylation and BDNF and DAT1 gene expression profiles in patients with drug addiction. Pathobiology: Journal of Immunopathology, Molecular and Cellular Biology. 2015;**82**(2):94-99

[21] Kalivas PW, O'Brien C. Drug addiction as a pathology of staged neuroplasticity. Neuropsychopharmacology. 2008;**33**(1):166-180. Epub 07-09-2007

[22] Kalivas PW, Churchill L, Klitenick MA. GABA and enkephalin projection from the nucleus accumbens and ventral pallidum to the ventral tegmental area. Neuroscience. 1993;**57**(4): 1047-1060. Epub 01-12-1993

[23] Koob GF, Volkow ND. Neurocircuitry of addiction. Neuropsychopharmacology. 2010;**35**(1): 217-238. Epub 28-08-2009

[24] Johnson ML, Ho CC, Day AE, Walker QD, Francis R, Kuhn CM. Oestrogen receptors enhance dopamine neurone survival in rat midbrain. Journal of Neuroendocrinology. 2010;**22**(4):226-237. Epub 09-02-2010

[25] Johnson ML, Day AE, Ho CC, Walker QD, Francis R, Kuhn CM. Androgen decreases dopamine neurone survival in rat midbrain. Journal of Neuroendocrinology. 2010;**22**(4): 238-247. Epub 09-02-2010

[26] Purves-Tyson TD, Owens SJ, Double KL, Desai R, Handelsman DJ, Weickert CS. Testosterone induces molecular changes in dopamine signaling pathway molecules in the adolescent male rat nigrostriatal pathway. PLoS One. 2014;**9**(3):e91151

[27] Lenz B, Muller CP, Stoessel C, Sperling W, Biermann T, Hillemacher T, et al. Sex hormone activity in alcohol addiction: Integrating organizational and activational effects. Progress in Neurobiology. 2012;**96**(1):136-163. Epub 26-11-2011

[28] Lenz B, Muhle C, Braun B, Weinland C, Bouna-Pyrrou P, Behrens J, et al. Prenatal and adult androgen activities in alcohol dependence. Acta Psychiatr Scand. 2017 Jul;**136**(1): 96-107. Doi: 10.1111/acps.12725

[29] Downing J, Bellis MA. Early pubertal onset and its relationship with sexual risk taking, substance use and anti-social behaviour: A preliminary cross-sectional study. BMC Public Health. 2009;**9**:446

[30] Parmigiani S, Palanza P, vom Saal FS. Ethotoxicology: An evolutionary approach to the study of environmental endocrine-disrupting chemicals. Toxicology and Industrial Health. 1998;**14**(1–2):333-339. Epub 14-02-1998

[31] Peper JS, van den Heuvel MP, Mandl RC, Hulshoff Pol HE, van Honk J. Sex steroids and connectivity in the human brain: A review of neuroimaging studies. Psychoneuroendocrinology. 2011;**36**(8):1101-1113. Epub 07-06-2011

[32] Yoest KE, Cummings JA, Becker JB. Estradiol, dopamine and motivation. Central Nervous System Agents in Medicinal Chemistry. 2014;**14**(2):83-89

[33] Becker JB, Hu M. Sex differences in drug abuse. Frontiers in Neuroendocrinology. 2008; **29**(1):36-47

[34] Schettler T. Toxic threats to neurologic development of children. Environmental Health Perspectives. 2001;**109**(Suppl 6):813-816. Epub 18-12-2001

[35] von Melchner L, Pallas SL, Sur M. Visual behaviour mediated by retinal projections directed to the auditory pathway. Nature 2000;**404**(6780):871-876. Epub 29-04-2000

[36] Stiles J, Jernigan TL. The basics of brain development. Neuropsychology Review. 2010;**20**(4): 327-348. Epub 03-11-2010

[37] Koob GF, Arends MA, Le Moal M. Drugs, Addiction, and the Brain. United States of America: Elsevier; 2014

[38] Volkow ND, Fowler JS. Addiction, a disease of compulsion and drive: Involvement of the orbitofrontal cortex. Cerebral Cortex. 2000;**10**(3):318-325. Epub 24-03-2000

[39] Bassareo V, Di Chiara G. Differential influence of associative and nonassociative learning mechanisms on the responsiveness of prefrontal and accumbal dopamine transmission to food stimuli in rats fed ad libitum. The Journal of Neuroscience. 1997;**17**(2):851-861. Epub 15-01-1997

[40] Pfaus JG, Damsma G, Nomikos GG, Wenkstern DG, Blaha CD, Phillips AG, et al. Sexual behavior enhances central dopamine transmission in the male rat. Brain Research. 1990; **530**(2):345-348. Epub 22-10-1990

[41] Di Chiara G, Imperato A. Drugs abused by humans preferentially increase synaptic dopamine concentrations in the mesolimbic system of freely moving rats. Proceedings of the National Academy of Sciences of the United States of America. 1988;**85**(14):5274-5278. Epub 01-07-1988

[42] Kalivas PW, Volkow ND. The neural basis of addiction: A pathology of motivation and choice. The American Journal of Psychiatry. 2005;**162**(8):1403-1413

[43] Graybiel AM, Moratalla R, Robertson HA. Amphetamine and cocaine induce drug-specific activation of the c-fos gene in striosome-matrix compartments and limbic subdivisions of the striatum. Proceedings of the National Academy of Sciences of the United States of America. 1990;**87**(17):6912-6916

[44] Shughrue PJ, Lane MV, Merchenthaler I. Comparative distribution of estrogen receptor-alpha and -beta mRNA in the rat central nervous system. The Journal of Comparative Neurology. 1997;**388**(4):507-525

[45] Morissette M, Di Paolo T. Effect of chronic estradiol and progesterone treatments of ovariectomized rats on brain dopamine uptake sites. Journal of Neurochemistry. 1993;**60** (5):1876-1883

[46] Bosse R, Rivest R, Di Paolo T. Ovariectomy and estradiol treatment affect the dopamine transporter and its gene expression in the rat brain. Brain Research Molecular Brain Research. 1997;**46**(1–2):343-346

[47] Le Saux M, Di Paolo T. Influence of oestrogenic compounds on monoamine transporters in rat striatum. Journal of Neuroendocrinology. 2006;**18**(1):25-32

[48] Chavez C, Hollaus M, Scarr E, Pavey G, Gogos A, van den Buuse M. The effect of estrogen on dopamine and serotonin receptor and transporter levels in the brain: An autoradiography study. Brain Research. 2010;**1321**:51-59. Epub 19-01-2010

[49] Graham MD, Gardner Gregory J, Hussain D, Brake WG, Pfaus JG. Ovarian steroids alter dopamine receptor populations in the medial preoptic area of female rats: Implications for sexual motivation, desire, and behaviour. The European Journal of Neuroscience. 2015;**42**(12):3138-3148

[50] Hser YI, Anglin MD, Booth MW. Sex differences in addict careers. 3. Addiction. The American Journal of Drug and Alcohol Abuse. 1987;**13**(3):231-251

[51] Zilberman M, Tavares H, El-Guebaly N. Gender similarities and differences: The prevalence and course of alcohol- and other substance-related disorders. Journal of Addictive Diseases. 2003;**22**(4):61-74

[52] Justice AJ, De Wit H. Acute effects of d-amphetamine during the early and late follicular phases of the menstrual cycle in women. Pharmacology, Biochemistry, and Behavior. 2000;**66**(3):509-515

[53] Justice AJ, de Wit H. Acute effects of estradiol pretreatment on the response to d-amphetamine in women. Neuroendocrinology. 2000;**71**(1):51-59

[54] Tian YH, Baek JH, Lee SY, Jang CG. Prenatal and postnatal exposure to bisphenol a induces anxiolytic behaviors and cognitive deficits in mice. Synapse. 2010;**64**(6):432-439. Epub 20-02-2010

[55] Silverman JL, Koenig JI. Evidence for the involvement of ERbeta and RGS9-2 in 17-beta estradiol enhancement of amphetamine-induced place preference behavior. Hormones and Behavior. 2007;**52**(2):146-155. Epub 12-05-2007

[56] Wang LJ, Wu CC, Lee SY, Tsai YF. Salivary neurosteroid levels and behavioural profiles of children with attention-deficit/hyperactivity disorder during six months of methylphenidate treatment. Journal of Child and Adolescent Psychopharmacology. 2014;**24**(6):336-340. Epub 24-06-2014

[57] Wang LJ, Chou MC, Chou WJ, Lee MJ, Lin PY, Lee SY, et al. Does methylphenidate reduce testosterone levels in humans? A prospective study in children with attention-deficit/hyperactivity disorder. Int J Neuropsychopharmacol. 2017 Mar 1;**20**(3):219-227. Doi: 10.1093/ijnp/pyw101

[58] Rosario ER, Chang L, Head EH, Stanczyk FZ, Pike CJ. Brain levels of sex steroid hormones in men and women during normal aging and in Alzheimer's disease. Neurobiology of Aging. 2011;**32**(4):604-613. Epub 12-05-2009

[59] Yue X, Lu M, Lancaster T, Cao P, Honda S, Staufenbiel M, et al. Brain estrogen deficiency accelerates Abeta plaque formation in an Alzheimer's disease animal model. Proceedings of the National Academy of Sciences of the United States of America. 2005;**102**(52):19198-19203. Epub 21-12-2005

[60] Pines A. Surgical menopause and cognitive decline. Climacteric: the Journal of the International Menopause Society. 2014;**17**(5):580-582. Epub 08-02-2014

[61] Bove R, Secor E, Chibnik LB, Barnes LL, Schneider JA, Bennett DA, et al. Age at surgical menopause influences cognitive decline and Alzheimer pathology in older women. Neurology. 2014;**82**(3):222-229. Epub 18-12-2013

[62] Wroolie TE, Kenna HA, Williams KE, Rasgon NL. Cognitive effects of hormone therapy continuation or discontinuation in a sample of women at risk for alzheimer disease. The American Journal of Geriatric Psychiatry: Official Journal of the American Association for Geriatric Psychiatry. 2015;**23**(11):1117-1126

[63] Pandey D, Banerjee S, Basu M, Mishra N. Memory enhancement by Tamoxifen on amyloidosis mouse model. Hormones and Behavior. 2016;**79**:70-73. Epub 06-10-2015

[64] Lv W, Du N, Liu Y, Fan X, Wang Y, Jia X, et al. Low testosterone level and risk of alzheimer's disease in the elderly men: A systematic review and meta-analysis. Molecular Neurobiology. 2016;**53**(4):2679-2684

[65] Petanceska SS, Nagy V, Frail D, Gandy S. Ovariectomy and 17beta-estradiol modulate the levels of Alzheimer's amyloid beta peptides in brain. Neurology. 2000;**54**(12):2212-2217. Epub 06-07-2000

[66] Jayaraman A, Carroll JC, Morgan TE, Lin S, Zhao L, Arimoto JM, et al. 17beta-estradiol and progesterone regulate expression of beta-amyloid clearance factors in primary neuron cultures and female rat brain. Endocrinology. 2012;**153**(11):5467-5479. Epub 11-09-2012

[67] Ramsden M, Nyborg AC, Murphy MP, Chang L, Stanczyk FZ, Golde TE, et al. Androgens modulate beta-amyloid levels in male rat brain. Journal of Neurochemistry. 2003;**87**(4): 1052-1055. Epub 19-11-2003

[68] Prokai D, Berga SL. Neuroprotection via reduction in stress: Altered menstrual patterns as a marker for stress and implications for long-term neurologic health in women. International Journal of Molecular Sciences. 2016;**17**(12)

[69] Stacy M. Medical treatment of Parkinson disease. Neurologic Clinics. 2009;**27**(3):605-631, v. Epub 27-06-2009

[70] Lang AE. The progression of Parkinson disease: A hypothesis. Neurology. 2007;**68**(12): 948-952. Epub 21-03-2007

[71] Smith KM, Dahodwala N. Sex differences in Parkinson's disease and other movement disorders. Experimental Neurology. 2014;**259**:44-56. Epub 01-04-2014

[72] Wooten GF, Currie LJ, Bovbjerg VE, Lee JK, Patrie J. Are men at greater risk for Parkinson's disease than women? Journal of Neurology, Neurosurgery & Psychiatry. 2004;**75**(4):637-639

[73] Baldereschi M, Di Carlo A, Rocca WA, Vanni P, Maggi S, Perissinotto E, et al. Parkinson's disease and parkinsonism in a longitudinal study: Two-fold higher incidence in men. Neurology. 2000;**55**(9):1358-1363

[74] Rocca WA, Bower JH, Maraganore DM, Ahlskog JE, Grossardt BR, de Andrade M, et al. Increased risk of parkinsonism in women who underwent oophorectomy before menopause. Neurology 2008;**70**(3):200-209

[75] Cereda E, Barichella M, Cassani E, Caccialanza R, Pezzoli G. Reproductive factors and clinical features of Parkinson's disease. Parkinsonism & Related Disorders. 2013;**19**(12): 1094-1099

[76] Litim N, Morissette M, Di Paolo T. Neuroactive gonadal drugs for neuroprotection in male and female models of Parkinson's disease. Neuroscience and Biobehavioral Reviews. 2016;**67**:79-88. Epub 29-12-2015

[77] Okun MS, Wu SS, Jennings D, Marek K, Rodriguez RL, Fernandez HH. Testosterone level and the effect of levodopa and agonists in early Parkinson disease: Results from the INSPECT cohort. Journal of Clinical Movement Disorders. 2014;**1**:8. Epub 01-01-2014

[78] Nitkowska M, Tomasiuk R, Czyzyk M, Friedman A. Prolactin and sex hormones levels in males with Parkinson's disease. Acta Neurologica Scandinavica. 2015;**131**(6):411-416. Epub 18-11-2014

[79] Kenangil G, Orken DN, Ur E, Forta H, Celik M. The relation of testosterone levels with fatigue and apathy in Parkinson's disease. Clinical Neurology and Neurosurgery. 2009; **111**(5):412-414. Epub 10-01-2009

[80] Shumaker SA, Legault C, Rapp SR, Thal L, Wallace RB, Ockene JK, et al. Estrogen plus progestin and the incidence of dementia and mild cognitive impairment in postmenopausal women: The Women's Health Initiative memory study: A randomized controlled trial. Journal of the American Medical Association. 2003;**289**(20):2651-2662. Epub 29-05-2003

8

Testosterone and Erectile Function

Tomoya Kataoka and Kazunori Kimura

Abstract

Androgens are essential for male physical activity and normal erectile function. Hence, age-related testosterone deficiency, known as late-onset hypogonadism (LOH), is considered a risk factor for erectile dysfunction (ED). This chapter summarizes relevant basic research reports examining the effects of testosterone on erectile function. Testosterone affects several organs and is especially active on the erectile tissue. The mechanism of testosterone deficiency effects on erectile function and the results of testosterone replacement therapy (TRT) have been well studied. Testosterone affects nitric oxide (NO) production and phosphodiesterase type 5 (PDE-5) expression in the corpus cavernosum through molecular pathways, preserves smooth muscle contractility by regulating both contraction and relaxation, and maintains the structure of the corpus cavernosum. Interestingly, testosterone deficiency has relationship to neurological diseases, which leads to ED. Testosterone replacement therapy is widely used to treat patients with testosterone deficiency; however, this treatment might also induce some problems. Basic research suggests that PDE-5 inhibitors, L-citrulline, and/or resveratrol therapy might be effective therapeutic options for testosterone deficiency-induced ED. Future research should confirm these findings through more specific experiments using molecular tools and may shed more light on endocrine-related ED and its possible treatments.

Keywords: testosterone, erectile dysfunction, endothelial function, testosterone replacement therapy, basic science

1. Introduction

Androgens are essential for male physical activity and normal erectile function [1–5]. Thus, age-related androgen deficiency, known as late-onset hypogonadism (LOH), is a risk factor for erectile dysfunction (ED) [1, 2]. Several studies have reported that androgen replacement therapy mitigates the symptoms of LOH and ED. In this context, bioidentical or synthetic testosterone facilitates erectile function by maintaining an adequate supply of nitric oxide (NO), penile structure, and the endothelial functioning of the corpus cavernosum. Thus, reduced NO bioavailability is believed to be the main cause of ED in individuals with testosterone deficiency [6]; however, the pathophysiological mechanisms underlying this process remain unclear and require further study. This chapter summarizes relevant basic research reports examining the effects of testosterone on erectile function.

2. Testosterone and erectile function

Androgens are well established as being essential for erectile function, and their deficiency is considered a risk factor for ED. LOH is a result of the normal aging process and is responsible for androgen deficiency [7, 8]. In recent years, epidemiologic studies have suggested that metabolic syndrome and diabetes mellitus are also associated with the development of androgen deficiency [9–12].

Erectile function is regulated by complex mechanisms [13]. When sexual stimulation occurs, NO is released in the penis, causing corporal smooth muscle relaxation through the activation of the cGMP/protein kinase G signaling cascade. ED results when the relaxant system is weakened; therefore, many studies have focused on smooth muscle relaxation. In contrast, in the flaccid state, corporal smooth muscle contraction is controlled by constrictors such as noradrenaline. Recent studies have indicated that the balance between smooth muscle relaxation and contraction is disturbed by abnormal activation of the RhoA/Rho-kinase signaling pathway. In some syndromes causing ED, such as diabetes mellitus or metabolic syndrome, the RhoA/Rho-kinase signaling pathway is enhanced [14–16]. Additionally, enhancement of the RhoA/Rho-kinase signaling pathway is known to occur in aged individuals, and a Rho-kinase inhibitor (Y-27632) has been shown to improve erectile function in aged rats [17, 18]. As contractility may play a significant role in erectile function, its role in ED should be considered along with contraction. Thus, the balance between smooth muscle contraction and relaxation is important for normal erectile function.

3. Testosterone deficiency and ED

Most animal studies have shown that castration causes ED by reducing arterial inflow [19]. Further, endothelial nitric oxide synthase (eNOS) and neuronal NOS (nNOS) are important in erectile functioning. In castrated animals, testosterone administration restores the erectile response and NOS expression in the penis [20]. Li et al. showed that testosterone deficiency decreases eNOS activity (phosphor-eNOS/eNOS ratio) by upregulating reactive oxygen species production [21], and the decreased eNOS activity decreases cGMP levels in the penis.

Some studies found that testosterone changes phosphodiesterase type 5 (PDE-5) expression in the penis. Traish et al. showed that castration decreased PDE-5 activity in rabbit penises [22], whereas Zhang et al. showed that testosterone deficiency decreased PDE-5 expression in the rat penis and that testosterone administration increased PDE-5 expression [23]. These results suggest that testosterone is essential not only for regulating eNOS activity but also for regulating PDE-5 activity. Traish et al. also suggested that while these actions may seem paradoxical, in which androgens are upregulating both signal initiators (NOS) and signal terminators (PDE-5), they may be interpreted to be part of a homeostatic mechanism that maintains a relatively constant ratio of critical pathway enzymes [3]. They also postulated that PDE-5 expression may be controlled by NO. Androgen-mediated upregulation of NOS may lead to increased NO synthesis, which may then upregulate PDE-5 expression and activity. Conversely, androgen deprivation-mediated NOS downregulation also results in the downregulation of PDE-5 expression and activity. More studies are needed to define this delicate and crucial mechanism of testosterone action.

Testosterone also affects the smooth muscle of the corpus cavernosum. Reilly et al. showed that castration reduced the number of α-adrenergic-1 receptors on smooth fascia [24]. They also showed that testosterone modulated the adrenergic response of the corpus cavernosum vascular smooth muscle [25]. Their results indicate that when testosterone levels decrease, smooth muscle contractility also decreases. On the other hand, Wingard et al. showed that castration increased the levels of Rho-A and Rho-kinase proteins in rats. RhoA, a small monomeric GTPase, activates the Rho-associated protein kinase, a serine/threonine kinase, which phosphorylates the myosin-binding subunit of myosin light chain phosphatase, thereby deactivating it and promoting contraction [26]. Their results indicate that when testosterone levels decline, smooth muscle contractility increases, leading not only to the development of ED but also to the hypertension. Thus, although testosterone deficiency might increase contraction, additional research is required to fully elucidate its impact on smooth muscle contraction.

Interestingly, testosterone also directly affects smooth muscle relaxation. Yue et al., using an isometric tension study, showed that testosterone relaxed the smooth muscle of rabbit coronary arteries and aortas [27]. Others also showed that testosterone induces the relaxation of isolated human corpora cavernosa strips by activating smooth muscle ATP-sensitive K^+ channels [28]. These findings suggest that testosterone, in addition to its known endothelial action, might regulate erectile function locally by acting on human corpus cavernosum smooth muscle. These results indicate that testosterone might affect both the genomic and nongenomic actions of erectile function.

Some studies demonstrated that testosterone also impacts the structure of the penis. One group showed that castrated rats show smooth muscle loss and fibrosis [29], and another group reported that castration increases the collagen content of the internal pudendal arteries and decreases α-actin expression [30]. These testosterone effects suggest that testosterone deprivation results in programmed trabecular smooth muscle cell death (apoptosis) and increased development of extracellular matrix [22]. Traish et al. also proposed that testosterone deprivation is associated with the accumulation of fat-containing cells (fibroblasts or preadipocyte-like cells), especially in the subtunical region of the corpus cavernosum, contributing to impaired veno-occlusion [31]. Interestingly, Wang et al. showed that castration attenuates erectile function and induces corporeal fibrosis by inhibiting autophagy and promoting apoptosis of the corpus cavernosum smooth muscle cells in rats [32]. Their study has limitations, but they highlighted the important role of androgens in maintaining the structural integrity and functioning of the corpus cavernosum. This resulted from androgens mediating the counter-regulation of autophagy and apoptosis through regulation of the BECN 1-Bcl-2 (key dual regulators of autophagy and apoptosis) interaction [33, 34].

4. Testosterone and neurogenic factors

ED has relationships between not only cardiovascular diseases but also neurological diseases. Yang et al. found the hazard risk for Alzheimer's disease and non-Alzheimer dementia to be greater in patients with ED [35]. They also found that log-rank test revealed that patients with ED had significantly higher cumulative incidence rates of dementia than those without. Yang et al. found the incidence density rate of Parkinson's disease (PD) was higher in the ED cohort than in the non-ED cohort [36]. Balsamo et al. reported that men with multiple sclerosis had high risk of ED [37]. Interestingly, testosterone deficiency is often observed in these neurological disease patients relative to age-matched controls [38–40].

In basic study, there are some reports on the relationship between testosterone deficiency and neurogenic factors. Baba et al. reported the mean number of NOS-containing nerve fibers in the corpora cavernosa and in both dorsal nerves of castrated rats [41]. Others also showed that castration decreased nNOS protein expression in the corpus cavernosum [32]. However, reports regarding nNOS responses differ significantly; some studies show increased activity but no change in protein expression [42] in rats, whereas others report no effects in rabbits [43]. Thus, more research into the relationship between nNOS and testosterone is required.

On the other hand, Suzuki et al. measured the ICP during electrical stimulation of the preoptic area and cavernous nerve in castrated male rats with and without testosterone replacement [44]. They showed the actions of testosterone and its metabolites on both the central and peripheral neural pathways are crucial for maintaining and restoring erectile capacity. Syme et al. reported that castration resulted in a decreased erectile response to electrostimulation following nerve grafting due to decreased graft neuronal nitric oxide synthase-positive axonal regeneration [45]. Armagan et al. indicated that testosterone had a neuroprotective role in the nerve fibers of the dorsal nerve and testosterone deficiency led to different forms of nerve degeneration resulting in anatomic alterations [46]. Baba et al. also reported that castration decreased the number of nicotinamide adenine dinucleotide phosphate diaphorase-staining nerve fibers not only in corpus cavernosum but also in dorsal nerve [47]. These results indicate that testosterone deficiency would cause neurogenic dysfunction of erectile tissues; however, future study needs to unravel the mechanism of testosterone action to the nerve systems.

5. Testosterone and metabolic syndrome

Obesity has become a major public health issue that is associated with increased mortality primarily due to increased risks of cardiovascular disease and type 2 diabetes mellitus

(T2DM) [1, 48, 49]. Obesity is also considered a strong risk factor for ED [4, 5]. In men, visceral adipose tissue causes arteriosclerosis and vessel endothelial dysfunction [12]. Therefore, men with T2DM have a high incidence of ED [5, 48, 50, 51].

In recent years, epidemiologic studies have suggested that obesity is also associated with multiple alterations in the gonadal endocrine system, including low testosterone levels [1, 48, 52, 53]. Low testosterone levels have also been reported in animals with T2DM, including two seminal research papers that reported testosterone replacement therapy (TRT) in such animal models [54, 55]. Davis et al. administered TRT to obese Zucker rats, resulting in improved cholesterol parameters and insulin sensitivity [54]. On the other hand, others administered TRT to rabbits with high-fat diet-associated hypogonadotropic hypogonadism [55]. TRT partially ameliorated the animals' blood glucose levels and improved CC sensitivity to acetylcholine and eNOS.

We also reported that T2DM increased inflammatory biomarker (inducible NO synthase, interleukin-6, and tumor necrosis factor alpha) mRNA expression levels in the CC, but TRT decreased them [56]. Ota et al. reported an in vitro study that demonstrated testosterone prevented inflammation caused by hydrogen peroxide in blood vessel cells by upregulating the sirtuin-1 (Sirt1)/eNOS pathway [57, 58]. In one of our studies, testosterone administration upregulated Sirt1 and eNOS mRNA transcription, possibly preventing CC inflammation in T2DM rats (**Figures 1** and **2**). Interestingly, serum asymmetric dimethylarginine (ADMA) levels were also increased in T2DM rats, and rats receiving TRT were observed to have decreased ADMA levels. ADMA is an endogenous arginine compound that rises in individuals demonstrating some disease states [59]; in particular, several reports have suggested a potential relationship between ADMA levels and ED [60, 61]. ADMA has NOS inhibitory activity, and the elevation of ADMA levels contributes to decreased NO bioactivity and decreased endothelial functioning of vessel tissues. Zhang

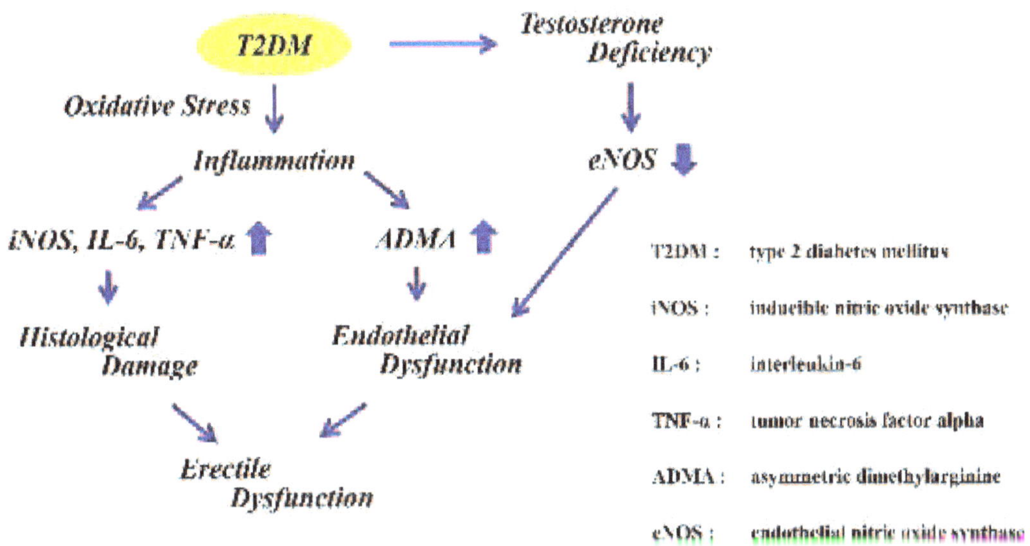

Figure 1. The mechanism of erectile dysfunction caused by T2DM.

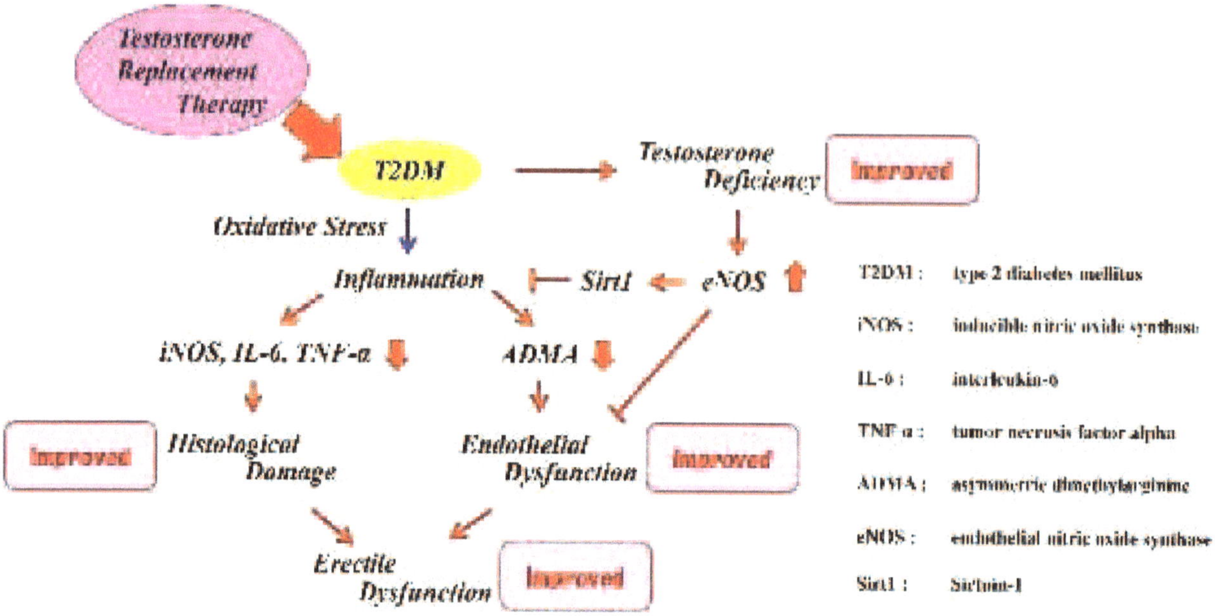

Figure 2. The mechanism of ART for T2DM.

et al. also reported that testosterone treatment improved nNOS activity using streptozotocin-induced diabetic rat [62].

6. TRT limitations

TRT is widely used to effectively treat patients with testosterone deficiencies. It has also been applied to animal models for investigating the mechanisms of testosterone action. However, Burns-Cox et al. pointed out that testosterone (testosterone enanthate) injections cause extremely high levels of testosterone after a few days [63]. Similarly, we injected testosterone enanthate into rats, and the animals demonstrated serum testosterone level increases that rose in a dose-dependent manner (**Figure 3**).

Amano et al. reported that the therapeutic administration of testosterone ointment to patients with LOH successfully kept testosterone at normal levels [64]. We administered low-dose testosterone (similar to applying testosterone ointment) to rats, as previous report [65], 4 weeks after castration. Interestingly, this TRT did not improve erectile functioning over the first 4 weeks of administration. However, after 8 weeks of TRT, partial ED improvements were observed (**Figure 4**). Baba et al. reported that delayed TRT improved ED, in rats, for 4 weeks [41]. However, they used high-dose testosterone administrations and the testosterone levels were ≥10 times normal. These results suggest that low-dose testosterone treatments may require longer treatment periods to overcome testosterone deficiency. Currently, testosterone undecanoate, a drug that is applied over a long period (about 3 months), is widely used in European countries. The medication has been shown to be a safe and effective treatment for patients with testosterone deficiencies [66]. However, some countries have not approved

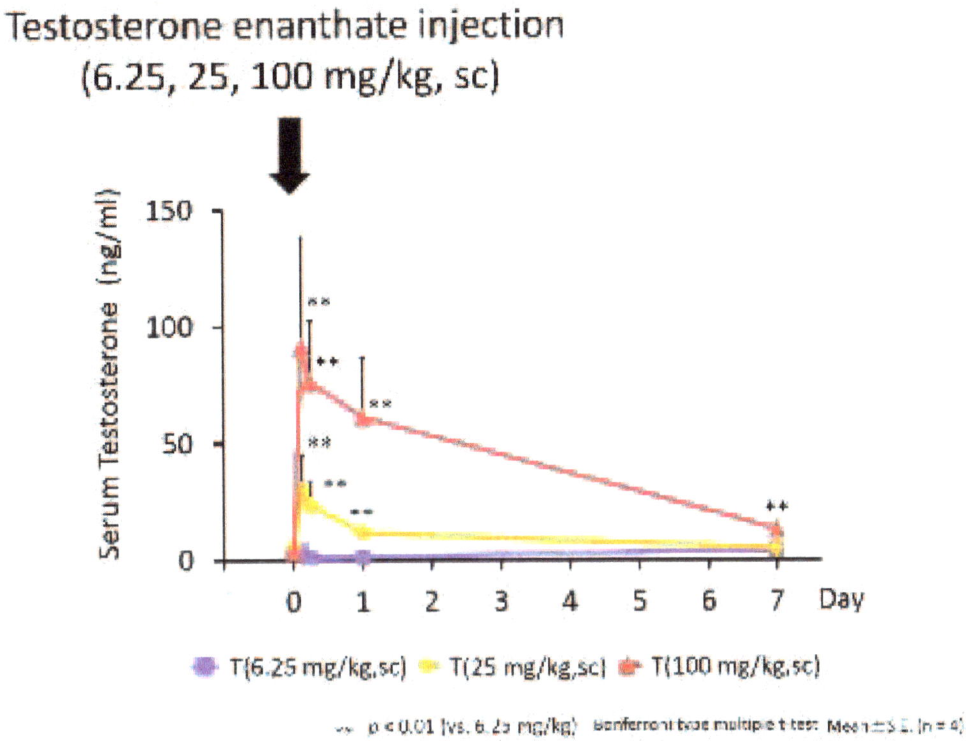

Figure 3. Testosterone levels after testosterone injection in rat.

the medication, and there are no basic science reports addressing its use. These results demonstrate the need to investigate differences between various testosterone administration methods.

Erectile functioning is a complex process, with an underlying mechanism that is affected by several factors [4, 67–69]. Recent studies have suggested that one of these factors may be endogenous estrogen levels [70–77]. For example, Baser et al. suggested that serum estrogen levels are correlated with aging in men and that estrogen may, therefore, play an important role in the expression of the symptoms of aging [70]. Further, Greco et al. reported that tadalafil treatment suppresses estrogen levels in some obese men and improved their erectile function domain scores [71]. Another group reported high estrogen levels in elderly patients with ED and sexual disinterest; therefore, they suggested that pathophysiological estrogen-testosterone imbalance is involved in these conditions among elderly men [72, 73]. In a basic study, Goyal et al. reported that estrogen caused developmental disorders of the rat penis and that it decreased penile testosterone levels [74, 75]. Others reported that estrogen caused pathophysiological changes in the corpus cavernosum and a decline in erectile function in rats [76]. These authors also reported that estrogen induction enhanced corpus cavernosum smooth muscle contraction and decreased smooth muscle relaxation in rabbits [77]. We reported the use of TRT in a rat model of testosterone deficiency induced by estrogen injections. Interestingly, TRT is not an effective ED treatment in the high-estrogen level model [78]. Thus, attention needs to be given not only to the testosterone levels but also to the levels of other hormones.

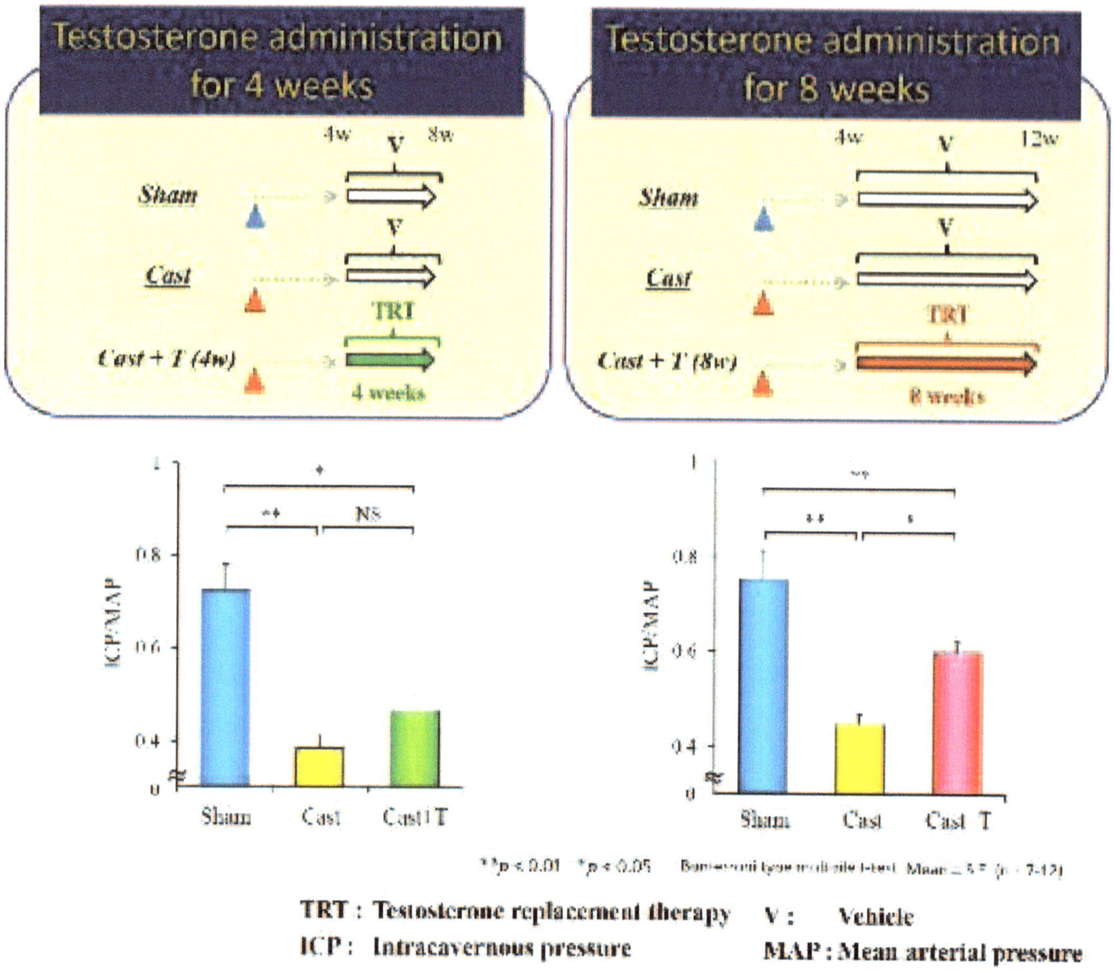

Figure 4. Different effects of TRT periods for delayed treatment.

7. New approaches for testosterone deficiency treatment

Although TRT is an effective treatment for testosterone deficiency, some reports have reported a new treatment approach based on the use of testosterone deficiency models that consider the mechanism of testosterone action on erectile function. PDE-5 inhibitors are the first choice for ED patients, but they are not always effective in patients with testosterone deficiencies [79, 80]. One of the reasons for the lack of efficacy might be the PDE-5 expression changes induced by testosterone. A combination therapy involving both testosterone and PDE-5 inhibitors is one choice, but it is the one that is being vigorously debated, with strong reasons being presented for and against its use. PDE-5 inhibitors are also effective, but regardless of their pharmacokinetics or the regimen used, none has been shown to cure ED [2].

Moody et al. showed that L-arginine administration also improves ED in castrated rats [81]. Similarly, we demonstrated that L-citrulline supplementation improves erectile function and penile structure in castrated rats [82]. L-arginine and L-citrulline are amino acids present in free form in the human body. When L-citrulline is orally administered, it is converted to L-argininosuccinate and, subsequently, to L-arginine by renal argininosuccinate lyase [83]. L-arginine is then converted to NO and L-citrulline by NOS [84]. Orally administered L-arginine is known to be extensively metabolized by autochthonous gut bacteria and by arginases in the gut and liver [3]. However, oral L-citrulline administrations were shown to avoid such metabolism [85]. Accordingly, oral L-citrulline supplementation was reported to increase L-arginine levels more efficiently than oral L-arginine administration; L-citrulline also increased NO production [86]. In addition, we conducted a similar study using an acute arteriogenic ED model [87]. In that study, oral L-citrulline supplementation improved erectile function and increased NO production, without side effects (e.g., decreased mean arterial pressure) [87].

Fukuhara et al. showed that resveratrol and vardenafil improved erectile responses in rats with streptozotocin-induced diabetes [88]. Recently, Dalaklioglu et al. also reported that resveratrol improved sildenafil-induced corpus cavernosum relaxation in both diabetic and non-diabetic aged rats, probably by potentiating NOS activity [89]. Oral supplementation might improve the vasculogenic condition, considering our previous study, though this is just speculation and needs to be examined.

8. Conclusions

Testosterone levels affect several organs, including the functioning of male erectile tissue. Many studies have described the mechanism of testosterone deficiency effects on erectile function as well as the impact of TRT. Testosterone affects NO production and PDE-5 expression in the corpus cavernosum through molecular pathways. It also preserves smooth muscle contractility by regulating both contraction and relaxation. Further, testosterone maintains the structure of the corpus cavernosum. TRT is widely used to treat patients with testosterone deficiencies; however, the present discussion has also documented some problems associated with this therapeutic approach. Basic research has also identified other potentially effective therapeutic methods for treating testosterone deficiency. Among these, PDE-5 inhibitors, L-citrulline, and resveratrol might be options for treating testosterone deficiency-induced ED. Future research should confirm these findings in more specific experiments that use molecular tools. Such additional research may shed more light on possible treatments for endocrine-mediated ED and its treatment.

Author details

Tomoya Kataoka[1] and Kazunori Kimura[1,2]*

*Address all correspondence to: kkimura@med.nagoya-cu.ac.jp

1 Department of Clinical Pharmaceutics, Graduate School of Medical Sciences, Nagoya City University, Japan

2 Department of Hospital Pharmacy, Graduate School of Pharmaceutical Sciences, Nagoya City University, Japan

References

[1] Meldrum DR, Gambone JC, Morris MA, Esposito K, Giugliano D, Ignarro LJ. Lifestyle and metabolic approaches to maximizing erectile and vascular health. International Journal of Impotence Research. 2012;**24**:61-68

[2] Isidori AM, Buvat J, Corona G, Goldstein I, Jannini EA, Lenzi A, Porst H, Salonia A, Traish AM, Maggi M. A critical analysis of the role of testosterone in erectile function: from pathophysiology to treatment: A systematic review. European Urology. 2014;**65**:99-112

[3] Traish AM, Goldstein I, Kim NN. Testosterone and erectile function: From basic research to a new clinical paradigm for managing men with androgen insufficiency and erectile dysfunction. European Urology. 2007;**52**:54-70

[4] Shamloul R, Ghanem H. Erectile dysfunction. The Lancet. 2013;**381**:153-165

[5] Buvat J, Maggi M, Guay A, Torres LO. Testosterone deficiency in men: Systematic review and standard operating procedures for diagnosis and treatment. The Journal of Sexual Medicine. 2013;**10**:245-284

[6] Maiorino MI, Bellastella G, Esposito K. Lifestyle modifications and erectile dysfunction: What can be expected? Asian Journal of Andrology. 2015;**17**:5-10

[7] Wang C, Nieschlag E, Swerdloff R, Behre HM, Hellstrom WJ, Gooren LJ, Kaufman JM, Legros JJ, Lunenfeld B, Morales A, Morley JE, Schulman C, Thompson IM, Weidner W, Wu FC. Investigation, treatment and monitoring of late-onset hypogonadism in males. European Journal of Endocrinology. 2008;**159**:507-514

[8] Morales A, Buvat J, Gooren LJ, Guay AT, Kaufman JM, Tan HM, Torres LO. Endocrine aspects of sexual dysfunction in men. The Journal of Sexual Medicine. 2004;**1**:69-81

[9] Diaz-Arjonilla M, Schwarcz M, Swerdloff RS, Wang C. Obesity, low testosterone levels and erectile dysfunction. International Journal of Impotence Research. 2009;**21**:89-98

[10] Yassin A, Saad F, Gooren LJ. Metabolic syndrome, testosterone deficiency and erectile dysfunction never come alone. Andrologia. 2008;**40**:259-264

[11] Corona G, Mannucci E, Fisher AD, Lotti F, Petrone L, Balercia G, Bandini E, Forti G, Maggi M. Low levels of androgens in men with erectile dysfunction and obesity. The Journal of Sexual Medicine. 2008;**5**:2454-2463

[12] Shabsigh R, Arver S, Channer KS, Eardley I, Fabbri A, Gooren L, Heufelder A, Jones Z, Meryn S, Zitzmann M. The triad of erectile dysfunction, hypogonadism and the metabolic syndrome. International Journal of Clinical Practice. 2008;**62**:791-798

[13] Andersson KE, Wagner G. Physiology of penile erection. Physiological Reviews. 1995;**75**:191-236

[14] Wingard C, Fulton D, Husain S. Altered penile vascular reactivity and erection in the Zucker obese-diabetic rat. The Journal of Sexual Medicine. 2007;**4**:348-363

[15] Morelli A, Chavalmane AK, Filippi S, Fibbi B, Silvestrini E, Sarchielli E, Zhang XH, Vignozzi L, Vannelli GB, Forti G, Maggi M. Atorvastatin ameliorates sildenafil-induced penile erections in experimental diabetes by inhibiting diabetes-induced RhoA/Rho-kinase signaling hyperactivation. The Journal of Sexual Medicine. 2009;**6**:91-106

[16] Wingard CJ, Moukdar F, Prasad RY, Cathey BL, Wilkinson L. Reversal of voltage-dependent erectile responses in the Zucker obese-diabetic rat by rosuvastatin-altered RhoA/Rho-kinase signaling. The Journal of Sexual Medicine. 2009;**6**:269-278

[17] Rajasekaran H, White S, Baquir A, Wilkes N. Rho-kinase inhibition improves erectile function in aging male Brown-Norway rats. Journal of Andrology. 2005;**26**:182-188

[18] Jin L, Liu T, Lagoda GA, Champion HC, Bivalacqua TJ, Burnett AL. Elevated RhoA/Rho-kinase activity in the aged rat penis: Mechanism for age-associated erectile dysfunction. The FASEB Journal. 2006;**20**:536-538

[19] Mills TM, Lewis RW, Stopper VS. Androgenic maintenance of inflow and veno-occlusion during erection in the rat. Biology of Reproduction. 1998;**59**:1413-1418

[20] Armagan A, Kim NN, Goldstein I, Traish AM. Dose-response relationship between testosterone and erectile function: Evidence for the existence of a critical threshold. Journal of Andrology. 2006;**27**:517-526

[21] Li R, Meng X, Zhang Y, Wang T, Yang J, Niu Y, Cui K, Wang S, Liu J, Rao K. Testosterone improves erectile function through inhibition of reactive oxygen species generation in castrated rats. PeerJ. 2016;**4**:e2000

[22] Traish AM, Park K, Dhir V, Kim NN, Moreland RB, Goldstein I. Effects of castration and androgen replacement on erectile function in a rabbit model. Endocrinology. 1999;**140**:1861-1868

[23] Zhang XH, Morelli A, Luconi M, Vignozzi L, Filippi S, Marini M, Vannelli GB, Mancina R, Forti G, Maggi M. Testosterone regulates PDE5 expression and in vivo responsiveness to tadalafil in rat corpus cavernosum. European Urology. 2005;**47**:409-416

[24] Reilly CM, Stopper VS, Mills TM. Androgens modulate the alphaadrenergic responsiveness of vascular smooth muscle in the corpus cavernosum. Journal of Andrology. 1997;**18**:26-31

[25] Reilly CM, Lewis RW, Stopper VS, Mills TM. Androgenic maintenance of the rat erectile response via a non-nitric-oxide-dependent pathway. Journal of Andrology. 1997;**18**: 588-594

[26] Sopko NA, Hannan JL, Bivalacqua TJ. Understanding and targeting the Rho kinase pathway in erectile dysfunction. Nature Reviews. Urology. 2014;**11**:622-628

[27] Yue P, Chatterjee K, Beale C, Poole-Wilson PA, Collins P. Testosterone relaxes rabbit coronary arteries and aorta. Circulation. 1995;**91**:1154-1160

[28] Han DH, Chae MR, Jung JH, So I, Park JK, Lee SW. Effect of testosterone on potassium channel opening in human corporal smooth muscle cells. The Journal of Sexual Medicine. 2008;**5**:822-832

[29] Dai YT, Stopper V, Lewis R, Mills T. Effects of castration and testosterone replacement on veno-occlusion during penile erection in the rat. Asian Journal of Andrology. 1999;**1**:53-59

[30] Alves-Lopes RU, Neves KB, Silva MA, Olivon VC, Ruginsk SG, Antunes-Rodrigues J, Ramalho LN, Tostes RC, Carneiro FS. Functional and structural changes in internal pudendal arteries underlie erectile dysfunction induced by androgen deprivation. Asian Journal of Andrology. 2017;**19**:526-532

[31] Traish AM, Toselli P, Jeong SJ, Kim NN. Adipocyte accumulation in penile corpus cavernosum of the orchiectomized rabbit: A potential mechanism for veno-occlusive dysfunction in androgen deficiency. Journal of Andrology. 2005;**26**:242-248

[32] Wang XJ, Xu TY, Xia LL, Zhong S, Zhang XH, Zhu ZW, Chen DR, Liu Y, Fan Y, Xu C, Zhang MG, Shen ZJ. Castration impairs erectile organ structure and function by inhibiting autophagy and promoting apoptosis of corpus cavernosum smooth muscle cells in rats. International Urology and Nephrology. 2015;**47**:1105-1115

[33] Lian J, Karnak D, Xu L. The Bcl-2-Beclin 1 interaction in (−)-gossypol-induced autophagy versus apoptosis in prostate cancer cells. Autophagy. 2010;**6**:1201-1203

[34] Kang R, Zeh HJ, Lotze MT, Tang D. The Beclin 1 network regulates autophagy and apoptosis. Cell Death and Differentiation. 2011;**18**:571-580

[35] Yang CM, Shen YC, Weng SF, Wang JJ, Tien KJ. Increased risk of dementia in patients with erectile dysfunction: A population-based, propensity score-matched, longitudinal follow-up study. Medicine (Baltimore). 2015;**94**:e990

[36] Yang Y, Liu H, Lin T, Kuo Y, Hsieh T. Relationship between erectile dysfunction, comorbidity, and Parkinson's disease: Evidence from a population-based longitudinal study. Journal of Clinical Neurology. 2017;**13**:250-258

[37] Balsamo R, Arcaniolo D, Stizzo M, Illiano E, Autorino R, Natale F, Costantini E, Damiano R, De Sio M. Increased risk of erectile dysfunction in men with multiple sclerosis: An Italian cross-sectional study. Central European Journal of Urology. 2017;**70**:289-295

[38] Barron AM, Pike CJ. Sex hormones, aging, and Alzheimer's disease. Frontiers in Bioscience (Elite Edition). 2012;**4**:976-997

[39] Okun MS, McDonald WM, DeLong MR. Refractory nonmotor symptoms in male patients with Parkinson disease due to testosterone deficiency: A common unrecognized comorbidity. Archives of Neurology. 2002;**59**:807-811

[40] Bove R, Musallam A, Healy BC, Raghavan K, Glanz BI, Bakshi R, Weiner H, De Jager PL, Miller KK, Chitnis T. Low testosterone is associated with disability in men with multiple sclerosis. Multiple Sclerosis. 2014;**20**:1584-1592

[41] Baba K, Yajima M, Carrier S, Morgan DM, Nunes L, Lue TF, Iwamoto T. Delayed testosterone replacement restores nitric oxide synthase-containing nerve fibres and the erectile response in rat penis. BJU International. 2000;**85**:953-958

[42] Lugg J, Ng C, Rajfer J, Gonzalez-Cadavid N. Cavernosal nerve stimulation in the rat reverses castration-induced decrease in penile NOS activity. The American Journal of Physiology. 1996;**271**:E354-E361

[43] Giuliano F, Rampin O, Schirar A, Jardin A, Rousseau JP. Autonomic control of penile erection: Modulation by testosterone in the rat. Journal of Neuroendocrinology. 1993;**5**: 677-683

[44] Suzuki N, Sato Y, Hisasue S, Kato R, Suzuki K, Tsukamoto T. Effect of testosterone on intracavernous pressure elicited with electrical stimulation of the medial preoptic area and cavernous nerve in male rats. Journal of Andrology. 2007;**28**:218-222

[45] Syme DB, Corcoran NM, Bouchier-Hayes DM, Morrison WA, Costello AJ. The effect of androgen status on the structural and functional success of cavernous nerve grafting in an experimental rat model. The Journal of Urology. 2007;**177**:390-394

[46] Armagan A, Hatsushi K, Toselli P. The effects of testosterone deficiency on the structural integrity of the penile dorsal nerve in the rat. International Journal of Impotence Research. 2008;**20**:73-78

[47] Baba K, Yajima M, Carrier S, Akkus E, Reman J, Nunes L, Lue TF, Iwamoto T. Effect of testosterone on the number of NADPH diaphorase-stained nerve fibers in the rat corpus cavernosum and dorsal nerve. Urology. 2000;**56**:533-538

[48] Buvat J, Maggi M, Gooren L, Guay AT, Kaufman J, Morgentaler A, Schulman C, Tan HM, Torres LO, Yassin A, Zitzmann M. Endocrine aspects of male sexual dysfunctions. The Journal of Sexual Medicine. 2010;**7**:1627-1656

[49] García-Cruz E, Leibar-Tamayo A, Romero J, Piqueras M, Luque P, Cardeñosa O, Alcaraz A. Metabolic syndrome in men with low testosterone levels: Relationship with cardiovascular risk factors and comorbidities and with erectile dysfunction. The Journal of Sexual Medicine. 2013;**10**:2529-2538

[50] Esposito K, Giugliano F, Martedì E, Feola G, Marfella R, D'Armiento M, Giugliano D. High proportions of erectile dysfunction in men with the metabolic syndrome. Diabetes Care. 2005;**28**:1201-1203

[51] Ryan JG, Gajraj J. Erectile dysfunction and its association with metabolic syndrome and endothelial function among patients with type 2 diabetes mellitus. Journal of Diabetes and its Complications. 2012;**26**:141-147

[52] Wang C, Jackson G, Jones TH, Matsumoto AM, Nehra A, Perelman MA, Swerdloff RS, Traish A, Zitzmann M, Cunningham G. Low testosterone associated with obesity and the metabolic syndrome contributes to sexual dysfunction and cardiovascular disease risk in men with type 2 diabetes. Diabetes Care. 2011;**34**:1669-1675

[53] Zhang XH, Melman A, Disanto ME. Update on corpus cavernosum smooth muscle contractile pathways in erectile function: A role for testosterone? The Journal of Sexual Medicine. 2011;**8**:1865-1879

[54] Davis DD, Ruiz AL, Yanes LL, Iliescu R, Yuan K, Moulana M, Racusen LC, Reckelhoff JF. Testosterone supplementation in male obese Zucker rats reduces body weight and improves insulin sensitivity but increases blood pressure. Hypertension. 2012;**59**:726-731

[55] Filippi S, Vignozzi L, Morelli A, Chavalmane AK, Sarchielli E, Fibbi B, Saad F, Sandner P, Ruggiano P, Vannelli GB, Mannucci E, Maggi M. Testosterone partially ameliorates metabolic profile and erectile responsiveness to PDE5 inhibitors in an animal model of male metabolic syndrome. The Journal of Sexual Medicine. 2009;**6**:3274-3288

[56] Kataoka T, Hotta Y, Maeda Y, Kimura K. Assessment of androgen replacement therapy for erectile function in rats with type 2 diabetes mellitus by examining nitric oxide-related and inflammatory factors. The Journal of Sexual Medicine. 2014;**11**:920-929

[57] Ota H, Akishita M, Akiyoshi T, Kahyo T, Setou M, Ogawa S, Iijima K, Eto M, Ouchi Y. Testosterone deficiency accelerates neuronal and vascular aging of SAMP8 mice: Protective role of eNOS and SIRT1. PLoS One. 2012;**7**:e29598

[58] Yu J, Akishita M, Eto M, Ogawa S, Son BK, Kato S, Ouchi Y, Okabe T. Androgen receptor-dependent activation of endothelial nitric oxide synthase in vascular endothelial cells: Role of phosphatidylinositol 3-kinase/akt pathway. Endocrinology. 2010;**151**:1822-1828

[59] Bełtowski J, Kedra A. A symmetric dimethylarginine (ADMA) as a target for pharmacotherapy. Pharmacological Reports. 2006;**58**:159-178

[60] Ioakeimidis N, Vlachopoulos C, Rokkas K, Aggelis A, Terentes-Printzios D, Samentzas A, Alexopoulos N, Stefanadis C. Relationship of asymmetric dimethylarginine with penile Doppler ultrasound parameters in men with vasculogenic erectile dysfunction. European Urology. 2011;**59**:948-955

[61] Paroni R, Barassi A, Ciociola F, Dozio E, Finati E, Fermo I, Ghilardi F, Colpi GM, Corsi MM, Melzi d'Eril GV. Asymmetric dimethylarginine (ADMA), symmetric dimethylarginine (SDMA) and L-arginine in patients with arteriogenic and non-arteriogenic erectile dysfunction. International Journal of Andrology. 2012;**35**:660-667

[62] Zhang XH, Filippi S, Morelli A, Vignozzi L, Luconi M, Donati S, Forti G, Maggi M. Testosterone restores diabetes-induced erectile dysfunction and sildenafil responsiveness in two distinct animal models of chemical diabetes. The Journal of Sexual Medicine. 2006;**3**:2535-2545

[63] Burns-Cox N, Gingell JC. Erectile dysfunction: Endocrinological therapies risks and benefits of treatment. In: Carson CC, Kirby RS, editors. Textbook of Erectile Dysfunction. Oxford: Isis Medical Media; 1999. pp. 327-344

[64] Amano T, Imao T, Takemae K, Iwamoto T, Yamakawa K, Baba K, Nakanome M, Sugimori H, Tanaka T, Yoshida K, Katabami T, Tanaka M. Profile of serum testosterone levels after application of testosterone ointment (Glowmin) and its clinical efficacy in late-onset hypogonadism patients. The Journal of Sexual Medicine. 2008;**5**:1727-1736

[65] Kataoka T, Hotta Y, Maeda Y, Kimura K. Testosterone deficiency causes endothelial dysfunction via elevation of asymmetric dimethylarginine (ADMA) and oxidative stress in castrated rats. The Journal of Sexual Medicine. 2017;**14**:1540-1548

[66] Yassin AA, Nettleship J, Almehmadi Y, Salman M, Saad F. Effects of continuous long-term testosterone therapy (TTh) on anthropometric, endocrine and metabolic parameters for up to 10 years in 115 hypogonadal elderly men: Real-life experience from an observational registry study. Andrologia. 2016;**48**:793-799

[67] Keller J, Chen YK, Lin HC. Hyperthyroidism and erectile dysfunction: A population-based case-control study. International Journal of Impotence Research. 2012;**24**:242-246

[68] Andersen ML, Santos-Silva R, Bittencourt LR, Tufik S. Prevalence of erectile dysfunction complaints associated with sleep disturbances in Sao Paulo, Brazil: A population-based survey. Sleep Medicine. 2010;**11**:1019-1024

[69] Shaeer O, Shaeer K. The global online sexuality survey (GOSS): The United States of America in 2011. Chapter I: Erectile dysfunction among English-speakers. The Journal of Sexual Medicine. 2012;**9**:3018-3027

[70] Basar MM, Aydin G, Mert HC, Keles I, Caglayan O, Orkun S, et al. Relationship between serum sex steroids and aging male symptoms score and international index of erectile function. Urology. 2005;**66**:597-601

[71] Greco EA, Pili M, Bruzziches R, Corona G, Spera G, Aversa A. Testosterone:estradiol ratio changes associated with long-term tadalafil administration: A pilot study. The Journal of Sexual Medicine. 2006;**3**:716-722

[72] Srilatha B, Adaikan PG, Chong YS. Relevance of oestradiol-testosterone balance in erectile dysfunction patients' prognosis. Singapore Medical Journal. 2007;**48**:114-118

[73] Srilatha B, Adaikan PG. Endocrine milieu and erectile dysfunction: Is oestradiol-testosterone imbalance, a risk factor in the elderly? Asian Journal of Andrology. 2011;**13**:569-573

[74] Goyal HO, Braden TD, Williams CS, Williams JW. Estrogen-induced developmental disorders of the rat penis involve both estrogen receptor (ESR)- and androgen receptor (AR)-mediated pathways. Biology of Reproduction. 2009;**81**:507-516

[75] Simon L, Avery L, Braden TD, Williams CS, Okumu LA, Williams JW, et al. Exposure of neonatal rats to anti-androgens induces penile mal-developments and infertility comparable to those induced by oestrogens. International Journal of Andrology. 2012;**35**:364-376

[76] Adaikan PG, Srilatha B. Oestrogen-mediated hormonal imbalance precipitates erectile dysfunction. International Journal of Impotence Research. 2003;**15**:38-43

[77] Srilatha B, Adaikan PG. Estrogen and phytoestrogen predispose to erectile dysfunction: Do ER-alpha and ER-beta in the cavernosum play a role? Urology. 2004;**63**:382-386

[78] Kataoka T, Hotta Y, Ohno M, Maeda Y, Kimura K. Limited effect of testosterone treatment for erectile dysfunction caused by high-estrogen levels in rats. International Journal of Impotence Research. 2013;**25**:201-205

[79] Boloña ER, Uraga MV, Haddad RM, Tracz MJ, Sideras K, Kennedy CC, Caples SM, Erwin PJ, Montori VM. Testosterone use in men with sexual dysfunction: A systematic review and meta-analysis of randomized placebo-controlled trials. Mayo Clinic Proceedings. 2007;**82**:20-28

[80] Mäkinen JI, Huhtaniemi I. Androgen replacement therapy in late-onset hypogonadism: Current concepts and controversies—A mini-review. Gerontology. 2011;**57**:193-202

[81] Moody JA, Vernet D, Laidlaw S, Rajfer J, Gonzalez-Cadavid NF. Effects of long-term oral administration of L-arginine on the rat erectile response. The Journal of Urology 1997;**158**:942-947

[82] Hotta Y, Shiota A, Kataoka T, Motonari M, Maeda Y, Morita M, Kimura K. Oral L-citrulline supplementation improves erectile function and penile structure in castrated rats. International Journal of Urology. 2014;**21**:608-612

[83] Curis E, Nicolis I, Moinard C, Osowska S, Zerrouk N, Bénazeth S, Cynober L. Almost all about citrulline in mammals. Amino Acids. 2005;**29**:177-205

[84] Morris SM Jr. Enzymes of arginine metabolism. The Journal of Nutrition. 2004;**134**: 2743S-2747S

[85] Schwedhelm E, Maas R, Freese R, Jung D, Lukacs Z, Jambrecina A, Spickler W, Schulze F, Böger RH. Pharmacokinetic and pharmacodynamic properties of oral l-citrulline and l-arginine: Impact on nitric oxide metabolism. British Journal of Clinical Pharmacology. 2008;**65**:51-59

[86] Wijnands KA, Vink H, Briedé JJ, van Faassen EE, Lamers WH, Buurman WA, Poeze M. Citrulline a more suitable substrate than arginine to restore NO production and the microcirculation during endotoxemia. PLoS One 2012;**7**:e37439

[87] Shiota A, Hotta Y, Kataoka T, Morita M, Maeda Y, Kimura K. Oral l-citrulline supplementation improves erectile function in rats with acute arteriogenic erectile dysfunction. The Journal of Sexual Medicine. 2013;**10**:2423-2429

[88] Fukuhara S, Tsujimura A, Okuda H, Yamamoto K, Takao T, Miyagawa Y, Nonomura N, Okuyama A. Vardenafil and resveratrol synergistically enhance the nitric oxide/cyclic guanosine monophosphate pathway in corpus cavernosal smooth muscle cells and its therapeutic potential for erectile dysfunction in the streptozotocin-induced diabetic rat: Preliminary findings. The Journal of Sexual Medicine. 2011;**8**:1061-1071

[89] Dalaklioglu S, Bayram Z, Tasatargil A, Ozdem S. Resveratrol reverses diabetes-related decrement in sildenafil-induced relaxation of corpus cavernosum in aged rats. Aging Clinical and Experimental Research. 2017;**29**:345-351

9

New Insights for Hormone Therapy in Perimenopausal Women Neuroprotection

Manuela Cristina Russu and
Alexandra Cristina Antonescu

Abstract

Perimenopause is a mandatory period in women's life, when the medical staff may initiate hormone therapy with sex steroids for the delay of brain aging and neurodegenerative diseases, during the so-called "window of opportunity." Animals' models are helpful to sustain the still controversial results of human clinical observational and/or randomized controlled studies. Estrogens, progesterone, and androgens, with their nuclear and membrane receptors, genes, and epigenetics, with their connections to cholinergic, GABAergic, serotoninergic, and glutamatergic systems are involved in women's normal brain or in brain's pathology. The sex steroids are active through direct and/or indirect mechanisms to modulate and/or to protect brain plasticity, and vessels network, fuel metabolism—glucose, ketones, ATP, to reduce insulin resistance, and inflammation of the aging brain through blood-brain barrier disruption, microglial aberrant activation, and neural cell survival/loss.

Keywords: perimenopause, "window" of opportunity, neuroprotection, sex steroid hormones

1. Introduction

The months/years of perimenopause represent an important moment during women's aging, when sex steroids and their receptors decline are evident in the hippocampal and cortical neurons, after estrogen exposure during the reproductive years. The sex steroid hormones decline is associated/acts synergic to other factors as hypertension, diabetes, hypoxia/obstructive sleep apnea, obesity, vitamin B12/folate deficiency, depression, and traumatic brain injury to promote diverse pathological mechanisms involved in brain aging, memory impairment, and AD.

2. Sex steroid hormones involvement in aging brain. The perimenopausal "window" of opportunity for neuroprotection

Perimenopause represents the critical period during women's brain aging when it is possible to use the "window" of opportunity to delay/postpone the proved deleterious effects of sex steroids decline. The complex/complicated feedback loops between non-reproductive brain regions—prefrontal neocortex, hippocampus, amigdala, and brainstem, thalamus and hypothalamus, and the ovaries are made by sex steroid hormones, their network receptors through the entire brain, enzymes involved in their metabolism, their metabolites, neurotransmitters, cytokines, chemokines, and many other proteins/peptides. A multitude of studies are demonstrating the effects of estrogens (estradiol-E2, estetrol-E4, and in a less measure estrone-E1), progesterone, and androgens in brain during reproductive years, and have preventive functions to cognitive and memory performances, being involved in brain bioenergetic control by regulation of glucose transport, aerobic glycolysis coupled to the citric acid cycle, and mitochondrial respiration to generate ATP [1], and also in anti-inflammatory actions in the biology of neuroaging and neurodegenerative diseases. These effects of sex steroids are covering the two hypothesis of neurodegeneration discussed in the previous chapter.

Beside involvement in reproduction, sex steroids exert regulatory actions on the receptors in non-reproductive brain regions, including (but not limited to) prefrontal cortex and hippocampus, amigdala, thalamus, and brainstem, which occur *via* neural circuitry linking the hypothalamus to other CNS systems.

The steroid hormones are acting by indirect mechanisms on coagulation, metabolisms to prevent atherosclerosis, and to vasodilation of cerebral vessels, increasing the blood flow to the hippocampus and left superior temporal gyrus [2], and through direct cellular mechanisms on different types of neurons, microglia, and astroglia, on their synapses particularly in the brain regions that show preclinical abnormalities in individuals who are at risk for AD (**Table 1**).

Starting from basic science, preclinical and clinical studies, experimental, observational, and controlled trials are linked to estrogen-inducible neuroprotective, neurotrophic, and neurogenic actions. There are animal (rats, mice, non-human primates) and human evidences on cellular mechanisms of estrogen-regulated functions/systems, which are presented in **Table 2**.

2.1. Estrogens' involvement in brain aging

All types of studies have demonstrated that the neuroprotective effects of estrogens—mainly 17 β—and 17α-estradiol, progesterone, and androgens (DHEA mainly) are on the vessels, neurons, microglia, and astroglia. The vast majority of gynecological, endocrinological, and/or neurological research studies are about the thrombotic and ischemic stroke risks after the age of 50 years (median age of menopause).

Observational studies on large numbers of cases from North America as the Baltimore Longitudinal Study of Aging [3], the Manhattan Study of Aging [4] have associated HT/ET to significant prevention or delay onset of AD, or reduction risk of AD (9/156 [5.8%] estrogen

Author(s)/year	Type of study	Steroid	Action/Effect
Tang et al. [138]	Prospective observational (1–5 yrs. follow-up)	E2	Estrogen promotes the growth and survival of cholinergic neurons, and could decrease cerebral Aβ deposition, both of which may delay the onset or prevent AD.
Maki and Resnick [2]	Prospective (2 yrs. follow-up)	E2	Increasing the blood flow to the hippocampus and left superior temporal gyrus
McEwen et al. [79] Adams et al. [37]	Experimental Experimental	E2 E2	Estrogen synapses formation in the CA1 region of the dorsal hippocampus during the estrous cycle of the female rat E2 did not induced the increased synapses number in aged rats
Zhang et al., [34]	Experimental	17β E2, testosterone or methyl-testosterone	Estrogen & Androgen Protection of Human Neurons against Intracellular Amyloid Toxicity through Heat Shock Protein 70
Xu et al. [139]	Basic study	E2	Provides protection against β-amyloid-induced damage and tau-related changes
Norbury et al. [140]	RCT	E2	Maintenance of the cholinergic system in the hippocampus and frontal cortex
Persad et al. [141]	RCT	Ethinyl-E2 and progestin	Increased activation in brain regions associated with the left middle/superior frontal cortex, and left inferior parietal cortex during verbal memory encoding tasks on functional magnetic resonance imaging
Harburger et al. [64]	Experimental	E2 + progesterone	E2 alone and combined E2 + P4 may influence ERK activation in different time frames or enhance memory of objects recognition in young ovariectomized mice
Silverman et al. [142]	RCT	E2	Higher metabolism in language processing and auditory association areas compared to other HRT regimens (CEE or CEE + MPA)
Yao et al. [143]	Experimental	17β-E2	Early correction of bioenergetics deficits, and mitochondrial β-amyloid deposition when ovarian hormones decline
Zhao et al. [52]	Experimental	E2 + CyP4 vs. E2 + CoP4	Differential regulation of hippocampal gene expression according to P4 supplementation to E2
Tskitishvili et al. [46]	Experimental	E4	Antioxidative actions, neurogenesis and possibly promyelinating activities

Legend: E2: estradiol; Ethinyl-E2: ethinylestradiol; MPA: medroxyprogesterone acetate; CEE: conjugated equine estrogens; RCT: randomized control trial; CyP4: progesterone cylic; CoP4: progesterone continuous

Table 1. Actions/effects of sex steroid hormones on brain aging.

users vs. 158/968 [16.3%] nonusers; 0.40 [95% Cl 0.22–0.85], $p < 0.01$), and for a longer duration than 1 year, with no effect observed for the age of menopause. At that moment, the researchers considered the necessity of prospective studies for the establishment of the dose and duration of ET to provide this benefit and to assess the safety in elderly postmenopausal women.

The "healthy-cell bias" hypothesis demonstrated the E2 neural different effects at different ages, and at different stages of Aβ presence, making the explanations of different results

Estrogen-regulated functions/systems	Reference(s)
• Estrogens prevent apoptotic death cascades and neuronal death	Lebesgue et al. [40] Etgen et al. [144] Inagaki et al. [42]; Etgen and Inagaki [41]
• Estradiol rapidly stimulates signaling cascades: as the mitogen-activated protein (MAP) kinase family and the phosphatidylinositol 3-kinase (PI3K), pathway leading to the phosphorylation of Akt (a key signaling molecule), and Akt can promote local protein synthesis related to the formation of new spines through a non-genomic mechanism • Estradiol increases phosphorylated Akt (pAkt) present in CA1 dendrites, spines, and synapses	Cordey et al. [145] Znamensky et al. [90] Zhao et al. [146]; Mannella and Brinton [86];
• Estrogens increase the dendritic spine and synaptic density by 30% on CA1 pyramidal cells in the hippocampus • Estrogens provide potential to protect or have the capacity to alter synaptic and postsynaptic circuitry in hypothalamus, hippocampus, and neocortex	Gould et al. [36]; Adams et al. [147] Choi et al. [148].
• Estrogen- induced mitochondrial functions in brain bioenergetics • Estradiol promotes mitochondrial respiration and hence ATP generation and antioxidant enzymes that offset the increase in free radical generation induced by increased respiration • Estradiol significantly reduces mitochondrial lipid peroxidation	Nilsen and Brinton [149]. Nilsen et al. [150]. Simpkins et al. [151]
• Estrogen-induced calcium signaling pathways both promote neuronal function and can exacerbate neuronal demise in neurodegenerative disease states.	Brewer et al. [152]
• Estrogens augment the glutamatergic impact on hippocampal function	Zhao et al. [153];
• Estrogens exerts on the GABAergic and cholinergic systems in the hippocampus and frontal cortex	Rudick et al. [154] Tinkler et al. [155].

Table 2. Evidences on cellular mechanisms of estrogen-regulated functions/systems.

between experimental, observational studies and large RCT, that E2 is beneficial on rats' healthy hippocampal neurons before Aβ exposure [4–6]. More than this hypothesis on "healthy-cell bias," there are discussions and comments about the discrepancies between basic science and/or observational studies supporting estrogen neuroprotective effects and RCT results, focusing the attention to age, stage of reproductive aging, duration of hypogonadism, and the presence of symptoms of cognition or memory impairment, in the efforts for reconciliations [7] between HT and risk for AD [17]. If neurons are healthy at the time of estrogen exposure, their response to estrogen is beneficial for both neuronal survival and neurological function. In contrast, if neurological health is compromised, estrogen exposure over time exacerbates neurological demise. These last two statements represent the opinion of Brinton [8] from the Department of Pharmacology and Pharmaceutical Sciences of California University (USA). In concordance to these facts, the North American and Chinese researchers had elaborated, and tried to confirm the "hypothesis of critical period of estrogen neuroprotection," which appreciates the risk of duration of estrogen deprivation [9]. It was suggested as a "critical period" or a "critical window of opportunity" for the beneficial protective effect of E2 on the human brain [10, 11], and that estrogens have to be administered at perimenopause or earlier to observe a beneficial effect on the neural system [12, 13], as it is for the cardiovascular system.

A consensus began to emerge (although not without controversies) that HT/ET at the time of the menopause transition and afterward could have beneficial effects on several neurological symptoms [7, 14]. The actions of sex steroid hormones are bidirectional to the body periphery and to the brain, and today, there are current evidences that estrogen and progesterone may have beneficial, neutral, or detrimental effects on the brain, depending on age at therapy initiation, type of menopause (natural vs. induced), or stage of menopause, specificity of administered medication, mainly the association of E2 to progesterone (P4) (exogenous), active on cognition through its 5α-reduced metabolite, allopregnanolone [15].

There are characteristics that contribute to several discrepancies in the results: age, stage of reproductive aging, duration of hypogonadism, and symptoms presence. A better understanding of the nature of these discrepancies will be base for future studies of clinical relevance of ovarian steroids and hormone therapies in women.

The Canadian gynecologists [16] were the first who described neurological and psychological disturbances after oophorectomy, than the Italian gynecologists [17]. One may consider that these surgical circumstances are an abrupt, deep decline/withdrawal of steroids, different from the gradual decline in natural menopause, and the cognitive decline in surgical/chemical menopause is more severe [18]. In natural menopause, either premature or early or at the median age of 51 years, the hormonal decline is on a slow slope for E2 and E1, and the androgens (testosterone, androstenedione, and dehydroepiandrosterone) [19] are still present up to the age of 65 [20].

Professional organizations including the British Menopause Society [21], the International Menopause Society [22], and North American Menopause Society [23] recommend estrogen replacement therapy for women with premature menopause or premature ovarian failure. There are evidences, although not from RCT that restoring pathologically low estrogen levels will reduce the later development of cardiovascular disease, osteoporosis, and possibly dementia. This leads to the general recommendation that estrogen be continued in women who experience premature menopause or early menopause until at least around the median age of natural menopause (approximate age 51 years), effects which are evident up to 60 years for women in natural menopause treated for menopausal symptoms [10]. Different to this category of age, the initiation of ET alone or in combination with a progestin in the late postmenopausal stage (ages 65–79 years) induced an increased risk of dementia and cognitive decline regardless of the type of menopause ([10], citing WHIMS), as the "continuum of neurological health progresses from healthy to unhealthy so to do the benefits of ET/HT" [4].

2.1.1. *Animal models*

Experimental evidences support the favorable estrogen effect in neurons, on spinogenesis and synaptogenesis, and the rationale option for the prevention/reduction of the risk or the delay of the onset of AD in postmenopausal women. The North American experiments of McEwen at the Laboratory of Neuroendocrinology from The Rockefeller University, New York, on rats' brain in the years of 1990s' were a surprising discovery on the modulation of hippocampal structural plasticity done by estrogens, and it was considered as a "whole new field in the science" [24]. In the animal models, there are differences between species, regarding reproductive and brain aging scenarios, both changes precede natural reproductive failure [7]. There are some similarities between humans and rodents, and differences between rats and mice.

Estrogens influence the process of adult neurogenesis. E2 promotes the migration of newly generated neurons toward the damaged brain regions, facilitating brain remodeling, and repair after ischemic stroke injury [25].

E2 induces neuronal plasticity underlying cognitive function. Acute E2 treatment promotes hippocampal neurogenesis in the female rat [26], which has been linked to hippocampal-dependent learning and memory [27]. It was revealed on rats experiments [28] that different forms of estrogens modulate neuroplasticity and cognition in complex and intriguing ways. Estrogens specifically up-regulate adult hippocampal neurogenesis (*via* cell proliferation) and synaptic protein levels in the hippocampus in a time- and dose-dependent manner [29]. Low levels of E2 facilitate spatial working memory and contextual fear conditioning, while high levels of estradiol impair spatial working, spatial reference memory and contextual fear conditioning, and estrone (E1) impairs contextual fear conditioning. The rats' experiments show that only 17β-E2 and not E1 is increasing the survival and activation of new neurons in the hippocampus in response to spatial memory compared to controls [30].

The Chinese experiments on menopausal mice had identified morphological changes in the hippocampus mitochondrial damage, lipofuscin deposition and microtubule degradation, which were possible to be partially restored: mitochondrial damage and lipofuscin increase, not the microtubules degradation, and only in early postmenopausal stages [31].

Regarding the first hypothesis on bioenergetics failure in females' brain aging, animal models demonstrated estrogens effects on mitochondria energetic metabolism. E2 is regulating mitochondrial proteome, being a key metabolic control of enzymes including pyruvate dehydrogenase, aconitase, and ATP-synthetase, and so it is a high respiratory control ratio, elevated cytochrome-c oxidase activity and expression, and it is reduced brain free radical generation [32], according to the knowledge that in aging brain is a high lactate level [30].

E2 is able to mitigate negative effects of glucocorticoids, as animal and human researches indicate: E2-related mitigation of glucocorticoid damage and interference is one benefit of E2 supplementation during perimenopause or soon after menopause. The evidence for E2-related protection against glucocorticoids suggests that maintaining E2 levels in postmenopausal women could protect them from stress-induced declines in neural and cognitive integrity [33].

Physiological doses of 17β-E2, testosterone or methyl-testosterone reduce induced cell death by 50% in neurons treated after the injection and by 80–90% in neurons treated 1 h before the injection [34]. The effect is mediated by genomic mechanisms proved by the blockage of ERs and ARs, and by a proteomic mechanism—the increasing levels of heat shock protein 70 (Hsp70), and the hormones role is to protect from the development and toxicity of the intracellular Aβ (iA1–42), which induces neuronal apoptosis and death, being known that AD starts with intraneuronal iA1–42 accumulation in human brain [35].

The "estrogen action hypothesis" known as "healthy-cell bias" elaborated in the North American Laboratories for Neuroscience Research [4, 5, 8] tries to explain the differences between the effects of estrogens on normal/healthy neurons and aged/damaged neurons. It was demonstrated with different doses (low dose of 10 ng/ml and large dose of 200 ng/ml) and on different schedules (acute vs. continuous vs. intermittent) in experiments on rats' hippocampal neurons exposed to Aβ, that is possible to prevent neurodegeneration when E2 is administered before or during Aβ exposure, the strongest effect being on continuous administration, and the effects are worsened up to neuronal death when are large doses or when Aβ is already present. These results were obtained after previous studies regarding estrogen critical different effects on synaptic system at different rats' ages. Whereas, young rats displayed a 30% increase in axospinous synapse density in CA1 [36], fact which is absent in aged rats [37], as is mentioned in **Table 2**.

There are findings in rodents and monkeys providing evidences that the hippocampus (in rats) and the frontal cortex (in monkeys) remain responsive to E2 administered either *in vivo* or *in vitro* even after prolonged periods of hormone withdrawal [38, 39]. The physiological concentrations of E2 exert profound neuroprotective action on apoptotic death cascades and neuronal death from focal and global ischemia causing selective, delayed death of hippocampal CA1 neurons and associated cognitive deficits after a single injection in acute ischemia [40]. E2 administered at physiological levels for 2 weeks before ischemia rescues neurons destined to die in the hippocampal CA1, and ameliorates ischemia-induced cognitive deficits in ovariectomized female rats [41]. An acute post-ischemic infusion of E2 into the brain ventricles is neuroprotective in aged rats after 6 months of hormone deprivation, and E2 enhances synaptic transmission in CA1 pyramidal neurons of aged long-term hormone deprived females [42].

There are evidences about distinct estrogens effects on different cognitive aspects, anxiety-like, and depressive-like behaviors. There are comparisons regarding the subregion-specific effects on tryptophan hydroxylase-2 (TpH2, the brain-specific, rate-limiting enzyme for 5-HT biosynthesis, a serotonin precursor). The comparison of CEE and E2 treatments on behavior and TpH2 mRNA on female ovariectomized Sprague Dawley rats [43]. Both CEE and E2 exert beneficial behavioral effects, although efficacy depended on the distinct behavior and for cognition, on the task difficulty. Compared to CEE, E2 generally had more robust anxiolytic and antidepressant effects. E2 increased TpH2 mRNA in the caudal and mid dorsal raphe nucleus. The recent Chinese study on adult male Sprague Dawley rats [44] demonstrated that low dose E2 administered for the first 3-months after bilateral common carotid artery occlusion (BCCAO) exerted long-lasting beneficial effects, including significant neuroprotection of hippocampal CA1 neurons and preservation of hippocampal-dependent cognitive function when examined at 6 months after BCCAO.

Recent evidences demonstrate a *de novo* estradiol synthesis within the hippocampus and other brain regions, which seems highly likely that activity-dependent estradiol signaling can play an essential role in the modulation of discrete signaling units within individual cells, affording "fine- tuned" control of neuronal excitability [45].

Animals and *in vitro* studies are demonstrating the role of estetrol (E4) on nervous system. The antioxidative actions of E4 mostly depend on ER-α and ER-β, whereas neurogenesis and possibly promyelinating activities might be realized through ER-β, and the membrane GRP30 receptor for estrogens and progesterone is less important for LDH activity and cell survival in E4 actions [46].

The animal experiments reconcile the discordance between studies showing favorable steroids/estrogen effects in neurons to the results from former randomized trials, as the largest randomized clinical trial of HT ever conducted—Women's Health Initiative Memory Study

(WHIMS), which showed that women who initiated estrogen therapy alone or in combination with the progestin MPA after the age of 60 years had a twofold greater risk to develop dementia [47] or are affected regarding mean cognitive performance over periods of time ranging up to 5 years [10], or estrogen-containing hormone therapy initiated in the late postmenopausal stage (ages 65–79 years) is followed by an increased risk of dementia and cognitive decline regardless the type of menopause—naturally, medically, or surgically induced [48].

2.1.2. Human studies

The Mayo Clinic Cohort Studies of Oophorectomy and Aging—unilateral or bilateral oophorectomy [48–50] and estrogens, before the age of menopause. The risk of cognitive impairment/dementia is increased after either unilateral or bilateral oophorectomy compared to referent women (Hazard ratio [HR] of 1.46; 95% CI 1.13 to 1.90; adjusted for education, type of interview, and history of depression). These associations were similar regardless of oophorectomy indication, and for women who underwent unilateral or bilateral oophorectomy were considered separately. The risk increased with younger age at oophorectomy (test for linear trend; adjusted $p < 0.0001$). The same study group from the Mayo Clinic showed that women who underwent bilateral oophorectomy before menopause were at increased risk of Parkinsonism, and the risk increased with younger age at time of oophorectomy [49, 50]. Their conclusion was a sizeable neuroprotective effect of estrogen before the age of 50 years.

Some studies are sustaining that estrogen neuroprotective actions are modulated by progesterone/progestogens. Specifically, continuous progestogen exposure is associated with inhibition of estrogen actions, whereas cyclic delivery of progestogens may enhance neural benefits of estrogen [51]. In the next subchapter, more evidences on these findings are discussed. The North American study [52] provides evidence at the molecular level that different regimens of HT can induce disparate gene expression profiles in brain. From a translational perspective, confirmation of these results in a model of natural menopause would imply that the common regimen of continuous combined HT may have adverse consequences, whereas a cyclic combined regimen, which is more physiological, could be an effective strategy to maintain neurological health and function. It has to be remembered that different factors may determine the efficacy of ER/HT as age, menopausal status, route of administration and dose, the starting cognitive function, and the presence of pre-existing risk factors (smoking, apolipoprotein E genotype) [53].

2.2. Progesterone neuroprotective role in women's aging

During menopausal transition on assists at lowering progesterone (P4) values by luteal defect, and afterward in perimenopause P4 which is absent, and at the beginning of the history of HT recommendations, P4 administration was mandatory for women with intact uterus, fact that continues to be actual. There were intensive efforts to develop progesterone neurobiology in the hippocampus and cortex, and current discoveries are sustaining P4 administration for more than uterine protection from endometrial hyperplasia and cancer, but for brain aging protection, besides the much analyzed "therapeutic window" of progesterone in brain trauma. P4 is active on cognition through its 5α-reduced metabolite, allopregnanolone [15, 54], a fact that differentiates P4 from the progestin MPA, which proved as a jeopardizing drug for elder postmenopausal women. P4 has neuroprotective effects mediated by various mechanisms such as reduction of neuronal vulnerability to neurotoxic molecules, reduction of cell loss, inhibition of lipid peroxidation, and expression of pro-inflammatory genes [55–57]. P4 can exert protective effects through its metabolites—allopregnanolone or 3α, 5α-tetrahydroprogesterone, the best known, which can interact with membrane-associated receptors coupled to ion-channels, such as the $GABA_A$ receptor system. P4 and allopregnanolone, exert various effects on both cognitive and non-mnemonic functions in females. Allopregnanolone may also elicit its protective effects through its actions on the mitochondria [58]. Allopregnanolone is enhancing cognitive performances and placement memory in mice, by inducing higher levels of brain-derived neurotrophic factor (BDNF) in the prefrontal cortex and hippocampus, an effect that is contrary to the lowest levels among mice administered MPA [15]. MPA—the progestin used to balance CEE in WHIMS —was proved by *in vitro* studies to be the best antagonist to neurotrophic and neuroprotective estrogen actions in neurons, fact that makes it completely different to P4 which alone is neuroprotective [59], and acts synergistic with estradiol [60]. MPA (Provera®) metabolic involvement is also divergent from P4, regarding the action on nuclear mitogen-activated protein kinase signaling [61], and on the exacerbation of neuroexcitotoxicity of glutamate [62]. The well-known object recognition task is a valuable experimental paradigm that can be used to determine the effects and mechanisms of progestogens for mnemonic effects across the lifespan. Improvements in object recognition performance of rodents are often associated with higher hormone levels in the hippocampus and prefrontal cortex during natural cycles, with progesterone replacement following ovariectomy in young animals, or with aging [54].

The estrogens neuroprotective actions are modulated by progesterone. It was demonstrated [63] in young ovariectomized mice that E2 enhances object memory consolidation, which depends on dorsal hippocampal activation of the extracellular signal-regulated kinase/mitogen-activated protein kinase (ERK/MAPK) signaling pathway, and the questions were if the E2 actions need progesterone adding, which was latter demonstrated, and more than this the effect is E2 dose-dependent [64]. It was suggested that E2 alone, and combined with P4, may influence ERK activation in different time frames or enhance memory through different mechanisms. E2 alone significantly increased phospho-p42 ERK protein levels in the dorsal hippocampus relative to vehicle controls. In contrast, no combination of E2 and P4 affected dorsal hippocampal phospho-ERK levels.

2.3. Androgens neuroprotective role in women's aging

Recent studies on normal age-related testosterone and its androgen metabolite dihydrotestosterone (DHT) loss in plasma and brain in men are emerging AD risk, and the protective role of endogenous testosterone/DHT is not only to increase the neuronal resilience against AD-related insults, but also to reduce intracellular Aβ accumulation [34, 36, 52], testosterone actions are similar, but also cumulative to those of estrogens in perimenopausal women. In perimenopause, estrogens and androgens are still in physiological levels in plasma and brain, and their presence is considered to prevent the accumulation of intracellular amyloid 1-42 (iA1-42) in the hippocampus and the entorhinal cortex neurons, preceding amyloid plaque formation, and further induction of neuronal death [65]. Proteomic analyses are demonstrating increased levels of Hsp70 in testosterone- and estrogen-treated human neurons [15], which is a sign of Aβ toxicity inhibition.

Cell cultures are bringing strong evidences that both androgens and estrogens are neuroprotective, and many studies analyzed the different pathways for neural cells protection from Aβ toxicity. Testosterone is involved in regulation of spine synapse density in the CA1 region of hippocampus [66].

A special analysis is to be made on DHEA(S)—the "youth" hormone—for which human body does not have receptors, but it is a source of intracrinology, with different enzymes for steroid-forming and/or for steroid-inactivating, permitting each cell/tissue to synthesize a small amount of androgens and/or estrogens in order to meet the local physiological needs without affecting the other tissues of the organism [67]. Blood concentrations are not different from those observed in normal postmenopausal women having high serum DHEA concentrations, when DHES is supplemented to maintain serum estrogen level at sub-threshold or biologically inactive concentrations.

On the other hand, all androgens are made intracellularly from DHEA by the mechanisms of intracrinology, and are always maintained at very low levels in the blood in pre- and postmenopausal women [67]. According to this conceptus, it was proposed a short-term DHEA supplementation (5 mg/day × 7 days) in perimenopausal female rhesus macaques [68]. The comparison of serum and hippocampal levels in treated and controls of the same age revealed that despite lower concentrations of the estrogens in the serum of elder animals, their concentrations in the hippocampus did not show any obvious differences due to age or to DHEA supplementation. The results suggest that *de novo* estrogen synthesis in the brain may compensate for the perimenopausal loss of estrogens in the circulation even without supplemental DHEA.

3. Receptors mediators of sex steroid hormone signaling mechanisms of action in neuroprotection

The sex steroids can protect through the activation of transcriptional activity in the genomic mechanism or *via* signaling of neurons survival pathways [69–71] or *via* non-genomic mechanism through membrane receptors.

More and more studies/trials are presenting new insights of sex steroids involvement in hypothalamic, hippocampal, and other brain neurons, their actions being partially common to other organs/tissues effects, but with important peculiarities. The well-known mediation *via* intracellular receptor/transcription factors that interact with steroid response elements on target genes, regarding the genomic mechanism, is doubled or tripled in the speed of alterations of the neuronal activity within seconds, indicating that some cellular effects can occur *via* membrane delimited events. Sex steroid hormone ligands bind to membrane-associated G protein-coupled receptor (GPR 30) [72], and caveolin proteins have an essential role for membrane receptors [73]. In addition, estrogens can affect metabotropic glutamate receptors, and the second messenger systems, including calcium mobilization, and a plethora of kinases to alter cell signaling. This subchapter considers the current knowledge of rapid membrane-initiated and intracellular signaling by steroids in the brain, the nature of receptors involved, and how they contribute to homeostatic functions.

3.1. Estrogen receptors (ERs). Genetic polymorphism and epigenetics of ERs

The protective role of estrogens in the brain is sure, and the missing preventive effects revealed by RCT is connected to the age-related changes of ERs, as it is in the endometrium/uterus [74], suggesting that several key players in the local synaptic response to E2 are compromised in aging females. The brain has one of the most complex and complicated ERs network of the body, which is changing life-long. In addition to its well-documented hormonal action, E2 is considered as a neurotransmitter in the brain [75].

In the last 10 years, molecular and biochemical animal studies are demonstrating that the mechanisms used by estrogens are greatly influenced by brain cell type, ER type, and metabotropic glutamate receptors (mGluRs) independent of glutamate, and/or region of the brain-cortex and/or hippocampus, all these leading to differential regulation of neuronal circuitry in each area [45, 76]. The hippocampus cognitive performance is directly connected to ER-α, other ERs such as ER-β and GPR30 [8]. The ERs have similar distribution in female and male brains, but may differ in relative expression [77]. ER-α and ER-β expression patterns generally overlap, where ER-α is associated with reproductive behavior, whereas ER-β is associated with non-reproductive behaviors such as learning and memory [78] and anxiety-related behaviors. In hippocampus and cortical neurons, the estrogens—mainly E2 and other estrogenic ligands bind to membrane—associated and mitochondrial-associated G protein-coupled receptor (GPR 30), and activates the classical/canonical nuclear and extranuclear or intra-cytoplasmatic ER isoforms—α and β—functioning as transcription factors [79–81], and a new type of nuclear ER, the orphan estrogen-related receptor γ (ERR γ), which regulates dopaminergic neuronal phenotype [82], and IGF-1 receptor, which was recently recognized as a receptor for estrogens.

The nongenomic or alternative signaling pathways mechanism involving extranuclear ERs respond to physiological concentration of estrogens to elicit neuroprotection, resulting in the "fine tuning" of neuronal circuitry [45]. Often, rapid activation of intracellular signalers such as mitogen-activated protein kinase (MAPK) or phosphatidylinositol-3-kinase (PI3K) underlie alternative estrogen-induced neuroprotection upon activation of specific binding sites at the plasma membrane. The plasma membrane ER (mER) originates from, or is related to canonical nuclear ERs, and GPR30 mimics short latency E2 facilitation of synaptic transmission in the hippocampus, to enhance memory and cognition [83]. The activation of GPR30 by G-1 (its specific ligand) is associated with a mobilization of calcium in dissociated and cultured rat hypothalamic neurons [80, 84, 85]. There were elaborated cellular models of Aβ toxicity where classical and alternative pathways activated by estrogens seem to coexist to orchestrate neuroprotection, fact that is a unique signaling profile of estrogen neuroprotection, dependent upon activation of the MAPK signaling [86].

ER-α and ER-β mediate the effects of E2 on both intracellular signaling and gene transcription, sharing similar domain organization, and using almost identical DNA-binding elements, co-regulators, and transcription machinery. There are differences between ER-labeled regarding each female, species (rats, non-human primates, human), age (young, old), estrogen levels, brain reference area, vulnerability of spines/synapses based on size (large or small), or presynaptic/postsynaptic location of ER. Both, ER-α and ER-β are located predominantly at extranuclear sites; ER-α are found in dendritic spines, many originating from pyramidal cells, axons, terminals, astrocytes, and microglia [81], in symmetric and asymmetric synapses. ER-β is detected on or near the plasma membrane of somata and dendritic shafts and spines in hippocampal neurons [81], in axons and axon terminals and both in the cytoplasm and on endomembranes near mitochondria *in vivo* [81], and within mitochondria *in vitro*, in pyramidal cells, in newly generated cells in a few interneurons and in glia [81]. Changes in ER-β expression occur in the presynaptic membrane, cleft, and postsynaptic membranes, where neurotransmitter release and postsynaptic receptor binding occurs. Conversely, ER-α changes are detected presynaptically in synaptic vesicles and postsynaptically in plasmalemmal and cytoplasmic regions of spine heads where protein translation occurs. In aged animals, it was demonstrated for the first time [78] that the window for E2-mediated benefits on cognition and hippocampal E2 responsiveness can be reinstated by increased expression of ER-α.

Studies have determined that membrane-localized ER-α and ER-β are capable of activating multiple metabotropic glutamate receptors (mGluRs) independent of glutamate, leading to downstream second messenger signaling [73, 76]. The expression of ER-α and ER-β mRNA in the hippocampus is limited [87], and GPR30 may be the major receptor subtype by which estrogen produces its enhancing effects. The physiological consequence of activation of GPR30 can regulate local synthesis pathways in a novel direction of our understanding of rapid estrogen signaling within the brain and its ability to induce the "fine-tuning" of neuronal circuits [45]. E2 works as a neuroprotector by membrane receptors coupled to E2 induction of intracellular $Ca^{(2+)}$ influx *via* the L-type channels, connected to memory mechanisms, and through Src/ERK/cyclic AMP response element-binding protein activation in single hippocampal neurons [88]. The presence of the L-type Ca (2+) channel inhibitor, nifedipine (10 microM), partially inhibits 17 β E2 [89].

It was discovered an aging decrease of about 50% of ER-α-labeled synapses [37, 45], with alteration in the ratio of ER-β to ER-α, fact that contributes to age-related decreases in the capacity to form additional spines and synapses in response to E2 in rats. In addition, synaptic pAkt thought is activated by ER-α [90], which is also decreased dramatically in aged CA1 axospinous synapses [91], as is ER-β [92], suggesting that several key players in the local synaptic response to E2 are compromised with age in female rats.

It was reported for the first time in Mont Sinai University (New-York, USA) [93] that in the monkey's neocortex 46, approximately 50% of the axospinous synapses contains ER-α, with axon terminals more likely to have ER-α than spines, and that presynaptic ER-α was often associated with vesicles, whereas postsynaptic ER-α was widely distributed in the PSD, adjacent to the PSD, and in the spine core.

The duration of brain's estrogen deprivation is connected to C terminus of heat shock cognate protein (Hsc) 70-interacting protein (CHIP)-mediated proteasomal degradation of hippocampal estrogen receptor-α in conditions of rats' global ischemia, or of aging hippocampal CA1 region [9]. Natural aging is associated with increased ER-α and ER-β CHIP binding and ubiquitination, and with decreased ER-α and ER-β levels in the hippocampal CA1 region, fact that is different from the aging uterus in the rat model of long-term E2 deprivation (LTED) or after ovariectomy, where the level of ER *via* the ubiquitin-proteasome degradation pathway is increasing after estrogen exposure [9].

The studies on rats and monkeys [39] from Mount Sinai School of Medicine (New York, USA) have emerged three key findings: (1) synaptic ER-α is present in axospinous synapses in monkeys dorsolateral prefrontal cortex, in area 46; (2) it is stable across treatment and age groups (which is not the case in rat hippocampus); and (3) the abundance and distribution of synaptic ER-α is a key correlate of individual variation in cognitive performance in certain age and treatment groups.

Another interesting and important findings about rats cortex are that ER-α can modulate synaptic function and behavior even in the absence of circulating gonadal E2, in response to E2 synthesized within neurons [94], and that ER-α may initiates the non-genomic signaling mechanisms modulating synaptic plasticity in the hippocampus in response to either circulating or locally synthesized E2 [39, 93]. These findings are considered of great importance for the design of HT strategies for both surgically and naturally menopausal women.

The detected levels of ERs in postmortem brain tissue of AD patients is related to the severity of cognitive impairment assessed proximate to death, and only the reduction of ER-α from frontal cortex is correlated to Mini-Mental State Examination score, not the ER-β [95]. The spectrometry, immunohistochemistry, and quantitative real-time PCR of the autopsied Japanese AD patients compared to controls [96] have revealed a glial nuclear ER-β expression significantly lower in white matter in the AD group vs. controls, without any significant differences in estrogen concentrations, and the conclusion was that estrogens have effects on glias and neurons in the etiology of AD, and the correlation between BMI and estrogen concentrations in the frontal lobe suggests the importance of non-brain sources of estrogens particularly in controls.

Long-term E2 treatment initiated 14 days prior to global ischemia in ovariectomized female rats demonstrated that E2 at near physiological concentrations acts *via* the IGF-1 receptor to protect the functional integrity of hippocampal CA1 neurons and synapses in conditions of global ischemia, but not the classical ER-α or β. [97]. The transactivation of IGF-1 receptors and stimulation of ERK/MAPK signaling pathway maintains CREB activity in the ischemic CA1.

All three types of ERs cooperate in neuroprotection against AD [98], in association to intracellular calcium signaling cascade, which is very important, and the ER-α is the central key, for maintaining channel inactivation and may be relevant in neuronal preservation against Aβ injury. It was demonstrated that combination of ERm and caveolin in caveolae, and ER-α-mediated inhibition of Death domain-associated protein translocation may protect neurons against Aβ injury. ER-α and IGF-IR co-activation may mediate neuroprotection, and many other growth factors and intracellular signaling responses triggered by ER-α may play important roles in the process [98].These data are crucial for contemporary societies, with high risks for diabetes mellitus, in all populations. A very recent study from the University of Missouri,

St. Louis (USA) [99] demonstrated the neuroprotection of the coupling of IGF1 to estrogens and/androgens. It is considered that both steroids are involved in many neuroprotective processes that operate on similar signaling cascades [100].

Another tested hypothesis is upon GPR30 that act together with intracellular estrogen receptors to activate cell signaling pathways to promote hippocampal neuron survival after global ischemia [101]. E2 at physiological concentrations intervenes in apoptotic death cascades and ameliorates neuronal death, increasing BCL-2 expression in rat hippocampal neurons [88] (in experimental models of focal and global ischemia), but the proper mechanism is still unclear.

Regarding ERs, there are new details about the genes, and mRNA variants of ER-α expressed in different parts of the human brain, and there are specific ER-α mRNA splice variants or isoforms of ER-α in the medial mammillary nucleus (MMN) in AD [102] or in the frontal cortex in AD patients [95], and their relationship to cognitive impairment.

There are some therapeutic indications for cognition and memory support, which are partially controversial. The first is regarding the benefits from the upregulation of the expression of ER-α, but not of ER-β, in the hippocampus of aged animals, in order to restore the potential of E2 treatments and rejuvenate E2-induced hippocampal plasticity [78]. The second are from the results of a multinational study [103] sustaining the beneficial effects of long-term treatment with diarylpropionitrile (DPN, 0.05 mg/kg/day, sc.), a selective ER-β agonist, on the hippocampal transcriptome in ovariectomized, middle-aged (13 months) rats. The results reveal the contribution of ER-β-mediated processes to the regulation of transcription, translation, neurogenesis, neuromodulation, and neuroprotection in the hippocampal formation, and the authors concluded that the findings are supporting the notion that selective activation of ER-β may be a viable approach for treating the neural symptoms of E2 deficiency in menopause. There are studies suggesting that DPN—a selective ER-β agonist—mimics many basic effects of E2 in the hippocampus and enhance mice's hippocampus-dependent spatial memory [104, 105].

Recent studies are involving the genetic polymorphism of ERs, especially of ER-β in cognitive impairment and increased risk for AD predominantly in women [106]. It was examined that the role of single nucleotide polymorphisms (SNP) in the ERs genes: rs9340799, rs2234693, rs2228480 (in the ESR1 gene), and rs4986938 (in the ESR2 gene) as a risk factor for amnesic mild cognitive impairment (MCI) and AD. The less represented alleles of SNPs studied are associated with MCI and AD in women APOEε4 allele carriers [107, 108]. Some studies are focusing the association of Eε4 allele of apolipoprotein E gene to obesity, inflammation, and the risk of AD. Although, the pathways underlying this relationship are unclear the sex steroid hormones may be the connection [109, 110].

The epigenetic processes are associated to brain aging. The post-translational histone changes and DNA methylation are modulating the hippocampal memory-enhancing effects of E2 [111, 112].

3.2. Progesterone receptors

P4 has neuroprotective effects mediated by various mechanisms P4 or its metabolites-regulated neural responses are mediated by an array of progesterone receptors (PRs) which are broadly expressed throughout the brain, inclusive the hippocampus, and can be detected in every neural cell type [113]. There are known the classic nuclear PR-A (the N-terminally truncated form of PR-B) and PR-B receptors, and splice variants of each, explaining the P4 genomic mechanism of action through specific progesterone response elements (PRE) within the promoter region of target genes to regulate transcription of the genes [114], and the two types of cell surface-associated proteins [membrane PRs (mPRs) and the progesterone membrane receptor component (PGMRC)].These PRs induce classic regulation of gene expression while also transducing signaling cascades that originate at the cell membrane and ultimately activate transcription factors. As for estrogens the genomic and non-genomic mechanisms of P4 are coupled, so the distinctions are not as clear-cut as was first thought [115]. The nuclear PRs are up-regulated by E2 in glial and neural cells, but more in the glial cells, implicating crucial progenitor cells, as preferential targets of P4 [116] (**Figures 1** and **2**).

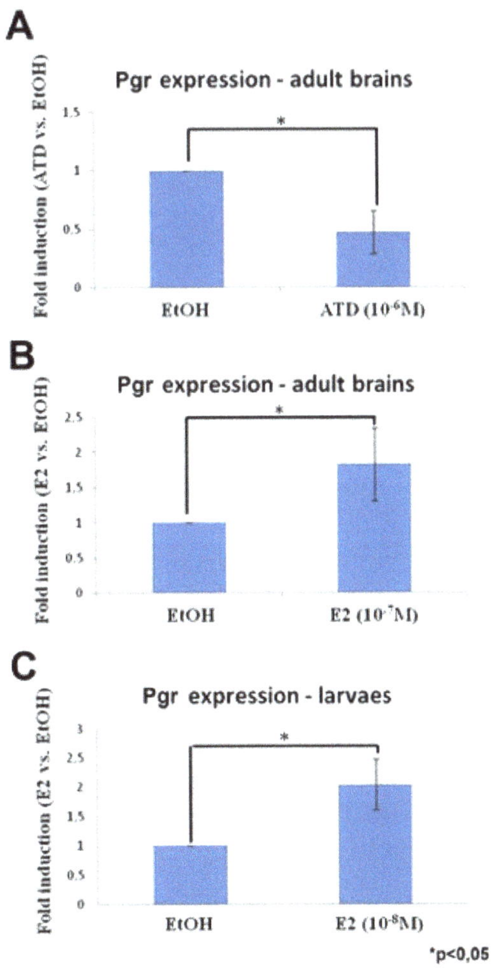

Figure 1. Progesterone nuclear receptor (pgr) is upregulated by estrogen. Experiments on developing and adult brain of zebrafish, and larvae. Legend: Fold induction of P4 expression after treatment of adult zebrafish with an aromatase inhibitor (A, 10^{-6} M of ATD) or estradiol (B, 10^{-7} M of 17β-estradiol), and larvae with E2 (C, 10^{-8} M of 17β-estradiol). The graphs present the mean value +/– the standard deviation. Asterisk (*) indicates significant differences ($p < 0.05$, Student's t test). **Panel A:** the aromatase inhibitor (ATD) leads to a significant decrease of *pgr* expression in individual brains of adult zebrafish (n = 4). **Panel B**, the estrogenic treatment leads to a significant increase of *pgr* expression in pools of 5 brains of adult zebrafish (n = 3). **Panel C**: the estrogenic treatment leads to a significant increase of *pgr* expression in pool of 20 larvae (n = 2).

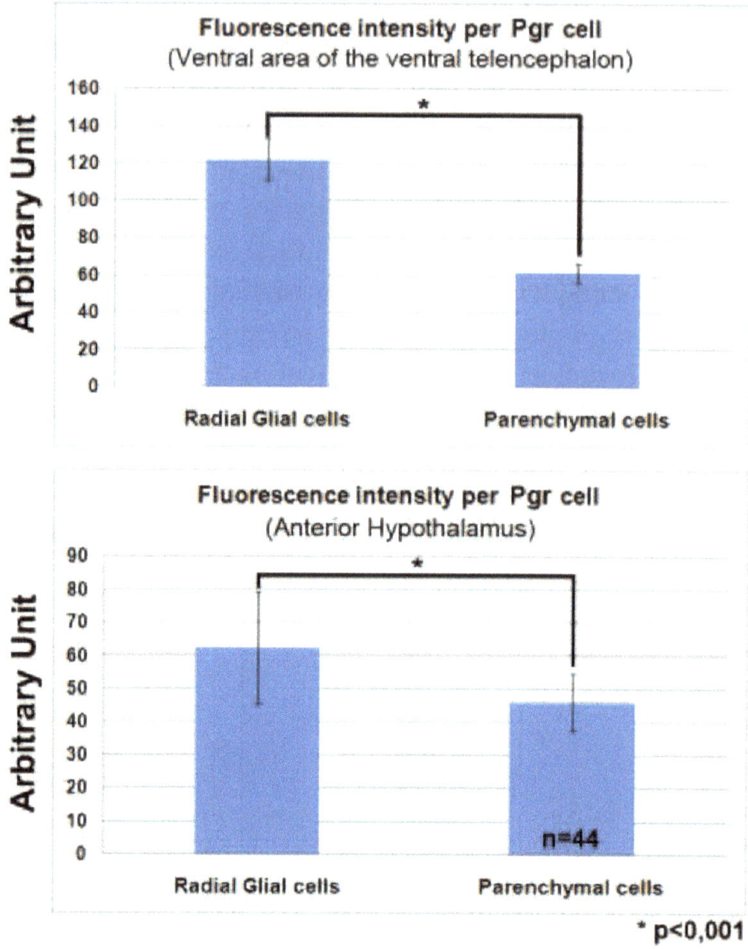

Figure 2. Experiments on Zebrafish hypothalamicP4 receptors. *Legend*: Analysis of the P4 staining intensity in the ventral subpallium and in the anterior hypothalamus revealing a stronger intensity (mean value +/− the standard deviation).in the radial cells than neural cells ($p < 0.001$ Student's t test). **Figures 1** and **2** are adapted from [116].

PR-A is exerting a negative control on PR-B-mediated transcription, and the mediated transcription of the ER and glucocorticoid receptors [117], fact that may underlie, at least in part, the mechanism by which progesterone functionally antagonize the effects of estrogen. PRA and PRB can interact as dimers with DNA progesterone responsive element, and with signaling proteins of the Src/Ras/Erk pathway outside the nucleus [118]. The "non-genomic" mechanisms explains the non-reproductive P4 actions, the rapid activation of cytoplasmic kinase signaling that can result in both transcription-independent and transcription-dependent effects. These "non-genomic" actions can be partially explained by membrane transport *via* nuclear receptor [119]. The mPRs (molecular mass of approximately 40 kDa) had thought to be comprised of three subtypes, mPR α, β, and γ, which belong to the seven-transmembrane domain adiponectin Q receptor (PAQR) family, plus two newly discovered subtypes (mPRδ, and mPRε) [120]. It was shown that cDNAs for the mPRα subtypes of spotted seatrout (st-mPRalpha) and humans (hu-mPRα-) encode progesterone/progestin receptors that display many functional characteristics of G protein-coupled receptors [121], and that mPRβ promotes progesterone-dependent neurite outgrowth in PC12 neuronal cells *via* non-G protein-coupled receptor (GPCR) signaling [122]. Progesterone receptor membrane component-1 (PGRMC-1) and PGRMC-2, with a single-transmembrane domain protein, are mediating the rapid non-genomic effects of E2 and P4, such as the activation of MAPK signaling and intracellular Ca^{2+} increase [123, 124] mPRβ activates also MAPK cascade, without GPCR signaling, and progesterone-stimulated mPRβ activation did not exhibit the elevation of $[Ca^{2+}]$ [121]. In comparison to the mPRs, the single-transmembrane protein Pgrmc1 (molecular mass 25–28 kDa) and the related Pgrmc2 are a part of a multi-protein complex that binds to P4, other steroids, and to pharmaceutical compounds [123]. Besides the location to membrane surface, Pgrmc1 was reported to have subcellular localization: in endoplasmic reticulum, Golgi apparatus, and nuclei [125].

PRs are differentially expressed in neurons, in oligodendrocytes, astrocytes, and reactive microglia, the mPRα expression is observed in oligodendrocytes, astrocytes, and reactive microglia. The increase in mPR expression was proposed to mediate the anti-inflammatory effects of progesterone under conditions of injury [126].

The classical PR and mPRs have overlapping regional expression (e.g., both are expressed in the hippocampus, cortex, hypothalamus, and cerebellum), but their profile of ligand specificity is not identical [126]. The "non-classical/non-genomic" effects of P4 can be initiated rapidly at the cell surface to activate intracellular signaling pathways, through modulation of putative cell surface receptors, ion channels, and cytoplasmic second messenger cascades, the rapid activation of cytoplasmic kinase signaling can result in both transcription-independent and transcription-dependent effects.

Among the rapid non-genomic signaling pathways activated by P4 are the extracellular signal-related kinase (ERK) pathways [127], cAMP/protein kinase A (PKA) signaling [128], PKG signaling [129], Ca^{2+} influx/PKC activation [130], phosphatidylinositol 3-kinases (PI3 K)/Akt pathway [124], and other signal transduction cascades. P4 or its metabolites can act directly and rapidly on neurotransmitter receptors as the GABA-A receptor [131] and Sigma-1/2 receptors [132] to regulate cellular function.

The consequences of activation of these signaling pathways are numerous and include influences on neurotrophin release [125], neural progenitor proliferation, regulation of intracellular Ca^{2+} levels, and regulation of cell viability [57, 127, 131] all of which can contribute to the overall health and function of the brain.

3.3. Androgens mechanisms in neuroprotection

Androgen neuroprotective effects are mediated both directly by activation of androgen receptors (ARs) pathways, and indirectly by aromatization to estradiol and initiation of protective estrogen signaling mechanisms, but this last action is not totally accepted [133–135]. The knowledge on the effects of testosterone on women cognitive capacities are few.

Testosterone protects primary human neurons against serum deprivation [134], cultured rat hippocampal neurons against extracellular Aβ toxicity [136], rat neurons against heat shock-mediated hyperphosphorylation of tau by modulating glycogen synthase kinase 3 activation [85], cerebellar granule neurons against oxidative stress [133], and rat hippocampal neurons against kainic acid-induced toxicity [135] transiently activate mitogen-activated protein kinase (MAPK) in cultured hippocampal neurons, as evidenced by phosphorylation of extracellular signal-regulated kinase (ERK)-1 and ERK-2 and by this effect subsequently drives neuroprotection [137].

4. Perspectives

Brain aging and neurodegenerative diseases have a multifactorial nature, metabolic and inflammatory changes from the moment of transition to menopause, blood-brain barrier disruption, and aberrant microglial activation can be modulated or prevented in a moment prior to their onset in the "critical period of opportunity," if the clinicians and the patients are both interested and have a good understanding of very early perimenopausal symptoms. The differences between estrogen types, between progesterone and progestins, between the classes of steroid receptors agonists—NeuroSERMs (novel neuro-selective estrogen receptor modulator) and PhytoSERMs (phyto-selective estrogen receptor modulator), and the new molecules tested in high-tech laboratories, will help the clinicians to recommend the best neurotrophic, neuroprotective molecule without any breast or uterine harmful action.

Author details

Manuela Cristina Russu[1]* and Alexandra Cristina Antonescu[2]

*Address all correspondence to: manuela_russu@yahoo.com

1 "Dr. I. Cantacuzino" Clinic of Obstetrics and Gynecology, "Carol Davila" University of Medicine and Pharmacy, Bucharest, Romania

2 Intromed Laboratories, Bucharest, Romania

References

[1] Rettberg JR, Yao J, Brinton RD. Estrogen: A master regulator of bioenergetic systems in the brain and body. Frontiers in Neuroendocrinology. 2014;**35**(1):8-30. DOI: 10.1016

[2] Maki PM, Resnick SM. Longitudinal effects of estrogen replacement therapy on PET cerebral blood flow and cognition. Neurobiology of Aging. 2000;**21**(2):373-383

[3] Kawas C, Resnick S, Morrison A, et al. A prospective study of estrogen replacement therapy and the risk of developing Alzheimer's disease: The Baltimore Longitudinal Study of Aging. Neurology. 1997;**48**(6):1517-1521

[4] Brinton RD. Investigative models for determining hormone therapy-induced outcomes in brain: Evidence in support of a healthy cell bias of estrogen action. Annals of the New York Academy of Sciences. 2005;**1052**:57-74

[5] Chen S, Nilsen J, Brinton RD. Dose and temporal pattern of estrogen exposure determines neuroprotective outcome in hippocampal neurons: Therapeutic implications. Endocrinology. 2006;**147**(11):5303-5313. DOI: 10.1210/en.2006-049

[6] Barha CK, Galea LA. Influence of different estrogens on neuroplasticity and cognition in the hippocampus. Biochimica et Biophysica Acta. 2010;**1800**(10):1056-1067. DOI: 10.1016/j.bbagen.2010.01.006 S632–S633

[7] Morrison JH, Brinton RD, Schmidt PJ, Gore AC. Estrogen, menopause, and the aging brain: How basic neuroscience can inform hormone therapy in women. The Journal of Neuroscience. 2006;**26**:10332-10348

[8] Brinton RD. Estrogen regulation of glucose metabolism and mitochondrial function: Therapeutic implications for prevention of Alzheimer's disease. Advanced Drug Delivery Reviews. 2008;**60**(13–14):1504-1511. DOI: 10.1016/j.addr.2008.06.003

[9] Zhang QG, Han D, Wang R, Dong Y, Yanf F, Vadlamudi KR, Brann WD. C terminus of Hsc70-interacting protein (CHIP)-mediated degradation of hippocampal estrogen receptor-α and the critical period hypothesis of estrogen neuroprotection. Proceedings of the National Academy of Sciences of the United States of America. 2011;**108**:E617-E624

[10] Henderson VW. Cognition and cognitive aging. Climacteric. 2007;**10**(Suppl 2):88-91

[11] Scott E, Zhang QG, Brann D, et al. Estrogen neuroprotection and the critical period hypothesis. Frontiers in Neuroendocrinology. 2012;**33**(1):85-104. DOI: 10.1016/j.yfrne.2011.10.001

[12] Sherwin BB. Estrogen therapy: Is time of initiation critical for neuroprotection? Nature Reviews. Endocrinology. 2000;**5**:620-627

[13] Sherwin BB. The critical period hypothesis: Can it explain discrepancies in the oestrogen-cognition literature? Journal of Neuroendocrinology. 2007;**19**:77-81

[14] Dye VR, Miller JK, Singer JE, Levine JA Hormone replacement therapy and risk for neurodegenerative diseases. International Journal of Alzheimer's Disease 2012; 18 pgs; Ed: K. S. Jagannatha Rao. Article ID 258454, doi.org/10.1155/2012/258454

[15] Frye CA, Koonce CJ, Walf AA. Progesterone, compared to medroxyprogesterone acetate, to C57BL/6, but not 5α-reductase mutant, mice enhances object recognition and placement memory and is associated with higher BDNF levels in the hippocampus and cortex. Neuroscience Letters. 2013;**551**:53-57. DOI: 10.1016/j.neulet.2013.07.002

[16] Sherwin BB, Phillips SJ. Estrogen and cognitive functioning in surgically menopausal women. Annals of the New York Academy of Sciences. 1990;**592**:474-475

[17] Nappi ER, Sinforiani E, Nappi G, et al. Memory functioning at menopause: Impact of age in ovariectomized women. Gynecologic and Obstetric Investigation. 1999;**47**:29-36

[18] Vearncombe KJ, Pachana NA. Is cognitive functioning detrimentally affected after early, induced menopause? Menopause. 2009;**16**(1):188-198. DOI: 10.1097

[19] Fogle RH, Stanczyk FZ, Zhang X, Paulson RJ. Ovarian androgen production in postmenopausal women. The Journal of Clinical Endocrinology and Metabolism. 2007;**92**: 3040-3043

[20] Davison SL, Bell R, Davis SR, et al. Androgen levels in adult females: Changes with age, menopause, and oophorectomy. The Journal of Clinical Endocrinology and Metabolism. 2005;**90**:3847-3853

[21] Pitkin J, Rees MC, Stevenson JC, et al. Management of premature menopause. Menopause International. 2007;**13**:44-45

[22] Pines A, Sturdee DW, Birkhauser MH, Schneider HP, Gambacciani M, et al. For the Board of the International Menopause S—IMS updated recommendations on postmenopausal hormone therapy. Climacteric. 2007;**10**:181-194

[23] Utian WH, Archer DF, Heiman JR, et al. Estrogen and progestogen use in postmenopausal women: July 2008 position statement of The North American Menopause Society. Menopause. 2008;**15**:584-602

[24] Dumitriu D, Rapp PR, BS ME, Morrison JH. Estrogen and the aging brain: An elixir for the weary cortical network. Annals of the New York Academy of Sciences. 2010;**1204**: 104-112. DOI: 10.1111/j.1749-6632.2010.05529

[25] Suzuki S, Gerhold LM, Wise PM, et al. Estradiol enhances neurogenesis following ischemic stroke through estrogen receptors alpha and beta. The Journal of Comparative Neurology. 2007;**500**(6):1064-1075

[26] Barker JM, Galea LA. Repeated estradiol administration alters different aspects of neurogenesis and cell death in the hippocampus of female, but not male, rats. Neuroscience. 2008;**152**:888-902

[27] Shors TJ, Townsend DA, Gould E, et al. Neurogenesis may relate to some but not all types of hippocampal-dependent learning. Hippocampus. 2002;**12**:578-584

[28] Barha CK, Dalton GL, Galea LA. Low doses of 17alpha-estradiol and 17beta-estradiol facilitate, whereas higher doses of estrone and 17alpha- and 17beta-estradiol impair, contextual fear conditioning in adult female rats. Neuropsychopharmacology. 2010; **35**(2):547-559. DOI: 10.1038/npp.2009.161

[29] McClure RE, Barha CK, Galea LA. 17β-Estradiol, but not estrone, increases the survival and activation of new neurons in the hippocampus in response to spatial memory in adult female rats. Hormones and Behavior. 2013;**63**(1):144-157. DOI: 10.1016/j.yhbeh.2012.09.011

[30] Ross JM, Oberg J, Terzioglu M, et al. High brain lactate is a hallmark of aging and caused by a shift in the lactate dehydrogenase A/B ratio. Proceedings of the National Academy of Sciences of the United States of America. 2010;**107**(46):20087-20092. DOI: 10.1073/ pnas.1008189107

[31] Yan Y, Cheng L, Chen X, Ai J, et al. Estrogen deficiency is associated with hippocampal morphological remodeling of early postmenopausal mice. Oncotarget. 2017;**8**(13):21892-21902. DOI: 10.18632

[32] Nilsen J, Irwin RW, Brinton RD, et al. Estradiol in vivo regulation of brain mitochondrial proteome. The Journal of Neuroscience. 2007;**27**(51):14069-14077. DOI: 10.1523

[33] Herrera AY, Mather M. Actions and interactions of estradiol and glucocorticoids in cognition and the brain: Implications for aging women. Neuroscience and Biobehavioral Reviews. 2015;**55**:36-52

[34] Zhang Y, Champagne N, Beitel KL, Goodyer GC, Trifiro M, LeBlanc A. Estrogen and androgen protection of human neurons against intracellular amyloid toxicity through heat shock protein 70. The Journal of Neuroscience. 2004;**24**(23):5315-5321

[35] Gouras GK, Tsai J, Relkin NR, et al. Intraneuronal Abeta 42 accumulation in human brain. The American Journal of Pathology. 2000;**156**:15-20

[36] Gould E, Woolley CS, McEwen BS, et al. Gonadal steroids regulate dendritic spine density in hippocampal pyramidal cells in adulthood. The Journal of Neuroscience. 1990;**10**:1286-1291

[37] Adams MM, Fink SE, Milner TA, McEwen BS, Morrison JH, et al. Estrogen and aging affect the subcellular distribution of estrogen receptor-alpha in the hippocampus of female rats. The Journal of Neuroscience. 2002;**22**:3608-3614

[38] Markowska AL, Savonenko AV. Effectiveness of estrogen replacement in restoration of cognitive function after long-term estrogen withdrawal in aging rats. The Journal of Neuroscience. 2002;**22**:10985-10995

[39] Bailay ME, Wang AC, Morrison JH, et al. Interactive effects of age and estrogen on cortical neurons: Implications for cognitive aging. Neuroscience. 2011;**191**:148-158. DOI: 10.1016/j.neuroscience.2011.05.045

[40] Lebesgue D, Chevalevre V, Zukin RS, Etgen AM. Estradiol rescues neurons from global ischemia-induced cell death: multiple cellular pathways of neuroprotection. Steroids. 2009;**74**(7):555-561. DOI: 10.1016

[41] Etgen AM, Inagaki T. Neuroprotective action of acute estrogens: Animal models of brain ischemia and clinical implications. Steroids. 2013;**78**(6):597-606. DOI: 10.1016

[42] Inagaki T, Kanedo N, Etgen AM, et al. Estradiol attenuates ischemia-induced death of hippocampal neurons and enhances synaptic transmission in aged, long-term hormone-deprived female rats. PLoS One. 2012;**7**(6):e38018. DOI: 10.1371

[43] Hiroi R, Weyrich G, Bimonte- Nelson HA, et al. Benefits of hormone therapy estrogens depend on estrogen type: 17β-estradiol and conjugated equine estrogens have differential effects on cognitive, anxiety-like, and depressive-like behaviors and increase tryptophan hydroxylase-2 mRNA levels in dorsal raphe nucleus subregions. Frontiers in Neuroscience. 2016;**10**:517. DOI: 10.3389/fnins.2016.00517

[44] Zhu Y, Zhang Q, Wang R, et al. Protective effect of 17β-estradiol upon hippocampal spine density and cognitive function in an animal model of vascular dementia. Scientific Reports. 2017;**7**:42660. DOI: 10.1038/srep42660

[45] Srivastava PD, Waters ME, Liu F, et al. Rapid estrogen signaling in the brain: Implications for the fine-tuning of neuronal circuitry. The Journal of Neuroscience. 2011;**31**(45): 16056-16063

[46] Tskitishvili E, Pequeux C, Foidart JM, et al. Estrogen receptors and estetrol-dependent neuroprotective actions: a pilot study. The Journal of Endocrinology. 2017;**232**(1):85-95

[47] Shumaker SA, Legault C, Wactawski-Wende J, et al. Estrogen plus progestin and the incidence of dementia and mild cognitive impairment in postmenopausal women: The Women's Health Initiative Memory Study: A randomized controlled trial. JAMA. 2003; **289**:2651-2662

[48] Rocca WA, Grossardt BR, Shuster LT. Oophorectomy, estrogen, and dementia: A 2014 update. Molecular and Cellular Endocrinology. 2014;**389**(1–2):7-12. DOI: 10.1016/j.mce.2014.01.020

[49] Rocca WA, Bower JH, Melton LJ 3rd, et al. Increased risk of cognitive impairment or dementia in women who underwent oophorectomy before menopause. Neurology. 2007;**69**(11):1074-1083

[50] Rocca WA, Shuster LT, Grossardt BR, et al. Long-term effects of bilateral oophorectomy on brain aging: Unanswered questions from the Mayo Clinic Cohort Study of Oophorectomy and Aging. Women's Health (London, England). 2009;**5**:39-48

[51] Pike CJ, Carroll JC, Rosario ER, Barron AM. Protective actions of sex steroid hormones in Alzheimer's disease. Frontiers in Neuroendocrinology. 2009;**30**(2):239-258. DOI: 10.1016/j.yfrne.2009.04.015

[52] Zhao L, Morgan ET, Brinton RD, et al. Continuous versus cyclic progesterone exposure differentially regulates hippocampal gene expression and functional profiles. PLoS One. 2012;**7**:e31267. DOI: 10.1371

[53] MacLusky NJ. Estrogen and Alzheimer's disease: The apolipoprotein connection. Endocrinology. 2004;**145**:3062-3064

[54] Walf AA, Koonce CJ, Frye CA. Progestogens' effects and mechanisms for object recognition memory across the lifespan. Behavioural Brain Research. 2015;**294**:50-61. DOI: 10.1016/j.bbr.2015.07.057

[55] Goodman Y, Bruce AJ, Cheng B, Mattson MP. Estrogens attenuate and corticosterone exacerbates excitotoxicity, oxidative injury, and amyloid beta-peptide toxicity in hippocampal neurons. Journal of Neurochemistry. 1996;**66**:1836-1844

[56] Schumacher M, Guennoun R, Stein DG, De Nicola AF. Progesterone: Therapeutic opportunities for neuroprotection and myelin repair. Pharmacology & Therapeutics. 2007;**116**:77-106

[57] Pluchino N, Cubeddu A, Giannini A, Merlini S, Cela V, et al. Progestogens and brain: An update. Maturitas. 2009;**62**:349-355

[58] Robertson CL, Puskar A, Hoffman GE, Murphy AZ, et al. Physiologic progesterone reduces mitochondrial dysfunction and hippocampal cell loss after traumatic brain injury in female rats. Experimental Neurology. 2006;**197**:235-243. DOI: 10.1016

[59] Brinton RD, Nilsen J. Effects of estrogen plus progestin on risk of dementia. JAMA. 2003; **290**:1706

[60] Nilsen J, Deng J, Brinton RD. Impact of clinically relevant progestins on the neural effects of estradiol and the signaling pathways involved. Drug News & Perspectives. 2005;**18**: 545-553

[61] Nilsen J, Brinton RD. Divergent impact of progesterone and medroxyprogesterone acetate (Provera) on nuclear mitogen-activated protein kinase signaling. Proceedings of the National Academy of Sciences of the United States of America. 2003;**100**:10506-10511

[62] Nilsen J, Morales A, Brinton RD. Medroxyprogesterone acetate exacerbates glutamate excitotoxicity. Gynecological Endocrinology. 2006;**22**:355-361

[63] Fernandez SM, Lewis MC, Frick KM, et al. Estradiol-induced enhancement of object memory consolidation involves hippocampal extracellular signal-regulated kinase activation and membrane-bound estrogen receptors. The Journal of Neuroscience. 2008;**28**: 8660-8667

[64] Harburger LL, Saadi A, Frick KM. Dose-dependent effects of post-training estradiol plus progesterone treatment on object memory consolidation and hippocampal extracellular signal-regulated kinase activation in young ovariectomized mice. Neuroscience. 2009; **160**(1):6-12. DOI: 10.1016/j.neuroscience.2009.02.024

[65] Takahashi RH, Milner TA, Li F, Gouras GK, et al. Intraneuronal Alzheimer abeta 42 accumulates in multivesicular bodies and is associated with synaptic pathology. The American Journal of Pathology. 2002;**161**:1869-1879

[66] Leonard TS, Winsauer JP. The effects of gonadal hormones on learning and memory in male mammals: A review. Current Zoology. 2011;**57**(4):543-558

[67] Labrie E. All sex steroids are made intracellularly in peripheral tissues by the mechanisms of intracrinology after menopause. The Journal of Steroid Biochemistry and Molecular Biology. 2015;**145**:133-138. DOI: 10.1016

[68] Urbanski HF, Sorwell KG, Prokai L, Kohama SG. Effect of short-term DHEA supplementation on serum and hippocampal estrogen concentrations in perimenopausal female rhesus macaques. Neurobiology of Aging. 2017;**55**:172-174. DOI: 10.1016

[69] Segars JH, Driggers PH. Estrogen action and cytoplasmic signaling cascades. Part I: Membrane-associated signaling complexes. Trends in Endocrinology and Metabolism. 2002;**13**:349-354

[70] Driggers PH, Segars JH. Estrogen action and cytoplasmic signaling pathways. Part II: The role of growth factors and phosphorylation in estrogen signaling. Trends in Endocrinology and Metabolism. 2002;**13**:422-427

[71] Heinlein CA, Chang C. The roles of androgen receptors and androgen-binding proteins in nongenomic androgen actions. Molecular Endocrinology. 2002;**16**:2181-2187

[72] Rønnekleiv OK, Kelly MJ. Membrane-initiated effects of estrogen in the central nervous system. In: Chief Pfaff WD, Arnold PA, Fahrbach ES, Etgen MA, Rubin TR, editors. Hormones, Brain and Behavior. 2nd ed. Elsevier Inc.; 2009. pp. 1099-1122. ISBN: 978-0-08-088783-8

[73] Boulware MI, Kordasiewicz H, Mermelstein PG. Caveolin proteins are essential for distinct effects of membrane estrogen receptors in neurons. The Journal of Neuroscience. 2007;**27**:9941-9950

[74] Russu M, Terzea D, Hudiţă D. Endometrial immunohistochemistry on Hormone Replacement Therapy. Climacteric, Book of Abstracts. 2002;**5**(Suppl. 2):67

[75] Balthazart J, Ball GF. Is brain estradiol a hormone or a neurotransmitter? Trends in Neurosciences. 2006;**29**:241-249

[76] Grove-Strawser D, Boulware MI, Mermelstein PG. Membrane estrogen receptors activate the metabotropic glutamate receptors mGluR5 and mGluR3 to bidirectionally regulate CREB phosphorylation in female rat striatal neurons. Neuroscience. 2010;**170**:1045-1055

[77] Tronson NC, Collette KM. (Putative) sex differences in neuroimmune modulation of memory. Journal of Neuroscience Research. 2017;**95**(1–2):472-486. DOI: 10.1002

[78] Bean LA, Kumar A, Rani A, Foster TC, et al. Re-opening the critical window for estrogen therapy. The Journal of Neuroscience. 2015;**35**(49):16077-16093. DOI: 10.1523

[79] McEwen BS, Akama KT, Alves SE, Milner TA, et al. Tracking the estrogen receptor in neurons: Implications for estrogen-induced synapse formation. Proceedings of the National Academy of Sciences of the United States of America. 2001;**98**:7093-7100

[80] Wu T, Chen S, Brinton RD. Estrogen membrane receptor imaging coupled with estradiol activation of intracellular calcium rise and ERK activation in single neurons. Society for Neuroscience – Abstracts. 2004;**30**:659.20

[81] Milner TA, Ayoola K, Alves SE, et al. Ultrastructural localization of estrogen receptor beta immunoreactivity in the rat hippocampal formation. The Journal of Comparative Neurology. 2005;**491**:81-95

[82] Heard DJ, Norby PL, Holloway J, Vissing H. Human ERRgamma, a third member of the estrogen receptor-related receptor (ERR) subfamily of orphan nuclear receptors: Tissue-specific isoforms are expressed during development and in the adult. Molecular Endocrinology. 2000;**14**:382-392

[83] Kim J, Szinte JS, Bonlware MI, Frick KM. 17β-Estradiol and agonism of G-protein-coupled estrogen receptor enhance hippocampal memory via different cell-signaling mechanisms. The Journal of Neuroscience. 2016;**36**(11):3309-3321. DOI: 10.1523

[84] Bologa CG, Revankar CM, Sklar LA, et al. Virtual and biomolecular screening converge on a selective agonist for GPR30. Nature Chemical Biology. 2006;**4**:207-212

[85] Brailoiu E, Dun SL, Brailoiu GC, Dun NJ, et al. Distribution and characterization of estrogen receptor G protein-coupled receptor 30 in the rat central nervous system. The Journal of Endocrinology. 2007;**193**:311-321

[86] Mannella P, Brinton RD. Estrogen receptor protein interaction with PI3K leads to activation of pAkt and pERK in the same population of cortical neurons: A unified mechanism of estrogen action. The Journal of Neuroscience. 2006;**26**:9439-9447

[87] Laflamme N, Nappi RE, Rivest S, et al. Expression and neuropeptidergic characterization of estrogen receptors (ERα and ERβ) throughout the rat brain: Anatomical evidence of distinct roles of each subtype. Journal of Neurobiology. 1998;**36**:357-378

[88] Wu TW, Wang JM, Chen S, Brinton RD. 17beta-estradiol induced Ca^{2+} influx via L-type calcium channels activates the Src/ERK/cyclic-AMP response element binding protein signal pathway and BCL-2 expression in rat hippocampal neurons: A potential initiation mechanism for estrogen-induced neuroprotection. Neuroscience. 2005;**135**:59-72

[89] Zhao L, Brinton RD. Estrogen receptor alpha and beta differentially regulate intracellular Ca(2+) dynamics leading to ERK phosphorylation and estrogen neuroprotection in hippocampal neurons. Brain Research. 2007;**1172**:48-59

[90] Znamensky V, Akama KT, BS ME, Milner TA. Estrogen levels regulate the subcellular distribution of phosphorylated Akt in hippocampal CA1 dendrites. The Journal of Neuroscience. 2003;**23**:2340-2347

[91] Yildirim M, Janssen WG, Morrison JH, et al. Effects of estrogen and aging on distribution of pAkt in CA1 of rat hippocampus. Society for Neuroscience – Abstracts. 2006;**32**: 659.1

[92] Janssen WG, Yildirim M, Lou WWY, McEwen BS, Milner TA, Morrison JH. Estrogen receptor β is affected by estrogen and aging in CA1sr region of female rat hippocampus. Society for Neuroscience – Abstracts. 2006;**32**:659.17

[93] Morrison J, Wang CJA, Hara Y, Janssen GMW, Rapp PR. Synaptic estrogen receptor-alpha levels in prefrontal cortex in female rhesus monkeys and their correlation with cognitive performance. The Journal of Neuroscience. 2010;**30**(38):12770-12776

[94] Hojo Y, Murakami G, Mukai H, Kawato S, et al. Estrogen synthesis in the brain—Role in synaptic plasticity and memory. Molecular and Cellular Endocrinology. 2008;**290**:31-43

[95] Kelly JF, Bienias JL, Bennett DA, et al. Levels of estrogen receptors alpha and beta in frontal cortex of patients with Alzheimer's disease: Relationship to mini-mental state examination scores. Current Alzheimer Research. 2008;**5**(1):45-51

[96] Honma N, Saji S, Harada N, et al. Estrogen-related factors in the frontal lobe of Alzheimer's disease patients and importance of body mass index. Scientific Reports. 2017;**7**:726. DOI: 10.1038/s41598-017-00815

[97] Takeucki K, Yang Y, Zukin RS, et al. Estradiol pretreatment ameliorates impaired synaptic plasticity at synapses of insulted CA1 neurons after transient global ischemia. Brain Research. 2015;**1621**:222-230. DOI: 10.1016

[98] Lan YL, Zhao J, Li S. Update on the neuroprotective effect of estrogen receptor alpha against Alzheimer's disease. Journal of Alzheimer's Disease. 2015;**43**(4):1137-1148. DOI: 10.3233

[99] Huffman J, Huffman C, Taylor GT. Integrating insulin-like growth factor 1 and sex hormones into neuroprotection: Implications for diabetes. World Diabetes. 2017;**8**(2):45-55. DOI: 10.4239

[100] Mendez P, Wandosell F, Garcia-Segura LM. Cross-talk between estrogen receptors and insulin-like growth factor-I receptor in the brain: Cellular and molecular mechanisms. Frontiers in Neuroendocrinology. 2006;**27**:391-403

[101] Miller NR, Joyer T, Etgen AM, et al. Estrogen can act via estrogen receptor alpha and beta to protect hippocampal neurons against global ischemia-induced cell death. Endocrinology. 2005;**146**(7):3070-3079

[102] Ishunina TA, Swaab DE, Fisher DF. Estrogen receptor-alpha splice variants in the medial mamillary nucleus of Alzheimer's disease patients: Identification of a novel MB1 isoform. The Journal of Clinical Endocrinology and Metabolism. 2005;**90**(6):3757-3765

[103] Sarvari M, Kallo I, Liposits Z, et al. Long-term estrogen receptor beta agonist treatment modifies the hippocampal transcriptome in middle-aged ovariectomized rats. Frontiers in Cellular Neuroscience. 2016;**10**:149. DOI: 10.3389

[104] Pisani SL, Neese SL, Korol DL, et al. Acute genistein treatment mimics the effects of estradiol by enhancing place learning and impairing response learning in young adult female rats. Hormones and Behavior. 2012;**62**:491-499. DOI: 10.1016/j.yhbeh.2012.08.006

[105] Pisani SL, Neese SL, Korol DL, et al. Estrogen receptor-selective agonists modulate learning in female rats in a dose- and task-specific manner. Endocrinology. 2016;**157**: 292-303. DOI: 10.1210/en.2015-1616

[106] Zhao L, Woody SK, Chhibber A. Estrogen receptor β in Alzheimer's disease: From mechanisms to therapeutics. Ageing Research Reviews. 2015;**24**(Pt B):178-190. DOI: 10.1016/j.arr.2015.08.001

[107] Elcoroaristizabal Martin X, Fernandez- Martinez M, de Pancorbo M, et al. Progression from amnesic mild cognitive impairment to Alzheimer's disease: ESR1 and ESR2 polymorphisms and APOE gene. Dementia and Geriatric Cognitive Disorders. 2011;**32**(5): 332-341. DOI: 10.1159/000335541

[108] Fernandez-Martinez M, Elcoroaristizabal Martin X, de Pancorbo M, et al. Oestrogen receptor polymorphisms are an associated risk factor for mild cognitive impairment and Alzheimer disease in women APOE {varepsilon}4 carriers: A case-control study. BMJ Open. 2013;**3**(9):e003200. DOI: 10.1136

[109] Moser VA, Pike CJ. Obesity and sex interact in the regulation of Alzheimer's disease. Neuroscience and Biobehavioral Reviews. 2016;**67**:102-118. DOI: 10.1016

[110] Uchoa MF, Moser VA, Pike CJ. Interactions between inflammation, sex steroids, and Alzheimer's disease risk factors. Frontiers in Neuroendocrinology. 2016;**43**:60-82. DOI: 10.1016

[111] Frick KM. Epigenetics, estradiol and hippocampal memory consolidation. Journal of Neuroendocrinology. 2013;**25**:1151-1162

[112] Fortress AM, Frick KM. Epigenetic regulation of estrogen-dependent memory. Frontiers in Neuroendocrinology. 2014;**35**:530-549

[113] Brinton RD, Thompson RF, Nilsen J, et al. Progesterone receptors: Form and function in brain. Frontiers in Neuroendocrinology. 2008;**29**(2):313-339. DOI: 10.1016/j.yfrne.2008.02.001

[114] Conneely OM, Lydon JP. Progesterone receptors in reproduction: Functional impact of the A and B isoforms. Steroids. 2000;**65**:571-577. DOI: 10.1016/S0039-128X(00)00115-X

[115] Vasudevan N, Pfaff DW. Non-genomic actions of estrogens and their interaction with genomic actions in the brain. Frontiers in Neuroendocrinology. 2008;**29**:238-257. DOI: 10.1016

[116] Diotel N, Servili A, Gueguen M-M, Mironov S, Pellegrini E, Vaillant C, Zhu Y, Kah O, Anglade I. Nuclear progesterone receptors are up-regulated by estrogens in neurons and radial glial progenitors in the brain of Zebrafish. PLoS. 30 Nov 2011;**6**(11):e28375. DOI: 10.1371

[117] Vegeto E, Shahbaz MM, Wen DX, Goldman ME, O'Malley BW, DP MD. Human progesterone receptor a form is a cell- and promoter-specific repressor of human progesterone receptor B function. Molecular Endocrinology. 1993;**7**:1244-1255. DOI: 10.1210/me.7.10.1244

[118] Boonyaratanakornkit V, McGowan E, Sherman L, Mancini MA, Cheskis BJ, et al. The role of extranuclear signaling actions of progesterone receptor in mediating progesterone regulation of gene expression and the cell cycle. Molecular Endocrinology. 2007;**21**:359-375

[119] Di Donato M et al. Cross-talk between androgen receptor/filamin A and TrkA regulates neurite outgrowth in PC12 cells. Molecular Biology of the Cell. 2015;**26**:2858-2872. DOI: 10.1091

[120] Pang Y, Dong J, Thomas P. Characterization, neurosteroid binding and brain distribution of human membrane progesterone receptors delta and {epsilon} (mPRdelta and mPR{epsilon}) and mPRdelta involvement in neurosteroid inhibition of apoptosis. Endocrinology. 2013;**154**:283-295. DOI: 10.1210/en.2012-1772

[121] Thomas P, Pang Y, Tubbs C, et al. Steroid and G protein binding characteristics of the seatrout and human progestin membrane receptor alpha subtypes and their evolutionary origins. Endocrinology. 2007;**148**(2):705-718

[122] Kasubuchi M, Watanabe K, Kimura I, et al. Membrane progesterone receptor beta (mPRβ/Paqr8) promotes progesterone-dependent neurite outgrowth in PC12 neuronal cells via non-G protein-coupled receptor (GPCR) signaling. Scientific Reports. 2017;**7**(1): 5168. DOI: 10.1038/s41598-017-05423-9

[123] Thomas P. Characteristics of membrane progestin receptor alpha (mPRalpha) and progesterone membrane receptor component 1 (PGMRC1) and their roles in mediating rapid progestin actions. Frontiers in Neuroendocrinology. 2008;**29**:292-312. DOI: 10.1016

[124] Singh M. Ovarian hormones elicit phosphorylation of Akt and extracellular-signal regulated kinase in explants of the cerebral cortex. Endocrine. 2001;**14**:407-415. DOI: 10.1385

[125] Su C, Cunningham RL, Rybalchenko N, Singh M. Progesterone increases the release of brain-derived neurotrophic factor from glia via progesterone receptor membrane component 1 (Pgrmc1)-dependent ERK5 signaling. Endocrinology. 2012;**153**:4389-4400. DOI: 10.1210/en.2011-2177

[126] Meffre D, Labombarda F, Delespierre B, Stein DG, et al. Distribution of membrane progesterone receptor alpha in the male mouse and rat brain and its regulation after traumatic brain injury. Neuroscience. 2013;**231**:111-124. DOI: 10.1016

[127] Nilsen J, Brinton RD. Impact of progestins on estrogen-induced neuroprotection: Synergy by progesterone and 19-norprogesterone and antagonism by medroxyprogesterone acetate. Endocrinology. 2002;**143**:205-212. DOI: 10.1210/en.143.1.205

[128] Petralia SM, Frye CA. In the ventral tegmental area, cyclic AMP mediates the actions of progesterone at dopamine type 1 receptors for lordosis of rats and hamsters. Journal of Neuroendocrinology. 2006;**18**:902-914. DOI: 10.1111/

[129] Peluso JJ. Progesterone as a regulator of granulosa cell viability. The Journal of Steroid Biochemistry and Molecular Biology. 2003;**85**:167-173. DOI: 10.1016/S0960-0760(03)00192-4

[130] Swiatek-De Lange M, Stampfl A, Hauck SM, Deeg CA, et al. Membrane-initiated effects of progesterone on calcium dependent signaling and activation of VEGF gene expression in retinal glial cells. GLIA. 2007;**55**:1061-1073. DOI: 10.1002/glia.20523

[131] Ishihara Y, Kawami T, Ishida A, Yamazaki T. Allopregnanolone-mediated protective effects of progesterone on tributyltin-induced neuronal injury in rat hippocampal slices. The Journal of Steroid Biochemistry and Molecular Biology. 2013;**135**:1-6. DOI: 10.1016

[132] Xu J, Zeng C, Chu W, Pan F, Rothfuss M, Zhang F, et al. Identification of the PGRMC1 protein complex as the putative sigma-2 receptor binding site. Nature Communications. 2011;**2**:380. DOI: 10.1038

[133] Ahlbom E, Prins GS, Ceccatelli S. Testosterone protects cerebellar granule cells from oxidative stress-induced cell death through a receptor mediated mechanism. Brain Research. 2001;**892**:255-262

[134] Hammond J, Le Q, Goodyer C, Gelfand M, Trifiro M, LeBlanc A. Testosterone-mediated neuroprotection through the androgen receptor in human primary neurons. Journal of Neurochemistry. 2001;**77**:1-9

[135] Ramsden M, Shin TM, Pike CJ. Androgens modulate neuronal vulnerability to kainate lesion. Neuroscience. 2003;**122**:573-578

[136] Pike CJ. Testosterone attenuates beta-amyloid toxicity in cultured hippocampal neurons. Brain Research. 2001;**919**:160-165

[137] Nguyen VVT, Yao M, Pike JC. Androgens activate mitogen-activated protein kinase signaling: Role in neuroprotection. Journal of Neurochemistry. 2005;**94**:1639-1651

[138] Tang MX, Jacobs D, Stern Y, Marder K, Schofield P, Gurland B, Andrews H, Mayeux R. Effect of oestrogen during menopause on risk and age at onset of Alzheimer's disease. The Lancet. 1996;**348**(9025):429-432

[139] Xu H, Wang R, Zhang YW, Zhang X. Estrogen, β-amyloid metabolism/trafficking, and Alzheimer's disease, Annals of the New York Academy of Sciences. 2006;**1089**:324-342

[140] Norbury R, Travis MJ, Erlandsson K, Waddington W, Ell PJ, Murphy DGM. Estrogen therapy and brain muscarinic receptor density in healthy females: A SPET study. Hormones and Behavior. 2007;**51**(2):249-257

[141] Persad CC, Zubieta JK, Love T, Wang H, Tkaczyk A, Smith YR. Enhanced neuroactivation during verbal memory processing in postmenopausal women receiving short-term hormone therapy. Fertility and Sterility. 2009;**92**(1):197-204

[142] Silverman DHS, Geist CL, Kenna HA, et al. Differences in regional brain metabolism associated with specific formulations of hormone therapy in postmenopausal women at risk for AD. Psychoneuroendocrinology. 2010;**36**:502-513

[143] Yao J, Irwin R, Chen S, Hamilton R, Cadenas E, Brinton RD. Ovarian hormone loss induces bioenergetic deficits and mitochondrial beta-amyloid. Neurobiology of Aging. 2012;**33**:1507-1521

[144] Etgen AM, Jover Mengual T, Zukin RS. Neuroprotective actions of estradiol and novel estrogen analogs in ischemia: Translational implications. Frontiers in Neuroendocrinology. Aug 2011;**32**(3):336-352. DOI: 10.1016

[145] Cordey M, Gundimeda U, Gopalakrishna R, Pike CJ. Estrogen activates protein kinase C in neurons: Role in neuroprotection. The Journal of Neurochemistry 2003;**84**:1340-1348

[146] Zhao L, Chen S, Wang JM, Brinton RD. 17 beta-estradiol induces Ca^{2+} influx, dendritic and nuclear Ca^{2+} rise and subsequent cyclic AMP response element-binding protein activation in hippocampal neurons: a potential initiation mechanism for estrogen neurotrophism. Neuroscience. 2005;**132**:299-311

[147] Adams MM, Shah RA, Janssen WG, Morrison JH. Different modes of hippocampal plasticity in response to estrogen in young and aged female rats. Proceedings of the National Academy of Sciences of the United States of America. 2001;**98**:8071-8076

[148] Choi JM, Romeo RD, Brake WG, Bethea CL, Rosenwaks Z, McEwen BS. Estradiol increases pre- and post-synaptic proteins in the CA1 region of the hippocampus in female rhesus macaques (*Macaca mulatta*) Endocrinology. 2003;**144**:4734-4738

[149] Nilsen J, Brinton RD. Mitochondria as therapeutic targets of estrogen action in the central nervous system. Curr Drug Targets CNS Neurol Disord. 2004;**3**:297-313

[150] Nilsen J, Irwin RW, Brinton RD. Brain mitochondria as therapeutic target for the prevention of Alzheimer's pathology. Alzheimer's and Dementia. 2006;**2**[Suppl 3]

[151] Simpkins JW, Wang J, Wang X, Perez E, Prokai L, Dykens JA. Mitochondria play a central role in estrogen-induced neuroprotection. Curr Drug Targets CNS Neurol Disord 2005;**4**:69-83

[152] Brewer GJ, Reichensperger JD, Brinton RD. Prevention of age-related dysregulation of calcium dynamics by estrogen in neurons. Neurobiology of Aging. 2006;**27**:306-317

[153] Zhao L, Wu T-W, Brinton RD. Estrogen receptor subtypes alpha and beta contribute to neuroprotection and increased Bcl-2 expression in primary hippocampal neurons. Brain Research. 2004;**1010**:22-34

[154] Rudick CN, Gibbs RB, Woolley CS. A role for the basal forebrain cholinergic system in estrogen-induced disinhibition of hippocampal pyramidal cells. The Journal of Neuroscience. 2003;**23**:4479-4490

[155] Tinkler GP, Tobin JR, Voytko ML. Effects of two years of estrogen loss or replacement on nucleus basalis cholinergic neurons and cholinergic fibers to the dorsolateral prefrontal and inferior parietal cortex of monkeys. The Journal of Comparative Neurology. 2004; **469**:507-521

10

Clinical Use of Progesterone and its Relation to Oxidative Stress in Ruminants

Mushap Kuru, Abdulsamed Kükürt, Hasan Oral and Metin Öğün

Abstract

Studies to determine the physiological effects and functions of progesterone started in the twentieth century. Progesterone is a steroid-structured hormone with 21 carbon atoms originating from cholesterol. The corpus luteum, formed after ovulation in ruminants, secretes progesterone, which plays a role in the continuity of the pregnancy. Progestagens can be used for estrus synchronization in cows and heifers. Similarly, they are used for estrus synchronization during the breeding season or outside the breeding season by taking advantage of the negative feedback effect of progesterone in small ruminants. It is applied for the treatment of embryonic deaths due to luteal insufficiency in cows with high milk yield. In anovulatory anestrus, exogenous progesterone applications can be very useful. Progesterone treatment contributes to the resolution of the anestrus by rearranging hypothalamic functions in cattle with follicular cysts. The oxidative stress index in the luteal phase, when progesterone is high in ruminants, is higher than in the follicular phase. In the critical period of pregnancy, a high index of oxidative stress-induced progesterone causes embryonic death. Factors that cause stress in high milk-yielding cows can affect the amount of progesterone synthesis by inhibiting luteal cell function due to excessive free radical production.

Keywords: progesterone, ruminants, oxidative stress, estrus synchronization, embryonic death

1. Introduction

Many methods have been developed for controlling reproduction in farm animals. Among these methods, synchronization protocols to increase reproductive efficiency have an important place. The desired level of pregnancy rates is often not obtained because of the difficulty of following the estrus cycle in each animal on large farms. For this reason, estrus synchronization use in large farms becomes inevitable. Thus, progesterone-assisted estrus synchronizations are implemented intensively in farm animals. In addition, progesterone can also be used for the treatment of reproductive problems such as anestrus, cystic ovarian disease, and luteal insufficiency [1, 2].

This section provides information on the structure of progesterone, its role in physiological events in ruminants, its use in clinical practice, and its relation to oxidative stress.

2. The structure and biochemical synthesis of progesterone

Steroid hormones are lipophilic organic compounds with a low-molecular weight derived from cholesterol (**Figure 1**). Steroid hormones are synthesized in the mitochondria and smooth endoplasmic reticulum in gonads, such as the ovary and testis, and then released into the bloodstream. The steroid hormones are broadly classified into three categories based on their physiological functions: glucocorticoids, mineralocorticoids, and sex steroids [3]. Cholesterol is an obligate intermediate used for steroid hormone synthesis by the adrenal gland, ovary, testis, and placenta that can be obtained from three principal sources: de novo synthesis of cholesterol from acetate, cholesterol from circulating high-density lipoproteins, and cholesterol

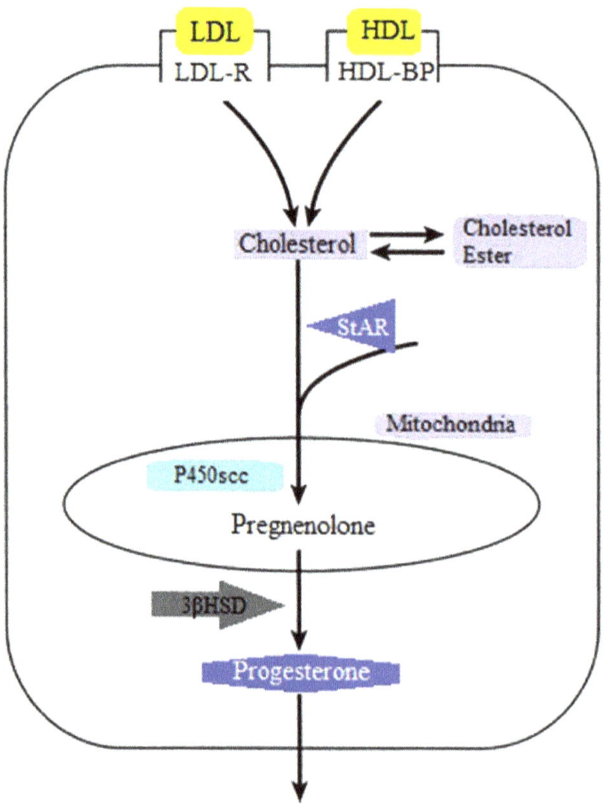

Figure 1. Sources of cholesterol for progesterone biosynthesis.

stored in plasma membranes. The major source of cholesterol for luteal cells in ruminants is circulating high-density lipoproteins [3, 4].

Cholesterol is primarily a hydrophobic molecule, and this makes it difficult for cholesterol to diffuse freely through hydrophilic environments such as the cytoplasm. In addition, cholesterol has a hydroxyl group at the 3 position that produces a discrete hydrophilic region making it difficult for the "flip-flop" of cholesterol between membrane surfaces within the lipid bilayer of cellular membranes. Therefore, movement of cholesterol in the circulatory system (lipoproteins) or within the cell is dependent upon transport proteins. Addition of another hydroxyl group at the other end of the cholesterol molecule alleviates the need for transport proteins [5].

Progesterone is a steroid hormone primarily secreted by the corpus luteum and placenta. Production of progesterone in luteal cells is dependent more on transport of cholesterol within the cell than to changes in the activity of steroidogenic enzymes. The P450 cholesterol side chain cleavage enzyme (P450scc) is located on the inner mitochondrial membrane and catalyzes the conversion of cholesterol to pregnenolone [6]. This enzyme catalyzes three oxidation steps: hydroxylations at the 20 and 22 positions and then cleavage between these two carbons. Pregnenolone has two hydrophilic residues that increase mobility through cellular membranes. Pregnenolone diffuses from the mitochondria to the smooth endoplasmic reticulum where it is converted to progesterone by the enzyme 3-β hydroxysteroid dehydrogenase (3β-HSD). This final reaction produces a double bond between the 4 and 5 carbon of the molecule and is the basis for the abbreviation of pregnenolone as progesterone (**Figures 1** and **2**). Progesterone then diffuses from the luteal cells to the bloodstream for transport to target tissues [7, 8].

Progesterone is synthesized from pregnenolone in the corpus luteum, the placenta during pregnancy, and the adrenals as a step in androgen and mineralocorticoid synthesis. Its actions are primarily mediated by an intracellular progesterone receptor, whose numbers increase in the presence of estrogen [9].

The products of hormone synthesis vary with the menstrual cycle; estradiol is the main product during follicular maturation, whereas progesterone is the main product in the luteal phase following ovulation. Progesterone is secreted by ovarian follicular cells prior to ovulation; it is also secreted in larger amounts by the corpus luteum, which forms from follicular granulosa cells following ovulation. The corpus luteum will grow for 10–12 days and then regress if fertilization does not occur; if fertilization does occur, the corpus luteum is maintained for the first 2–3 months of pregnancy. Progesterone plays several important actions in the normal female reproductive cycle. Progesterone prepares the uterus for pregnancy by shifting the endometrium from proliferation to secretion. Withdrawal of progesterone in the absence of pregnancy leads to organized shedding (menstruation) and it helps to mediate sexual response in the brain. After fertilization, progesterone organizes the vasculature of the endometrium to prepare for implantation. It promotes enzymatic digestion of the zona pellucida to allow the oocyte to implant into the uterine wall. In addition, it inhibits contractions of the uterine myometrium (smooth muscle layer) and counteracts the effects of oxytocin on contractility. Progesterone promotes lobuloalveolar growth in the breasts to prepare for lactation, but suppresses premature milk protein synthesis prior to parturition. Some of the effects of progesterone may be related to its ability to antagonize estrogen by decreasing expression of estrogen receptors, e.g. the ability of progesterone to inhibit estrogen-mediated endometrial proliferation. It also has a potent effect as a mineralocorticoid

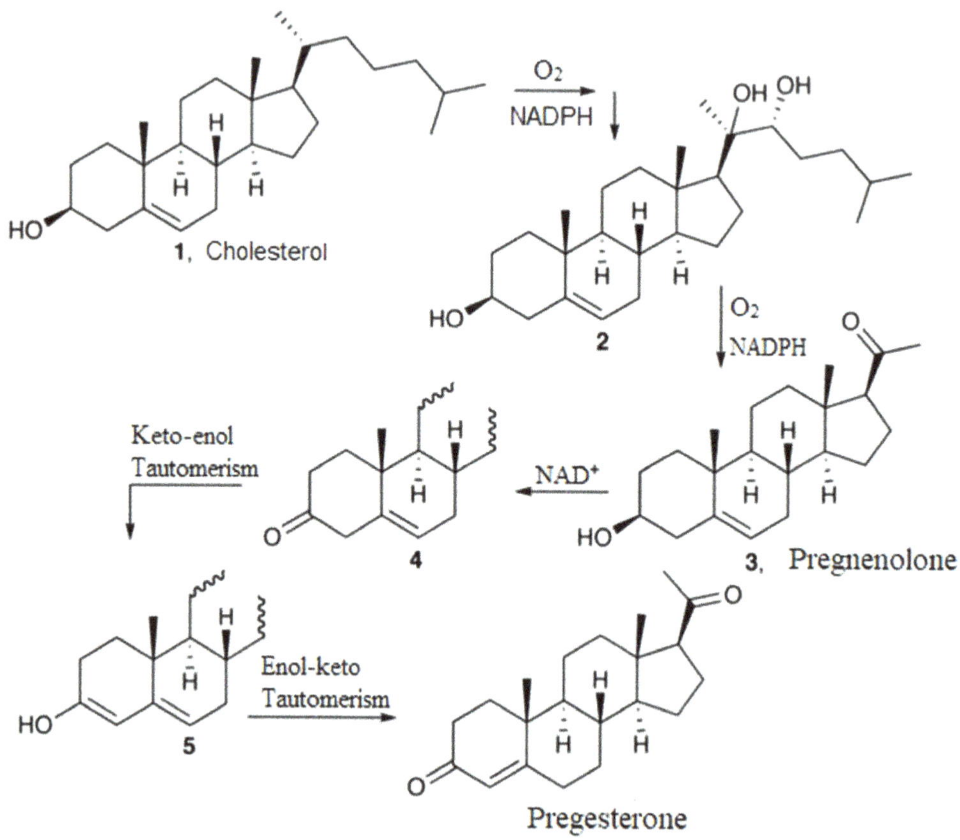

Figure 2. Pathway synthesis of progesterone from cholesterol.

receptor antagonist that reduces sodium retention when present and increases sodium retention when progesterone is withdrawn [8, 9].

The role of progesterone in males is less clear, but it is believed to play a role in activating sperm in the female reproductive tract. It has also been implicated as a modulator of male sexual response and behavior [7].

3. Progesterone synthesis and secretion during the sexual cycle and pregnancy in ruminants

The corpus luteum formed after ovulation in ruminants is a functional structure formed by membrane granulosa in the wall of Graaf follicles. Hypertrophy and luteinization of the theca interna cells play a role in the continuity of the pregnancy, secrete progesterone for a temporary period, and have endocrine activity. In particular, there is a close correlation between corpus luteum development and blood progesterone levels [10, 11].

Progesterone levels in the proestrus and estrus stages of the estrous cycle in cattle are very low. Newly developing corpus luteum cannot produce sufficient progesterone after ovulation (in the period of metaestrus). Therefore, a significant increase in blood progesterone levels cannot be detected. In the diestrus period, the corpus luteum acquires a functional structure and synthesizes >2 ng/mL progesterone. The progesterone level is highest during days 8–10 of the estrous cycle in cows. If pregnancy does not occur, prostaglandin F2 alpha (PGF2α), which is synthesized in the uterus, passes to the ovarian arteries from the uterine vein inducing corpus luteum degeneration. As a result, the blood progesterone level decreases rapidly to less than 0.5 ng/mL [11]. If pregnancy occurs, blood progesterone levels in the cows can be 6–8 ng/mL on day 21 of pregnancy [12, 13].

In sheep, the corpus luteum following ovulation begins to secrete progesterone after the third day of the estrous cycle. Because the corpus luteum formation is rapid, the blood progesterone level rises rapidly and reaches measurable levels [13]. The progesterone level is the highest (4 ng/mL) between days 9 and 13 of the cycle. If there is no pregnancy, the corpus luteum starts to shrink and the amount of PGF2α in the blood starts to increase on the 12th day of the cycle. On the 14th day of the cycle, the progesterone level is 10 ng/mL but is <0.2 ng/mL on the 16th day of the cycle [14]. Pregnancy in sheep is maintained by the corpus luteum until the 50th day and later by placenta-derived progesterone. Progesterone levels are highest between 60 and 130 days of gestation. As long as pregnancy continues, the concentration of progesterone never falls below 1 ng/mL [12].

The corpus luteum forms after ovulation and progesterone levels begin to increase in goats. Maximum levels of progesterone (6–10 ng/mL) are found in the middle of the cycle. This level starts to decrease on the 15th day of the cycle and descends to basal levels on the 19th day [15, 16].

4. Clinical use of progesterone in ruminants

4.1. Use of progesterone for estrus synchronization in cattle

Progestagens (ear implants and intravaginal devices [progesterone-releasing intravaginal device (PRID) and controlled internal drug release (CIDR)]) can be administered for 5–20 days for the purpose of estrus synchronization in cows and heifers without uterine infection. Progesterone applications can stimulate puberty in some heifers and initiate normal cyclic activities in anestrus cows. In addition, following the first ovulation after progesterone treatment, normal length sexual activities may continue [2, 17–24].

After the end of progesterone application, synchronized estrus is observed within 3 days [2, 17]. However, when progesterone is used for a prolonged period, the fertility rates decrease due to the persistence of the follicle. In addition, when melengestrol acetate (MGA) is used for estrus synchronization, subfertile estrus occurs initially because of the persistent follicles and artificial insemination is not recommended [24]. Long-term use negatively affects the intrauterine environment and spermatozoon transport. For this reason, estrus synchronization with progesterone for 5–9 days is more suitable for increasing fertility [25, 26].

According to studies conducted in recent years, the pregnancy rate may be 10–15% higher in short-term progesterone use protocols than long-term protocols. However, other researchers argue that there is no difference between pregnancy rates [2, 26–28].

4.1.1. *Estrus synchronization with progestagens + prostaglandins*

Progesterone administration allows the synchronization of estrus in ruminants in different stages of the cycle. PGF2α may be injected on the last day of progesterone administration (5–10 days) or 1–2 days before the end of progesterone. After the application of progesterone, estrus occurs and artificial insemination is done [21, 29–31]. Some researchers obtained 54% pregnancy rates in the first estrus in dairy cows (n = 102) given progesterone for 7 days (CIDR) with PGF2α administered on day 6. In addition, 49% pregnancy rates were obtained when a similar protocol was applied to non-cyclic and cyclic heifers [29]. In a similar study, the pregnancy rate was 47% in beef heifers (n = 247) and 59% in dairy heifers (n = 129) [32].

In some studies, artificial insemination was performed according to PGF2α injection and estrus follow-up (4–6 days) 17–19 days after 14 days of MGA application [25, 28]. In this protocol, the purpose of PGF2α injection is to lyse the corpus luteum that can be formed at the end of 14 days of MGA application [33].

4.1.2. *Ovulation synchronization protocols + progesterone*

Progesterone is administered as an ear implant or an intravaginal device between days 0 and 7 in order for the Ovsynch (GnRH/PGF2α/GnRH) protocol to be successful and the pregnancy rate to increase [27]. In a study performed on heifers (n = 383), a 47% pregnancy rate was obtained [34]. In another study, progesterone administration in Ovsynch did not increase the pregnancy rate in cows with corpus luteum [35]. Others reported that premature estrus was not observed due to progesterone used between 0 and 7 days for ovulation synchronization protocols and full synchronization was achieved [36, 37].

Progesterone administration is also performed in the Cosynch protocol. On day 0, the progesterone device is inserted and gonadotropin-releasing hormone (GnRH) is injected. Progesterone devices are removed during PGF2α injection (day 7). Fixed-time artificial insemination is performed in 48, 56, or 60 hours after GnRH is injected [38–40]. Such protocols may be applied for 12–14 days with progesterone [41, 42].

4.1.3. *Five-day Cosynch + progesterone protocols in the heifer*

Ovulation synchronization methods have a high pregnancy rate, especially in cows, although this rate is lower in heifers [2]. Synchronization protocols have been developed to stimulate ovulation, which do not require heat detection. Progesterone administration occurs for 5 days. During progesterone removal, PGF2α is administered. GnRH is administered 72 hours later and fixed-time artificial insemination is performed [19, 21, 22, 26, 27]. A 10.5% higher pregnancy rate can be obtained with this protocol [43]. The pregnancy rate improves between 45.9 and 54.2% in the 5-day Cosynch + PRID protocol and fixed-time artificial insemination with sexed semen in cyclic heifers [26].

It was determined that vaginitis and mucopurulent discharge were observed after use of intravaginal progesterone devices in heifers. The incidence of vaginitis in the heifers may be around 70% or more [22, 23, 26, 44].

4.2. Use of progesterone in estrus synchronization in small ruminants

In small ruminants, progesterone suppresses GnRH and luteinizing hormone (LH) release by negative feedback [45]. There may be up to 30-fold increases in LH concentration with a decrease in the plasma level of progesterone. In addition, the dominant follicular LH receptors are sensitive and thus ovulation occurs. As a general principle, these effects of progesterone can be used in estrus synchronization protocols [46–48]. Medroxyprogesterone acetate (MAP), fluorogestone acetate (intravaginal sponge), melengestrol acetate, levonorgestrel, and intravaginal progesterone-releasing devices (CIDR and DICO) are used for estrus synchronization in sheep and goats [48–55].

In sheep, progestagens are used effectively in the control and synchronization of estrus. Equine chorionic gonadotropin (eCG) injection is performed in addition to progestagen administration for 12–14 days in order to obtain high estrus rates and ovulation, especially during anestrus. Nevertheless, these types of manipulations may also vary depending on nutrition, body condition score, lactation, age, temperature, light, and breed [56–60].

In sheep synchronized with MAP during the breeding season, follicle size and LH pulse increase after ram introduction [61, 62]. Intravaginal CIDR or chronolone intravaginal sponge and 500 IU eCG did not affect the LH wave and peak in Tuj sheep outside the breeding season [63].

During the breeding season, estrus start and end times were different in sheep treated with MAP or CIDR for 12 days [64]. High estrus rates and similar fertility rates were determined in sheep that applied short-term (6 days) CIDR-G or fluorogestone acetate (FGA, intravaginal sponge) [52].

Short-term (5 day) FGA and eCG administration produce higher estrus rate than long-term FGA and eCG treatments in sheep during the breeding season [50]. Injections of eCG at different doses (300, 400, and 500 IU) to Awassi sheep in estrus synchronization with progesterone similarly affect fertility parameters [65]. The testosterone antibody, β-carotene, and vitamin E administration did not change the estrus and pregnancy rates 7 days before intravaginal 40 mg FGA administration in Tuj ewes during the non-breeding season [66].

Vaginal sponges with progesterone for 11–14 days were applied to Pirlak ewes during the non-breeding season and 92–100% entered estrus. The pregnancy rate was 37.7–44%. In the study, the fertility parameters did not change for 11 or 14 day vaginal sponge application. Progesterone administration at different day lengths may be effective for the onset of estrus [48].

Short or long-term progesterone treatment for estrus synchronization in goats can be done depending on the breeding season. At the end of progesterone treatment, the protocol is terminated by eCG administration [54, 58, 67–69].

Intravaginal levonorgestrel for 10 days and intramuscular PGF2α administration were used in goats causing high estrus rates (95%) during the breeding season [70]. In a study conducted on Abaza goats during the breeding season, the first estrus pregnancy rate was 73.3% and the pregnancy rate was 93.3% after estrus synchronization using CIDR for 11 days. In addition, the same pregnancy rate was achieved in goats that did not receive any intervention in the study. However, progesterone treatment and estrus synchronization contribute positively to reproductive parameters and increase twinning rates [55].

In sheep and goats, short-term progesterone-impregnated sponge therapy changed the microbial flora of the vagina and formed vaginitis. Staphylococcus is usually detected in these cases of vaginitis [13, 71, 72].

4.3. Use of progesterone to prevent embryonic death

Progesterone is the most important hormone for the continuity of pregnancy. Progesterone affects oocyte quality by affecting LH wave frequency and persistent follicle formation. Again, progesterone plays a vital role in influencing the endometrium and creating the appropriate environment for the survival of the embryo [73].

The rate of embryonic deaths in cows may range from 7 to 16% in the first week, 6–44% in the second week, 3–33% in the third week, and 19–42% after the fourth week. Embryonic deaths are caused by genetic and environmental factors. Most of the embryonic deaths, especially due to hormone insufficiency, are the result of luteal insufficiency. For this reason, progesterone or its analogues are applied to reduce embryonic losses before or after artificial insemination [74–76].

In ovulation synchronization protocols, such as Ovsynch and Cosynch, progesterone administration for 7 days between the first GnRH and PGF2α injections reduces the embryonic loss rate due to luteal phase deficiency [13]. Gestational losses were 3.6–6.8% after the 5-day Cosynch + progesterone protocol [26].

Progesterone-assisted estrus synchronization protocols can prevent early embryonic losses and increase the pregnancy rate. In many studies, there are reports that progesterone-assisted applications increase the pregnancy rate and decrease the embryonic loss rate. However, some researchers disagree [2, 35, 77, 78].

One of the most important causes of embryonic deaths in high milk-yielding cows is inadequate embryo development prior to implantation due to insufficient progesterone concentrations. Progesterone application performed between 3, 5, and 10 days after artificial insemination caused a statistically significant increase after CIDR administration compared with the control group. The pregnancy rate was 35% (22/63) in the control group and 48% (32/67) in the progesterone-treated group. The effect of exogenous progesterone is important for the development of pregnancy, especially in cows with first and second lactation [79].

Some researchers report an overall increase of 5% in pregnancy rates following progesterone administration. Progesterone administration time is critical to success. Progesterone treatment for 6 days after artificial insemination can increase pregnancy rates (10% more) [80].

Cows in the CIDR groups, which were administered progesterone for 6 or 12 days after the 5th and 7th days following artificial insemination, had higher pregnancy rates than the control group [81]. Intravaginal progesterone administration for 7 days starting 14 days after artificial insemination can reduce both embryonic deaths and fetal losses [77]. Similarly, post-mating treatment of FGA (intravaginal sponge) in sheep has been reported to reduce embryonic mortality [82].

4.4. Use of progesterone in anestrus or anovulatory anestrus

Anestrus is a situation in which a sign of heat cannot be detected in beef or dairy herds. Many forms of functional infertility result in anestrus in cows. This leads to serious economic losses for large farms [73].

Four different types of anovulatory anestrus may be encountered in the postpartum period. The first (type I) is characterized by follicle development remaining "emergent" (~ 4 mm) and not progressing to the "deviation" (~ 9 mm) phase. This type of anestrus is classically referred to as "inactive ovary." In type II, the "deviation" phase is passed, and after the "growth" phase, the follicle undergoes atresia. In type III, the follicle develops to the preovulatory stage but does not ovulate, thus becoming permanent follicles or follicular/luteal cysts. In type IV, the follicles develop and ovulate and the corpus luteum is formed, but the corpora lutea cannot regress and become permanent [13, 83].

In anovulatory anestrus, exogenous progesterone applications can be very useful [84]. The use of intravaginal progesterone devices, such as PRID or CIDR, may induce the restart of cyclic activity in the ovary [13]. Especially at the end of this application, the use of PGF2α and analogues may increase the pregnancy rate [73]. At the end of 10 days of progesterone therapy, injection of eCG, estradiol, or PGF2α is beneficial [83]. In this context, successful results were obtained after 9 days of PRID and intramuscular cloprostenol injection 1 day before PRID removal. Higher pregnancy rates can be achieved by adding progesterone to ovulation synchronization protocols in acyclic cows [13, 85].

4.5. Use of progesterone in cystic ovarian disease

Cystic ovarian follicles are non-ovulated preovulatory follicles that maintain long-lasting persistence without any luteal structure on the ovary. With progesterone administration, the number of LH pulses, and thus the LH level, is reduced and maintained at a luteal phase level throughout the cycle [73].

PRID or CIDR can be administered intravaginally for 7–14 days in cows with cystic ovarian disease [86]. In addition, progesterone is frequently used in the treatment of follicular cysts that cannot be mitigated with GnRH or human chorionic gonadotropin (hCG) injections. Progesterone therapy in cows with follicular cysts restarts hypothalamic functions and contributes to the resolution of the problem [83, 87].

Combination of progesterone administration for 9 days with GnRH and PGF2α may improve outcomes in cows with cystic ovarian disease. GnRH is injected and a progesterone-releasing device is applied intravaginally for 9 days. On day 7, PGF2α is administered intramuscularly, and 2 days later, the vaginal progesterone-releasing device is removed. Artificial insemination is done when the cows are in heat [88].

4.6. Use of progesterone to induction of lactation

The induction of lactation is a procedure that is applied to infertile heifers and non-lactating cows. The main purpose is to generate profit by initiating milk production. In particular, the combination of progesterone and estradiol in this type of cattle helps to develop the lobule alveolar system. Lactation can be successfully induced in 60% of cows treated with a combination of estrogen and progesterone for 7 or 10 days [89, 90].

When 50 mg progesterone and 20 mg 17β-estradiol are injected subcutaneously twice a day for 7 days in repeat breeders or aborted heifers, milk synthesis starts 10–21 days after the treatment [91]. In another study, lactation started 11–21 days after the first 17β-estradiol and progesterone injection. The highest milk yield was reached 30–35 days after the start of lactation [92].

Lactation can be induced in non-pregnant ewes using progesterone and estrogen treatment. Progesterone and 240 mg estradiol benzoate injection once every 3 days for 60 days increased udder size. At the same time, the development of the udder is stimulated daily by injecting 10 mg dexamethasone trimethylacetate or injecting 5 mg estradiol benzoate and 12.5 mg progesterone for 6 days. After this protocol, milk synthesis starts from the udder with physiological size [93].

5. Relationship between progesterone and oxidative stress in ruminants

Oxygen is necessary for metabolism in living organism, but oxygen can be damaging to the living organism when it generates reactive oxygen species [94]. Thus, living organism face an oxygen paradox. During vital biochemical reactions in living organisms, intermediate metabolic products called reactive oxygen species (ROS) are generated that cause oxidative damage in many tissues by reducing oxygen. Oxygen is a potentially toxic molecule that is necessary for aerobic organisms to survive. Oxygen species are called "oxidants" or "free radicals" because of the oxidative destruction they provoke. Free radicals occur in all living organisms that metabolize molecular oxygen [95]. Free radicals carry a single number of unshared electrons in their outer orbitals [96]. They are very short-lived reagents, which disrupt the structure of other electrons in the environment of highly energetic electrons. Therefore, free radicals are dangerous to the organism [97]. Free radicals can occur as a by-product in all parts of aerobic cells, during metabolism, or in pathological conditions and they can cause various changes in the cells. As a result, serious cell, tissue, and/or organ damage can occur [98].

Free radicals are highly reactive molecules. Electrons interact with other molecules in the cell generating oxidative damage. They also damage many biological materials such as proteins, lipids, DNA, and nucleotide coenzymes [99]. There are many defensive mechanisms in place to prevent the formation of ROS and damage to the organism. These mechanisms are generally referred to as "antioxidant defense systems" or "antioxidants" [100]. Antioxidants control the metabolism and free radical levels that occur in normal metabolic or pathological conditions and prevent or repair damage that may be caused by these radicals [101–103].

In the organism, the formation rate of free radicals and the rate of their removal are in balance. This condition, called "oxidative balance," prevents the organism from being affected by free radicals. An imbalance between free radical formation and the antioxidant defense mechanism in favor of free radicals is termed "oxidative stress," which in turn leads to tissue damage [104]. Antioxidants are known to have protective effects on lipids, proteins, nucleic acids, and other macromolecules. Antioxidants affect ROS in four ways: scavenger, quencher, restorative, and chain breaker [103]. All biomolecules are exposed to free radicals. However, lipids are most easily affected [105]. The membranes surrounding the cells and organelles contain a large amount of unsaturated fatty acids. The oxygen molecule has a high affinity for lipids in these unsaturated fatty acids in the cell membrane. The binding of oxygen to the double bonds in the unsaturated fatty acids found in tissues is the result of lipid peroxidation. Lipid peroxidation is the reaction of unsaturated fatty acids in the structure of phospholipids, glycolipids, glycerides, and steroids in the membrane by free oxygen radicals to various products such as peroxides, alcohols, aldehydes, hydroxy fatty acids, ethane, and pentane [106]. The major intracellular antioxidants found in organisms include superoxide dismutase (SOD), catalase (CAT), glutathione peroxidase (GPX), glutathione S transferase, glucose 6 phosphate dehydrogenase, and paraoxonase enzymes. Vitamin E, ferritin, transferrin, haptoglobin, uric acid, ceruloplasmin, glutathione, albumin, bilirubin, and β-carotene are antioxidant defenses in the extracellular environment [107].

Every month, the oocyte grows and begins to develop in the ovary. However, meiosis-I continues only in the dominant oocyte. This process is inhibited by antioxidants causing an increase in ROS. Thus, antioxidants promote meiosis-II [108]. The ROS produced by the preovulatory follicle is considered an important inducer of ovulation [109]. Thus, ROS do not always cause adverse effects [110]. Recently, ROS have been reported to regulate cell function by controlling the production or activation of substances with biological activity [111]. Oxygen deprivation stimulates follicular angiogenesis, which is important for the growth and development of the follicle in the ovary. While follicular ROS increases apoptosis, glutathione (GSH) and follicle stimulating hormone (FSH) act as a balance in the growing follicle. FSH increases in response to estrogen, which triggers catalase production in the dominant follicle, thereby preventing apoptosis [108].

After ovulation, the corpus luteum synthesizes progesterone. Likewise, ROS, which has a key role in reproduction, is also produced in the corpus luteum [108, 112], and antioxidants play an important role in corpus luteum physiology during the cycle [112–114]. When pregnancy does not occur, the corpus luteum shrinks. During pregnancy, progesterone is continuously synthesized [112].

In mammalian species, the main function of the corpus luteum (CL) is the synthesis of progesterone, which is required for the establishment of a uterine environment suitable for the development of the peri-implantation conceptus and the successful progression and maintenance of pregnancy. Progesterone acts on the endometrium to regulate the synthesis of growth factors, cytokines, transport and adhesion proteins, protease inhibitors, hormones, and enzymes, which are primary regulators of conceptus implantation, survival, and development. Thus, compromised CL progesterone production is a potential risk factor for prenatal development and pregnancy outcomes [114].

There should be a rapid decline in the progesterone level for good follicular growth. During the middle luteal phase, superoxide dismutase 1 (SOD1, cofactor Cu or Zn) increases in the CL and decreases during regression [108]. PGF2α is defined as luteolysin because it increases in the CL during regression [115] and inhibits progesterone production by luteal cells. The inhibitory effect of PGF2α on progesterone production by the CL is due in part to increased ROS. In addition, progesterone levels decrease due to the destructive effects of oxidative stressors on luteal cell steroidogenesis [116–118]. ROS can also inhibit progesterone synthesis through inhibition of cytochrome P450, mitochondrial intracellular transport of cholesterol, and degradation of LH receptors [112].

Although the mechanisms of CL rescue from cell death and maintenance of progesterone production are very complex and vary among mammalian species, substantial evidence suggests ROS are key factors in determining the CL lifespan and antioxidants play significant roles in CL physiology during the estrous/menstrual cycle. Luteal ROS production and propagation depend upon several regulating factors, including luteal antioxidants, steroid hormones and cytokines, and their crosstalk. However, it is unknown which of these factors have the greatest contribution to CL function. In addition, the sequence of events leading to the functional and structural luteal regression at the end of the estrous/menstrual cycle is still not clear. The scarce in-vivo reports studying the CL of rats and sheep have shown the importance of antioxidant enzymes in the control of CL function during the peri-implantation period. As a luteal phase defect can impact fertility by preventing implantation and early conceptus development in livestock and humans, this review attempts to address the importance of ROS-scavenging antioxidant enzymes in the control of mammalian CL function and integrity [119].

The production of ATP is derived from the mitochondrial respiratory chain oxidative phosphorylation, which is the main source of oxygen-free radicals and non-radical ROS. The ROS include superoxide anion (—O_2—), hydroxyl radical (—OH), nitric oxide (NO), hydrogen peroxide (H_2O_2), and peroxynitrite (ONOO—). ROS are also produced via enzymatic pathways, including the activity of membrane-bound NADH and NADPH oxidases, the activity of xanthine oxidase, the metabolism of arachidonic acid by lipoxygenases and cyclooxygenases (COX), and the mitochondrial cytochrome P450 [119].

The cause of the ROS concentration increase in the regression phase may be a decrease in the SOD1 concentration. A decrease in SOD1 concentration may be due to an increase in PGF2α or macrophages, or a decrease in blood flow to the ovaries [108]. In the CL, luteal cells and phagocytic leukocytes stimulate the production of a superoxide anion. With decreased blood flow to the ovaries, ROS production increases and causes tissue damage. Concentrations of superoxide dismutase 2 (SOD2, cofactor Mn) in the CL increase to clear the ROS produced in the mitochondria during regression. Along with the complete lysis of the CL, the regressor decreases significantly in the SOD2 cells [110]. The SOD1 enzyme is closely related to progesterone production. SOD2 protects luteal cells from oxidative stress induced inflammation [108].

Aerobic cells are equipped with antioxidant enzymes that control ROS production and prevent their propagation to toxic ROS. The conversion of —O_2— to H_2O_2 by superoxide dismutase (SOD) is the first enzymatic antioxidative pathway. Two different SOD enzymes were identified: copper-zinc-containing SOD (SOD1) is predominantly localized in the cytosol and can be found in mitochondria, and manganese-containing SOD (SOD2) localizes in the mitochondrial matrix. Glutathione peroxidase (GPX) is a group of selenium-containing enzymes that belong to the first antioxidant mechanism preventing the propagation of highly reactive ROS by catalyzing the conversion of H_2O_2 to H_2O and O_2. NADH and NADPH are key elements in the control of ROS production and maintenance of the cellular redox state. The mitochondrial NADP+-dependent isocitrate dehydrogenase generates NADPH via oxidative decarboxylation of isocitrate [119].

Like any aerobic cells, those of the CL produce ATP through the respiration of O_2 with the consequence of luteal ROS production. The rate-limiting step in steroidogenesis in all steroidogenic organs, including the CL, is the transfer of cholesterol from the outer to the inner mitochondrial membrane where it is converted into pregnenolone by the enzyme cytochrome

P450scc. Luteal ROS are generated via enzymatic pathways of the mitochondrial cytochrome P450. In the CL, macrophages and luteal cells produce ROS where they can affect progesterone production. Indeed, there is substantial evidence to indicate that ROS regulate steroid hormone biosynthesis in the CL. The induction of ovarian SOD by LH, which in turn could lead to the production of H_2O_2, suggests that this action is involved in the LH stimulation of progesterone secretion in the CL. Thus, ROS can function beneficially to control the production of progesterone by luteal cells over the course of the reproductive cycle and inhibit progesterone synthesis at the end of the cycle. The O_2— radical is reported to be involved in the mechanism by which LH stimulates progesterone secretion [94, 119].

Oxidative stress may affect various physiological functions, such as folliculogenesis and steroidogenesis, in the female reproductive system. High ROS levels may also cause adverse pregnancy outcomes or embryonic/fetal losses [120–122] and are implicated in the etiopathogenesis of cystic ovarian disease [123]. ROS and the oxidative stress index in cows may be higher in the luteal phase than follicular phase, especially when progesterone is high. Again, in the luteal phase, the antioxidant status can be high or low. Imbalances, especially in oxidant and antioxidant capacity, can cause cystic ovarian disease by disturbing physiological events necessary for ovulation [124].

High free radical and low progesterone concentrations were detected in cows identified as repeat breeders. Infertility problems such as repeat breeder are encountered due to a low progesterone level in the critical period of pregnancy and the short life of the CL. All kinds of stress factors cause excessive radical production in high milk-yielding cows. This may be a determining factor for the amount of progesterone synthesized by inhibiting luteal cell function [125, 126]. In another study, the complex arrangement of antioxidant enzymes and compounds in the bovine CL was discussed. In particular, the correlation between antioxidant capacity and progesterone concentration was determined in the luteal phase of the estrous cycle. Findings show that antioxidative mechanisms are activated to cope with oxidative stress, which has a negative effect on steroid hormone synthesis [127]. In support of the previous study, it has been suggested that an antioxidant substance (astaxanthin) promotes progesterone synthesis in bovine luteal cell culture. However, attention has been drawn to the fact that the use of antioxidant material at low doses is beneficial [128].

Anestrus is a problem of infertility in which cyclic activity is absent and therefore estrogen-progesterone hormones are not expressed. Non-cyclic Murrah buffaloes were found to have low concentrations of antioxidants such as β-carotene and vitamin E [129]. Oxidative stress biomarkers change in cow milk during the anovulatory and ovulatory estrous cycles. In particular, the SOD levels in cyclic cows are significantly higher than levels in the anovulatory cycle, while the concentrations of lipoperoxides, GSH-Px, and GSH are lower. A low level of lipoperoxides, GSH-Px, and GSH is assumed to be an important event prior to the ovulation response, with high levels of milk SOD concentration in the ovulatory cycle cows [130].

Nitric oxide is synergistic with progesterone and may reduce relaxation by relieving uterine contraction during the paracrine-style secretion phase. In sheep, the regulation of reproductive physiology is related to the effects of oxidative stress [117]. Increased levels of progesterone during pregnancy in sheep and goats as well as increased levels of malondialdehyde (MDA) in placentomas have been reported [131]. Significant reductions in antioxidant substances may occur in placentomas during early gestation in sheep. These changes in the antioxidant enzymatic defenses of the placenta are thought to be an adaptation to the oxidative stress caused by ROS in early pregnancy [132]. According to the results obtained, pregnancy may be a stressor and it may be beneficial to support progesterone production with antioxidants in order to mitigate oxidative stress effects [131, 132]. The application of antioxidant vitamins in estrus synchronization during the breeding season reduces free radical levels, increases pregnancy performance, and increases the litter size in Tuj sheep [133]. However, β-carotene and vitamin E applications before estrus synchronization did not cause significant changes in plasma MDA levels in sheep during the breeding season [66]. Serum progesterone concentration increases after administration of intravaginal progesterone-releasing devices for estrus synchronization in goats increases oxidants such as eNOS activity, NO, MDA, and total oxidation status total oxidation status decreased [68, 69]. Short-term PRID treatments increase serum progesterone levels but decrease total antioxidant capacity in dairy heifers [23].

6. Conclusion

Progesterone is synthesized in the luteal phase and is an important hormone required for the continuity of pregnancy in ruminants. It is widely used in cattle for the purpose of estrus synchronization. In addition, this hormone, which has many uses in clinical practice, continues to be explored in ruminants. As time progresses, more detailed facts about the complex effects of progesterone in the organism, its use in clinical practice in ruminants, and the relationship of progesterone to oxidative stress in ruminants will be revealed.

Author details

Mushap Kuru[1]*, Abdulsamed Kükürt[2], Hasan Oral[1] and Metin Öğün[2]

*Address all correspondence to: mushapkuru@hotmail.com

1 Department of Obstetrics and Gynecology, Faculty of Veterinary Medicine, Kafkas University, Kars, Turkey

2 Department of Biochemistry, Faculty of Veterinary Medicine, Kafkas University, Kars, Turkey

References

[1] Helbling IM, Luna JA. Progesterone administration in planned reproduction of cattle. In: Rivera C, editor. Progesterone: Functions, Uses and Research Insights. USA: Nova Science Publishers; 2017. pp. 69-125

[2] Kuru M. Holstein ırkı düvelerde progesteron ile kombine edilen Cosynch protokolünde ovulasyonun uyarılması amacıyla hCG veya GnRH hormonu kullanılmasının gebelik oranları üzerine etkisi [thesis in Turkish]. Kars: Kafkas University; 2015

[3] Salmon AB, Richardson A, Pérez VI. Update on the oxidative stress theory of aging: Does oxidative stress play a role in aging or healthy aging? Free Radical Biology and Medicine. 2010;**48**:642-655. DOI: 10.1016/j.freeradbiomed.2009.12.015

[4] Brewer GJ: Epigenetic oxidative redox shift (EORS) theory of aging unifies the free radical and insulin signaling theories. Experimental Gerontology. 2010;**45**:173-179. DOI: 10.1016/j.exger.2009.11.007

[5] Descamps A, Cespuglio R. Influence of aging on the sleep rebound induced by immobilization stress in the rat. Brain Research. 2010;**1335**:14-23. DOI: 10.1016/j.brainres.2010.03.087

[6] Garrido P, de Blas M, Del Arco A, Segovia G, Mora F. Aging increases basal but not stress-induced levels of corticosterone in the brain of the awakened rat. Neurobiology of Aging. 2010;**33**:375-382. DOI: 10.1016/j.neurobiolaging.2010.02.015

[7] Durieux J, Wolff S, Dillin A. The cell-non-autonomous nature of electron transport chain-mediated longevity. Cell. 2011;**144**:79-91. DOI: 10.1016/j.cell.2010.12.016

[8] Woo DK, Shadel GS. Mitochondrial stress signals revised an old aging theory. Cell. 2011;**144**:11-12. DOI: 10.1016/j.cell.2010.12.023

[9] Huang N, Pandey AV, Agrawal V, Reardon W, Lapunzina PD, Mowat D, Jabs EW, Van Vliet G, Sack J, Flück CE, Miller WL. Diversity and function of mutations in P450 oxidoreductase in patients with Antley-Bixler syndrome and disordered steroidogenesis. American Journal of Human Genetics. 2005;**76**:729-749. DOI: 10.1086/429417

[10] Miyamoto A, Shirasuna K: Luteolysis in the cow: A novel concept of vasoactive molecules. Animal Reproduction. 2009;**6**:47-59

[11] Kuru M, Oral H, Kulaksiz R. Mechanism of luteolysis and vasoactive agents in cows. Atatürk Üniversitesi Veteriner Bilimleri Dergisi. 2014;**9**:141-148. DOI: 10.17094/avbd.01918

[12] Alaçam E, Saban E, Ay SS. The evaluation of various radioimmunoassay progesterone kits for different stage of reproductive period in the cow, sheep and bitch. Ankara Üniversitesi Veteriner Fakültesi Dergisi. 2009;**56**:37-41. DOI: 10.1501/Vetfak_0000002183

[13] Öcal H, Doğan H, Saat N, Aydin M. Progesterone, progestins and antiprogestins. Turkiye Klinikleri Journal of Veterinary Sciences – Obstetrics and Gynecology – Special Topics. 2015;**1**:60-86

[14] Alaçam E. Koyun ve keçilerde döl verimi. In: Aytuğ CN, Alaçam E, Özkoç Ü, Yalçın BC, Gökçen H, Türker H, editors. Koyun-Keçi Hastalıkları ve Yetiştiriciliği. İstanbul: TÜM VET Hayvancılık Hizmetleri Yayını, Teknografik Matbaası; 1990. pp. 355-366 (Book in Turkish)

[15] Kalkan C, Horoz H. Pubertas ve seksüel sikluslar. In: Alaçam E, editor. Evcil Hayvanlarda Doğum ve İnfertilite. Ankara: Medisan, 2015. pp. 23-40 (Book in Turkish)

[16] Canooğlu E, Sarıbay K. Koyun keçilerde üreme kanalının morfolojisi ve fizyolojisi. In: Semacan A, Kaymaz M, Fındık M, Rişvanlı A, Köker A, editors. Çiftlik Hayvanlarında Doğum ve Jinekoloji. Malatya: Medipres; 2012. pp. 467-490 (Book in Turkish)

[17] Hanlon DW, Williamson NB, Wichtel JJ, Steffert IJ, Craigie AL, Pfeiffer DU. The effect of estradiol benzoate administration on estrous response and synchronized pregnancy rate in dairy heifers after treatment with exogenous progesterone. Theriogenology. 1996;**45**: 775-785. DOI: 10.1016/0093-691X(96)00007-6

[18] Patterson DJ, Wood SL, Kojima FN, Smith MF. Current and emerging methods to synchronize estrus with melengestrol acetate (MGA). In: Fields MJ, Sand RS, Yelich JV, editors. Factors Effecting Calf Crop Biotechnology of Reproduction. London: CRC Press; 2002. pp. 57-86

[19] Kuru M, Merhan O, Kaya S, Oral H, Kükürt A. The effect of short time PRID application on acute phase proteins for Holstein heifers. Turkish Journal of Chemistry. 2015;**40** (Suppl 1):63-64

[20] Kuru M, Oral H, Çolak A, Gürbulak K, Bekyürek T. The effect of hCG or GnRH administration for induction of ovulation as part of a 5-day Cosynch + Progesterone protocol on the pregnancy rates of heifers. In: VI. National Congress of Turkish Society of Veterinary Gynaecology; October 15–18, 2015; Muğla, Turkey: Plaza Event Kongre; pp. 86-87

[21] Kuru M, Merhan O, Kaya S, Oral H, Kukurt A. The effect of short term progesterone-releasing intravaginal device treatment on acute inflammation markers for Holstein heifers. Revue de Medecine Veterinaire. 2015;**166**:336-340

[22] Kuru M, Kükürt A, Oral H, Karapehlivan M. Relationship between pregnancy rate and serum sialic acid levels and paraoxonase activity after synchronization with progesterone releasing intravaginal device protocol in heifers. Journal of Cellular Neuroscience and Oxidative Stress. 2016;**8**:556-557

[23] Oral H, Ögün M, Kuru M, Kaya S. Evaluation of certain oxidative stress parameters in heifers that were administered short term PRID. Kafkas Universitesi Veteriner Fakultesi Dergisi. 2015;**21**:569-573. DOI: 10.9775/kvfd.2015.12969

[24] Day ML, Geary TW: Handbook of Estrous Synchronization. Western Association of Agricultural Experiment Station Directors (WAAESD). California: Western Region Publication No. 014; 2005

[25] Dorsey BR, Kasimanickam R, Whittier WD, Nebel RL, Wahlberg ML, Hall JB. Effect of time from estrus to AI on pregnancy rates in estrous synchronized beef heifers. Animal Reproduction Science. 2011;**127**:1-6. DOI: 10.1016/j.anireprosci.2011.07.014

[26] Kuru M, Oral H, Çolak A, Gürbulak K, Bekyürek T. The effect of hCG or GnRH administration on pregnancy rates in Holstein heifers when used to induce ovulation as part of a 5-day Co-Synch + Progesterone-Releasing Intravaginal Device protocol. Revue de Medecine Veterinaire. 2017;**168**:38-45

[27] Semacan A, Pancarcı ŞM. Üremenin denetlenmesi. In: Semacan A, Kaymaz M, Fındık M, Rişvanlı A, Köker A, editors. Çiftlik Hayvanlarında Doğum ve Jinekoloji. Malatya: Medipres; 2012. pp. 99-124 (Book in Turkish)

[28] Funston RN, Ansotegui RP, Lipsey RJ, Geary TW. Synchronization of estrus in beef heifers using either melengestrol acetate (MGA)/prostaglandin or MGA/Select Synch. Theriogenology. 2002;**57**:1485-1491. DOI: 10.1016/S0093-691X(02)00654-4

[29] Lucy MC, Billings HJ, Butler WR, Ehnis LR, Fields MJ, Kesler DJ, Kinder JE, Mattos RC, Short RE, Thatcher WW, Wettemann RP, Yelich JV, Hafs HD. Efficacy of an intravaginal progesterone insert and an injection of PGF2alpha for synchronizing estrus and shortening the interval to pregnancy in postpartum beef cows, peripubertal beef heifers, and dairy heifers. Journal of Animal Science. 2001;**79**:982-995. DOI: 10.2527/2001.794982x

[30] Lamb GC, Larson JE, Geary TW, Stevenson JS, Johnson SK, Day ML, Ansotegui RP, Kesler DJ, DeJarnette JM, Landblom DG. Synchronization of estrus and artificial insemination in replacement beef heifers using gonadotropin-releasing hormone, prostaglandin F2α, and progesterone. Journal of Animal Science. 2006;**84**:3000-3009. DOI: 10.2527/jas.2006-220

[31] Richardson AM, Hensley BA, Marple TJ, Johnson SK, Stevenson JS. Characteristics of estrus before and after first insemination and fertility of heifers after synchronized estrus using GnRH, PGF2α and progesterone. Journal of Animal Science. 2002;**80**:2792-2800. DOI: 10.2527/2002.80112792x

[32] Chenault JR, Boucher JF, Hafs HD. Synchronization of estrus in beef cows and beef and dairy heifers with intravaginal progesterone inserts and prostaglandin F2α with or without gonadotropin-releasing hormone. The Professional Animal Scientists. 2003;**19**: 116-123. DOI: 10.15232/S1080-7446(15)31390-5

[33] Bridges GA, Portillo GE, de Araujo JW, Thatcher WW, Yelich JW. Efficacy of either a single or split treatment of PGF2α after a 14 day melengestrol acetate treatment to synchronize estrus and induce luteolysis in *Bos indicus* x *Bos taurus* heifers. Theriogenology. 2005;**64**:344-362. DOI: 10.1016/j.theriogenology.2004.12.003

[34] McDougall S, Rhodes FM, Compton CWR. Evaluation of three synchrony programs for pasture-based dairy heifers. Theriogenology. 2013;**79**:882-889. DOI: 10.1016/j.theriogenology.2012.12.013

[35] Bisinotto RS, Pansani MB, Castro LO, Narciso CD, Sinedino LD, Martinez N, Carneiro PE, Thatcher WW, Santos JE. Effect of progesterone supplementation on fertility responses of lactating dairy cows with corpus luteum at the initiation of the Ovsynch protocol. Theriogenology. 2015;**83**:257-265. DOI: 10.3168/jds.2014-9058

[36] Kim IH, Suh GH, Son DS. A progesterone – based timed AI protocol more effectively prevents premature estrus and incomplete luteal regression than Ovsynch protocol in lactating Holstein cows. Theriogenology. 2003;**60**:809-817. DOI: 10.1016/S0093-691X(03)00136-5

[37] Wheaton JE, Lamb GC. Induction of cyclicity in postpartum anestrous beef cows using progesterone, GnRH and estradiol cypionate (ECP). Animal Reproduction Science. 2007;**102**:208-216. DOI: 10.1016/j.anireprosci.2006.11.006

[38] Stevenson JL, Dalton JC, Santos JEP, Sartori R, Ahmadzadeh A, Chebel RC. Effect of synchronization protocols on follicular development and estradiol and progesterone concentrations of dairy heifers. Journal of Dairy Science. 2008;**91**:3045-3056. DOI: 10.3168/jds.2007-0625

[39] Howard JM, Falk DG, Carnahan KG, Dalton JC, Chebel RC, Ahmadzadeh A. The use of gonadotropin-releasing hormone in a progesterone-based timed artificial insemination protocol in replacement beef heifers. The Professional Animal Scientists. 2009;**25**:757-761. DOI: 10.15232/S1080-7446(15)30785-3

[40] Colazo MG, Ambrose DJ. Neither duration of progesterone insert nor initial GnRH treatment affected pregnancy per timed-insemination in dairy heifers subjected to a Co-synch protocol. Theriogenology. 2011;**76**:578-588. DOI: 10.1016/j.theriogenology.2011.03.013

[41] Busch DC, Wilson DJ, Schafer DJ, Leitman NR, Haden JK, Ellersieck MR, Smith MF, Patterson DJ. Comparison of progestin-based estrus synchronization protocols before fixed-time artificial insemination on pregnancy rate in beef heifers. Journal of Animal Science. 2007;**85**:1933, 1939. DOI: 10.2527/jas.2006-845

[42] Hyland A, Seidel GE Jr, Enns RM, Peel RK, Whittier JC. Intervals of five or seven days between controlled internal drug-release insertion, gonadotropin-releasing hormone, and prostaglandin F2α injections: Effects on pregnancy rate and follicular size. The Professional Animal Scientists. 2009;**25**:150-154. DOI: 10.15232/S1080-7446(15)30697-5

[43] Kasimanickam R, Day ML, Rudolph JS, Hall JB, Whittier WD. Two doses of prostaglandin improve pregnancy rates to timed-AI in a 5-day progesterone-based synchronization protocol in beef cows. Theriogenology. 2009;**71**:762-767. DOI: 10.1016/j.theriogenology.2008.09.049

[44] Bartolome JA, Silvestre FT, Kamimura S, Arteche ACM, Melendez P, Kelbert D, Mchale J, Swift K, Archbald LF, Thatcher WW. Resynchronization of ovulation and timed insemination in lactating dairy cows I: Use of the Ovsynch and Heatsynch protocols after non-pregnancy diagnosis by ultrasonography. Theriogenology. 2005;**63**:1617-1627. DOI: 10.1016/j.theriogenology.2004.07.016

[45] Goodman RL. Neuroendocrine control of the ovine estrous cycle. In: Knobil E, Neil JD, editors. The Physiology of Reproduction. New York: Raven Press; 1988. pp. 1929-1969

[46] Kaneko H, Nakanishi Y, Taya K, Kishi H, Watanabe G, Sasemoto S, Hasegawa Y. Evidence that inhibin is an important factor in the regulation of FSH secretion during the mid-luteal phase in cows. The Journal of Endocrinology. 1993;**136**:35-41. DOI: 10.1677/joe.0.1360035

[47] Kaçar C, Kaya S, Kuru M, Zonturlu AK. Contemporary methods for the control of reproduction in sheep and goats. Turkiye Klinikleri Journal of Veterinary Sciences – Obstetrics and Gynecology – Special Topics. 2016;**2**:29-37

[48] Kuru M, Sogukpinar O, Makav M, Cetin N. Effect of barium selenate injections on fertility of Pirlak ewes subjected to estrus synchronization during non-breeding season. Medycyna Weterynaryjna. 2017;**73**:479-482

[49] Jackson CG, Neville TL, Mercadante VRG, Waters KM, Lamb GC, Dahlen CR, Redden RR. Efficacy of various five-day estrous synchronization protocols in sheep. Small Ruminant Research. 2014;**120**:100-107. DOI: 10.1016/j.smallrumres.2014.04.004

[50] Martemucci G, D'Alessandro AG. Synchronization of oestrus and ovulation by short time combined FGA, PGF2α, GnRH, eCG treatments for natural service or AI fixed-time. Animal Reproduction Science. 2011;**123**:32-39. DOI: 10.1016/j.anireprosci.2010.11.007

[51] Vilarino M, Rubianes E, van Lier E, Menchaca A. Serum progesterone concentrations, follicular development and time of ovulation using a new progesterone releasing device (DICO®) in sheep. Small Ruminant Research. 2010;**91**:219-224. DOI: 10.1016/j.smallrumres.2010.02.014

[52] Fleisch A, Werne S, Heckendorn F, Hartnack S, Piechotta M, Bollwein H, Thun R, Janett F. Comparison of 6-day progestagen treatment with Chronogest® CR and Eazi-breedTM CIDR® G intravaginal inserts for estrus synchronization in cyclic ewes. Small Ruminant Research. 2012;**107**:141-146. DOI: 10.1016/j.smallrumres.2012.05.014

[53] Kuru M, Kükürt A, Oral H, Kulaksiz R, Karapehlivan M. The effects of the use of controlled internal drug release CIDR for estrus synchronization on paraoxonase activities and total sialic acid levels in Georgian goats. In: 12th International Conference on Goats; September 25–30, 2016; Antalya, Turkey: International Goat Association; p. 192

[54] Kuru M, Kükürt A, Kulaksiz R, Oral H, Çetin N, Karapehlivan M. Controlled internal drug release use for synchronization on paraoxonase activities and total sialic acid levels in Abasian goats. Journal of Cellular Neuroscience and Oxidative Stress. 2016;**8**:544

[55] Kuru M, Boga Kuru B, Kulaksiz R, Ari UÇ, Oral H. Effects of the progesterone-based estrus synchronization on some reproductive parameters in Abaza goats. Kocatepe Veterinary Journal. 2017;**10**:156-163. DOI: 10.5578/kvj.57526

[56] Gordon I. Controlled Reproduction in Sheep and Goats. United Kingdom: CABI Publishing; 1997

[57] Kulaksız R, Daşkın A, Dalcı T. Some reproductive traits of ewes from different breeds following oestrus synchronisation by flugeston acetate-eCG during the breeding season. Atatürk Üniversitesi Veteriner Bilimleri Dergisi. 2011;**6**:9-15

[58] Abecia JA, Forcada F, Gonzalez-Bulnes A. Hormonal control of reproduction in small ruminants. Animal Reproduction Science. 2012;**130**:173-179. DOI: 10.1016/j.anireprosci.2012.01.011

[59] Kulaksız R, Uçar Ö, Daşkın A. Effects of FGA sponge and Ovsynch based protocols on reproductive performance of fat tailed ewes during the breeding season. Kafkas Universitesi Veteriner Fakultesi Dergisi. 2013;**19**:629-633. DOI: 10.9775/kvfd.2013.8568

[60] Fentoni LS, Shackell GH, Ramsay ML, Dodds KG, Reid PJ, Mcleodi BJ. Influence of year, age, and geographical location on induced oestrus in ewes early in the breeding season. New Zealand Journal of Agricultural Research. 1997;**40**:69-74. DOI: 10.1080/00288233.1997.9513231

[61] Evans ACO, Duffy P, Crosby TF, Hawken PAR, Boland MP, Beard AP. Effect of ram exposure at the end of progestagen treatment on estrus synchronisation and fertility during the breeding season in ewes. Animal Reproduction Science. 2004;**84**:349-358. DOI: 10.1016/j.anireprosci.2003.12.013

[62] Ungerfeld R, Rubianes E. Estrous response to ram effect in Corriedale ewes primed with medroxyprogesterone during the breeding season. Small Ruminant Research. 1999;**32**: 89-91. DOI: 10.1016/S0921-4488(98)00164-3

[63] Gungor O, Cenesiz M, Pancarci SM, Yildiz S, Kaya M, Kacar C, Ozyurlu N, Gurbulak K. Effects of different intravaginal progesterone releasing devices on estrous synchronization and LH surge in fat-tailed ewes during non-breeding season. Medycyna Weteryn aryjna. 2007;**63**:1316-1319

[64] Hashemi M, Safdarian M, Kafi M. Estrous response to synchronization of estrus using different progesterone treatments outside the natural breeding season in ewes. Small Ruminant Research. 2006;**65**:279-283. DOI: 10.1016/j.smallrumres.2005.07.051

[65] Zonturlu AK, Özyurtlu N, Kaçar C. Effect of different doses PMSG on estrus synchronization and fertility in Awassi ewes synchronized with progesterone during the transition period. Kafkas Universitesi Veteriner Fakultesi Dergisi. 2011;**17**:125-129. DOI: 10.9775/kvfd.2010.2572

[66] Kaçar C, Kamiloğlu NN, Gürbulak K, Pancarcı ŞM, Güngör Ö, Güvenç K, Gürbulak K, Şaban E. The effect of administration of testosterone antibody, β-carotene and vitamin E on multiple pregnancy and MDA (malondialdehyde) in Tuj breed sheep in non-breeding season. Kafkas Üniversitesi Veteriner Fakültesi Dergisi. 2008;**14**:51-56. DOI: 10.9775/kvfd.2008.03-A

[67] Abecia JA, Forcada F, González-Bulnes A. Pharmaceutical control of reproduction in sheep and goats. The Veterinary Clinics of North America Food Animal Practice. 2011;**27**:67-79. DOI: 10.1016/j.cvfa.2010.10.001

[68] Kuru M, Ögün M, Oral H, Kükürt A, Makav M, Kulaksiz R. The use of controlled internal drug release for synchronization augmented oxidative and nitrosative stress and leptin levels in Georgian goats. Journal of Cellular Neuroscience and Oxidative Stress. 2016;**8**:541-542

[69] Kuru M, Ögün M, Oral H, Kükürt A, Erkiliç EE, Kulaksiz R. Synchronization with controlled internal drug release CIDR on exacerbate oxidative and nitrosative stress and leptin levels in Abasian goats. In: 12th International Conference on Goats; September 25–30, 2016; Antalya, Turkey: International Goat Association; p. 191

[70] Zhao Y, Zhang J, Wei H, Sun X, Mu B, Yu M, Wang L. Efficiency of methods applied for goat estrous synchronization in subtropical monsoonal climate zone of Southwest China. Tropical Animal Health and Production. 2010;**42**:1257-1262. DOI: 10.1007/s11250-010-9558-6

[71] Penna B, Libonati H, Director A, Sarzedas AC, Martins G, Brandão FZ, Fonseca J, Lilenbaum W. Progestin-impregnated intravaginal sponges for estrus induction and synchronization influences on goats vaginal flora and antimicrobial susceptibility. Animal Reproduction Science. 2013;**142**:71-74. DOI: 10.1016/j.anireprosci.2013.09.006

[72] Oliveira JK, Martins G, Esteves LV, Penna B, Hamond C, Fonseca JF, Rodrigues AL, Brandão FZ, Lilenbaum W. Changes in the vaginal flora of goats following a short-term protocol of oestrus induction and synchronisation with intravaginal sponges as well as their antimicrobial sensitivity. Small Ruminant Research. 2013;**113**:162-166. DOI: 10.1016/j.smallrumres.2013.02.011

[73] Şenünver A, Nak Y. İnfertilite. In: Semacan A, Kaymaz M, Fındık M, Rişvanlı A, Köker, editors. Çiftlik Hayvanlarında Doğum ve Jinekoloji. Malatya: Medipres; 2012. pp. 409-464 (Book in Turkish)

[74] Perry GA, Smith MF, Roberts AJ, MacNeil MD, Geary TW. Relationship between size of the ovulatory follicle and pregnancy success in beef heifers. Journal of Animal Science. 2007;**85**:684-689. DOI: 10.2527/jas.2006-519

[75] Diskin MG, Morris DG. Embryonic and early foetal losses in cattle and other ruminants. Reproduction in Domestic Animals. 2008;**43**(Suppl 2):260-267. DOI: 10.1111/j.1439-0531.2008.01171.x

[76] Diskin MG, Parr MH, Morris DG. Embryo death in cattle: An update. Reproduction, Fertility, and Development. 2011;**24**:244-251. DOI: 10.1071/RD11914

[77] Alnimer MA, Lubbadeh WF. Effect of progesterone (P4) intravaginal device (CIDR) to reduce embryonic loss and to synchronize return to oestrus of previously timed inseminated lactating dairy cows. Animal Reproduction Science. 2008;**107**:36-47. DOI: 10.1016/j.anireprosci.2007.06.018

[78] Mehni SB, Shabankareh HK, Kazemi-Bonchenari M, Eghbali M. The comparison of treating Holstein dairy cows with progesterone, CIDR and GnRH after insemination on serum progesterone and pregnancy rates. Reproduction in Domestic Animals. 2012;**47**:131-134. DOI: 10.1111/j.1439-0531.2011.01811.x

[79] Larson FS, Butler RW, Currie BW. Pregnancy rates in lactating dairy cattle following supplementation of progesterone after artificial insemination. Animal Reproduction Science. 2007;**102**:172-179. DOI: 10.1016/j.anireprosci.2007.02.023

[80] Mann GE, Lamming GE. The influence of progesterone during early pregnancy in cattle. Reproduction in Domestic Animals. 1999;**34**:269-274. DOI: 10.1111/j.1439-0531.1999.tb01250.x

[81] Macmillan KL, Taufa VK, Day AM, Peterson AJ. Effects of supplemental progesterone on pregnancy rates in cattle. Journal of Reproduction and Fertility. Supplement. 1991;**43**:304

[82] Ataman MB, Aköz M, Saribay MK, Erdem H, Bucak MN. Prevention of embryonic death using different hormonal treatments in ewes. Turkish Journal of Veterinary and Animal Sciences. 2013;**37**:6-8. DOI: 10.3906/vet-1102-795

[83] Peter AT, Vos PLAM, Ambrose DJ. Postpartum anestrus in dairy cattle. Theriogenology. 2009;**71**:1333-1342. DOI: 10.1016/j.theriogenology.2008.11.012

[84] Yániz J, Murugavel K, López-Gatius F. Recent developments in oestrous synchronization of postpartum dairy cows with and without ovarian disorders. Reproduction in Domestic Animals. 2004;**39**:86-93. DOI: 10.1111/j.1439-0531.2004.00483.x

[85] Stevenson JS, Tenhouse DE, Krisher RL, Lamb GC, Larson JE, Dahlen CR, Pursley JR, Bello NM, Fricke PM, Wiltbank MC, Brusveen DJ, Burkhart M, Youngquist RS, Garverick HA. Detection of anovulation by heatmount detectors and transrectal ultrasonography before treatment with progesterone in a timed insemination protocol. Journal of Dairy Science. 2008;**91**:2901-2915. DOI: 10.3168/jds.2007-0856

[86] Peter AT. An update on cystic ovarian degeneration in cattle. Reproduction in Domestic Animals. 2004;**39**:1-7. DOI: 10.1046/j.0936-6768.2003.00466.x

[87] Hatler TB, Hayes SH, Anderson LH, Silvia WJ. Effect of a single injection of progesterone on ovarian follicular cysts in lactating dairy cows. Veterinary Journal. 2006;**172**:329-333. DOI: 10.1016/j.tvjl.2005.04.020

[88] López-Gatius F, Santolaria P, Yániz J, Rutllant J, López-Béjar M. Persistent ovarian follicles in dairy cows: A therapeutic approach. Theriogenology. 2001;**56**:649-659. DOI: 10.1016/S0093-691X(01)00596-9

[89] Davis SR, Welch RAS, Pearce MG, Peterson AJ. Induction of lactation in nonpregnant cows by estradiol-17β and progesterone from an intravaginal sponge. Journal of Dairy Science. 1983;**66**:450-457. DOI: 10.3168/jds.S0022-0302(83)81813-X

[90] Mohan K, Shridhar NB, Jayakumar K, Honnappa TG, Madhusudhan HS. Lactation induction protocols and cost benefit analysis in repeat breeding cows. Indian Journal of Animal Research. 2010;**44**:44-47

[91] Öcal H, Apaydın AM, Timurkan H, Kalkan C, Deveci H, Çetin H, Kaygusuzoğlu E. Döl tutmayan ve yavru atan düvelerde laktasyonun uyarılması ve bunun gebe kalma üzerine etkisi. Fırat Üniversitesi Sağlık Bilimleri Veteriner Dergisi. 1994;**8**:76-82 (Article in Turkish)

[92] Larry Smith K, Schanbacher FL: Hormone induced lactation in the bovine. I. lactational performance following injections of 17β-estradiol and progesterone. Journal of Dairy Science. 1973;**56**:738-743. DOI: 10.3168/jds.S0022-0302(73)85243-9

[93] Fulkerson WJ, McDowell GH. Artificial induction of lactation in ewes. The Journal of Endocrinology. 1974;**63**:167-173. DOI: 10.1677/joe.0.0630167

[94] Takiguchi S, Sugino N. Esato Karube-Harada A, Sakata A, Nakamura Y, Ishikawa H, Kato H. Differential regulation of apoptosis in the corpus luteum of pregnancy and newly formed corpus luteum after parturition in rats. Biology of Reproduction. 2004;**70**: 313-318. DOI: 10.1095/biolreprod.103.018853

[95] Stolon I, Oros A, Moldaveanu E. Mineral view, apoptosis and free radicals. Biochemical and Molecular Medicine. 1996;**59**:93-97. DOI: 10.1006/bmme.1996.0072

[96] Valko M, Izakovic M, Mazur M, Rhodes CJ, Telser J. Role of oxygen radicals in DNA damage and cancer incidence. Molecular and Cellular Biochemistry. 2004;**266**:37-56. DOI: 10.1023/B:MCBI.0000049134.69131.89

[97] Ozcan A, Ogun M. Biochemistry of reactive oxygen and nitrogen species. In: Gowder SJT, editor. Basic Principles and Clinical Significance of Oxidative Stress. Croatia: InTech; 2015. DOI: 10.5772/61193

[98] Koch OR, Pani G, Borrello S, Colavitti R, Cravero A, Farre S, Galeotti T. Oxidative stress and antioxidant defenses in ethanol-induced cell injury. Molecular Aspects of Medicine. 2004;**25**:191-198. DOI: 10.1016/j.mam.2004.02.019

[99] Kopani M, Celec P, Danisovic L, Michalka P, Biro C. Oxidative stress and electron spin resonance. Clinica Chimica Acta. 2006;**364**:61-66. DOI: 10.1016/j.cca.2005.05.016

[100] Gutteridge JMC, Halliwell B. Antioxidants in Nutrition, Health and Disease. New York: Oxford University Press; 1994

[101] Gitto E, Pellegroni S, Gitto P, Barberi I, Reiter RJ. Oxidative stress of the newborn in the pre- and postnatal period and the clinical utility of melatonin. Journal of Pineal Research. 2009;**46**:128-139. DOI: 10.1111/j.1600-079X.2008.00649.x

[102] Naito Y, Lee MC, Kato Y, Nagai R, Yonei Y. Oxidative stress markers. Anti-Aging. Medicine. 2010;**7**:33-44. DOI: 10.3793/jaam.7.36

[103] Cherubini A, Ruggiero C, Polidori MC, Mecocci P. Potential markers of oxidative stress in stroke. Free Radical Biology & Medicine. 2005;**39**:841-852. DOI: 10.1016/j.freeradbiomed.2005.06.025

[104] Clarkson PM, Thompson HS. Antioxidants: What role do they play in physical activity and health? The American Journal of Clinical Nutrition. 2000;**72**:637-646

[105] Cheeseman KH, Slater TF. An introduction to free radical biochemistry. British Medical Bulletin. 1994;**49**:481-493. DOI: 10.1093/oxfordjournals.bmb.a072625

[106] Serarslan G, Altuğ E, Kontas T, Atik E, Avci G. Caffeic acid phenetyl ester accelerates cutaneous wound healing in a rat model and decreases oxidative stress. Clinical and Experimental Dermatology. 2007;**32**:709-715. DOI: 10.1111/j.1365-2230.2007.02470.x

[107] Lichtenthaler R, Marx F, Kind OM. Determination of antioxidative capacities using an enhanced total oxidant scavenging capacity (TOSC) assay. European Food Research and Technology. 2003;**216**:166-173. DOI: 10.1007/s00217-002-0635-6

[108] Behrman HR, Kodaman PH, Preston SL, Gao S. Oxidative stress and the ovary. Journal of the Society for Gynecologic Investigation. 2001;**8**:S40-S42. DOI: 10.1177/1071557601008001S13

[109] Ruder EH, Hartman TJ, Goldman MB. Impact of oxidative stress on female fertility. Current Opinion in Obstetrics & Gynecology. 2009;**21**:219-222

[110] Shkolnik K, Tadmor A, Ben-Dor S, Nevo N, Galiani D, Dekel N. Reactive oxygen species are indispensable in ovulation. Proceedings of the National Academy of Sciences of the United States of America. 2011;**108**:1462-1467. DOI: 10.1073/pnas.1017213108

[111] Ciani F, Cocchia N, d'Angelo D, Tafuri S. Influence of ROS on ovarian functions. In: Wu B, editor. New Discoveries in Embryology. Croatia: InTech; 2015. DOI: 10.5772/61003

[112] Sugino N. Roles of reactive oxygen species in the corpus luteum. Animal Science Journal. 2006;**77**:556-565. DOI: 10.1111/j.1740-0929.2006.00386.x

[113] Al-Gubory KH, Camous S, Germain G, Bolifraud P, Nicole A, Ceballos-Picot I. Reconsideration of the proposed luteotropic and luteoprotective actions of ovine placental lactogen in sheep: In vivo and in vitro studies. The Journal of Endocrinology. 2006;**188**: 559-568. DOI: 10.1677/joe.1.06550

[114] Brannstrom M. Potential role of cytokines in ovarian physiology: The case for interleukin-1. In: Leung PCK, Adashi EY, editors. The Ovary. New York: Elsevier Academic Press; 2004. pp. 261-265

[115] Olofsson J, Norjavaara E, Selstam G. In vivo levels of prostaglandin F2α, E2 and prostacyclin in the corpus luteum of pregnant and pseudopregnant rats. Biology of Reproduction. 1990;**42**:792-800. DOI: 10.1095/biolreprod42.5.792

[116] Tanaka M, Miyazaki T, Tanigaki S, Kasai K, Minegishi K, Miyakoshi K, Ishimoto H, Yoshimura Y. Participation of reactive oxygen species in PGF2α-induced apoptosis in rat luteal cells. Journal of Reproduction and Fertility. 2000;**120**:239-245. DOI: 10.1530/jrf.0.1200239

[117] Celi P. The role of oxidative stress in small ruminants' health and production. Revista Brasileira de Zootecnia. 2010;**39**(Suppl. spe):348-363. DOI: 10.1590/S1516-35982010001300038

[118] Hayashi K, Miyamoto A, Konari A, Ohtani M, Fukui Y. Effect of local interaction of reactive oxygen species with prostaglandin F2α on the release of progesterone in ovine corpora lutea in vivo. Theriogenology. 2003;**59**:1335-1344. DOI: 10.1016/S0093-691X(02)01173-1

[119] Sugino N, Karube-Harada A, Taketani T, Sakata A, Nakamura Y. Withdrawal of ovarian steroids stimulates prostaglandin F2α production through nuclear factor-κB activation via oxygen radicals in human endometrial stromal cells: Potential relevance to menstruation. The Journal of Reproduction and Development. 2004;**50**:215-225. DOI: 10.1262/jrd.50.215

[120] Agarwal A, Gupta S, Sharma R. Role of oxidative stress in female reproduction. Reproductive Biology and Endocrinology. 2005;**3**:1-21. DOI: 10.1186/1477-7827-3-28

[121] Celi P, Merlo M, Da Dalt L, Stefani A, Barbato O, Gabai G. Relationship between late embryonic mortality and the increase in plasma advanced oxidised protein products (AOPP) in dairy cows. Reproduction, Fertility, and Development. 2011;**23**:527-533. DOI: 10.1071/RD10268

[122] Celi P, Merlo M, Barbato O, Gabai G. Relationship between oxidative stress and the success of artificial insemination in dairy cows in a pasture-based system. Veterinary Journal. 2012;**193**:498-502. DOI: 10.1016/j.tvjl.2012.02.002

[123] Rizzo A, Minoia G, Trisolini C, Mutinati M, Spedicato M, Jirillo F, Sciorsci RL. Reactive oxygen species (ROS): Involvement in bovine follicular cysts etiopathogenesis. Immunopharmacology and Immunotoxicology. 2009;**31**:631-635. DOI: 10.3109/08923970902932962

[124] Talukder S, Ingenhoff L, Kerrisk KL, Celi P. Plasma oxidative stress biomarkers and progesterone profiles in a dairy cow diagnosed with an ovarian follicular cyst. The Veterinary Quarterly. 2014;**34**:113-117. DOI: 10.1080/01652176.2014.953264

[125] Rizzo A, Minoia G, Trisolini C, Manca R, Sciorsci RL. Concentrations of free radicals and beta-endorphins in repeat breeder cows. Animal Reproduction Science. 2007;**100**:257-263. DOI: 10.1016/j.anireprosci.2006.08.013

[126] Rizzo A, Roscino MT, Binetti F, Sciorsci RL. Roles of reactive oxygen species in female reproduction. Reproduction in Domestic Animals. 2012;**47**:344-352. DOI: 10.1111/j.1439-0531.2011.01891.x

[127] Rapoport R, Sklan D, Wolfenson D, Shaham-Albalancy A, Hanukoglu I. Antioxidant capacity is correlated with steroidogenic status of the corpus luteum during the bovine estrous cycle. Biochimica et Biophysica Acta. 1998;**1380**:133-140. DOI: 10.1016/S0304-4165(97)00136-0

[128] Kamada H, Akagi S, Watanabe S. Astaxanthin increases progesterone production in cultured bovine luteal cells. The Journal of Veterinary Medical Science. 2017;**79**:1103-1109. DOI: 10.1292/jvms.17-0044

[129] Ghosh M, Gupta M, Kumar R, Kumar S, Balhara AK, Singh I. Relation between antioxidant status and postpartum anestrous condition in Murrah buffalo. Veterinary World. 2015;**8**:1163-1166. DOI: 10.14202/vetworld.2015.1163-1166

[130] Talukder S, Kerrisk KL, Gabai G, Fukutomi A, Celi P. Changes in milk oxidative stress biomarkers in lactating dairy cows with ovulatory and an-ovulatory oestrous cycles. Animal Reproduction Science. 2015;**158**:86-95. DOI: 10.1016/j.anireprosci.2015.05.004

[131] Nawito MF, Hameed AR, Sosa AS, Mahmoud KG. Impact of pregnancy and nutrition on oxidant/antioxidant balance in sheep and goats reared in South Sinai, Egypt. Veterinary World. 2016;**9**:801-805. DOI: 10.14202/vetworld.2016.801-805

[132] Garrel C, Fowler PA, Al-Gubory KH. Developmental changes in antioxidant enzymatic defences against oxidative stress in sheep placentomes. The Journal of Endocrinology. 2010;**205**:107-116. DOI: 10.1677/JOE-09-0362

[133] Kamiloğlu NN, Kaçar C, Güven A, Yıldız B, Kuru M, Kaya S, Eroğlu HA, Koç E. Changes in lipid peroxidation, glutathione and fertility in Tuj sheep after combined administration of vitamin A and E and passive immunization with testosterone antibodies. Kafkas Universitesi Veteriner Fakultesi Dergisi. 2017;**23**:459-465. DOI: 10.9775/kvfd.2016.17053

11

Sex Hormones and Inner Ear

Zi-Yu He and Dong-Dong Ren

Abstract

There are increasing evidence of interactions between sex hormones and the structure and function of inner ear, especially in hearing impairment and balance disorders. In this chapter, we will discuss the mechanism of sex hormones on the inner ear, describe both clinical and basic research that has led us to our current understanding, and conclude with future perspectives on avenues of investigation that may lead to innovative treatments on the hearing loss, tinnitus, and dizziness resulted from the changes in estrogen and progesterone levels. The presence of estrogen receptors α and β has earlier been shown in the inner ear of mice. Expression of estrogen receptors (ER) correlates with the protection of auditory function. Estrogen may have certain protective effects on the hearing. Evidence for the treatment of sex hormone-induced symptoms is principally restricted to case reports and retrospective studies. Recognition and understanding of sex hormone-related inner ear problems will allow otologists to notice and manage these patients. Also, basic studies on the mechanism of how sex hormones act on inner ear provide the way to further prevent and treat on hearing impairment and balance disorders. High-quality evidence for their management is limited, with further research required.

Keywords: sex hormones, inner ear, hearing, balancing functions, mechanism, treatment methods

1. Introduction

Hearing loss, vertigo, dizziness, and tinnitus are the common symptoms in otology clinics. The cochlea and vestibule in the inner ear are filled with endolymph and perilymph, and the homeostasis of the water and blood circulation in the inner ear is essential for maintaining its hearing and equilibrium functions [1]. There are more evidence of interactions between sex hormones and the function of the inner ear, especially in the mechanism of hearing impairment and balance disorders in old women and pregnant women. Is the female sex steroid estrogen the key to preserved hearing in the aging human? Is the hearing loss more profound in elderly males than females? Is the hearing loss easier spontaneously recovered in pregnant women? All these questions remain unanswered. In this chapter, we will discuss the mechanism of sex hormones on the inner ear, describe both clinical and basic research that has led us to our current understanding, and conclude with future perspectives on avenues of investigation that will contribute to stratification strategies on the hearing loss, tinnitus, autophony, and dizziness resulted from the changes in sex hormone levels.

2. How the different sex hormones may influence the inner ear

The sex hormones, including estrogen, progesterone, and androgen, are known to be implicated in normal auditory function in different proportions [2]. It is the balance of all three hormones in the body that promotes human health and vitality, including inner ear functions. Estrogen is usually thought of a "female" hormone; it may act as an auditory protectant; it is made in the ovaries, adrenal glands, and fat cells; and its levels are higher in those of reproductive age, which is helpful to prevent bone loss and works toward maintaining good cholesterol levels. Estrogens are known to facilitate the loss of intravascular fluid into the extravascular space, producing edema; however, blood vessel permeability, blood circulation, or inflammation has been reported to be related to the inner ear diseases. Progesterone is the sex steroid frequently mentioned for sexual health. In women, it is produced in the ovaries and through ovulation, which performs different benefits in balancing the unwanted effects of estrogen, helping the body use fat for energy, maintaining healthy weight, promoting restful sleep, and protecting against breast and uterine cancer; however, it may have a negative effect on hearing [3]. Androgen is a "male" hormone, the primary and most well-known androgen is testosterone, produced in the testicles and to a lesser degree in the adrenal glands, which helps build muscle tome, increases energy, contributes to a healthy libido, and aids in sperm production [4]. Healthy levels are also important in women; testosterone is produced in the female ovaries and a small amount is made in the adrenal glands, which helps to increase libido, promote musculoskeletal tone and strength, and raise energy levels. When testosterone is too high, however, it can lead to acne, unwanted hair on the face and body, polycystic ovaries with resulting interference of ovulation, and aggression among other concerns. Getting all three sex hormones balanced can be helpful for both men and women, and the results often offer clues on how to prevent unwanted inner ear symptoms in the future.

2.1. Estrogen

Estrogens influence physiological functions of many organs and systems in both female and male, including the skeletal, cardiovascular, and nervous systems, as well as the male urogenital tracts, mammary glands, and female reproductive organs. Estrogen could lead to neural excitation and thus facilitate auditory transmission, but the possible increase in neurosteroids in the brainstem may counteract this effect. Estrogen may act as an auditory protectant, which influences the inner ear at different levels, at the cochlea, vestibular organs, and more proximal levels.

Estrogens are mediated through estrogen receptors (ERs). There are at least three and possibly four distinct estrogen receptors. The most common estrogen receptors are ERα, which is encoded by a gene on chromosome 6, and ERβ, encoded by a gene on chromosome 14. Other ERs include G protein-coupled receptor (GFER, GPR30, and a putative receptor (ER-X), which has been studied mostly in brain [5]. Estrogen receptors α and β containing cells were also found in the inner ear, with a specific distribution pattern, both in auditory pathways and in the water/ion regulating areas. The presence of ERs in the inner ear cell nuclei implies that estrogen may have an influence on the inner ear and auditory functions. Estrogen receptors have been found in the inner ear of rats and mice in different cell types, including inner and outer hair cells, stria vascularis, spiral ligament, Reissner's membrane, and spiral ganglion cells especially type I cells [5]. Moreover, estrogen receptors in the auditory epithelium of vertebrates also occur in fishes [6], cichlid [7], songbird [5], and rodents [8], which suggest a widespread occurrence of steroid-dependent auditory plasticity among the vertebrates.

But in adult human inner ear, ERα-containing cells were only found in the spiral ganglion, and ERβ-containing cells in the stria vascularis selectively, which are important for hearing transmission and inner ear homeostasis [8]. It has been shown that there is less expression of ERα in strial marginal cells, outer hair cells, and type II ganglion cells [9]. ERα and ERβ are regulated depending on the stage of maturation, development, and pregnancy, suggesting that estrogen may have an effect on the cochlea during different life time. ERs were not found in the cochlea of the growing fetus, which implied that estrogen does not have an influence on the cochlea during the period of gestation [10]. Estrogen receptor mRNA is expressed in supporting cells with similar functions within the saccular epithelium of midshipman fish [6].

The expression of ERα was found in forebrain nuclei, including anterior parvocellular (PPa) and anterior tuberal (AT), which are sites of the integration between auditory and vocal motor system [11], and anterior tuberal is densely innervated by the neuropeptides, arginine vasotocin and isotocin, which modulate vocal motor patterning in midshipman [12–14]. Also, in some gene knockout studies, estradiol plays an important role in the regulation of both vasopressin and oxytocin, especially by ERα in limbic regions [15, 16] and by ERβ in hypothalamic areas [17].

The expression of ERs in known target organs is influenced by the amount of estrogen in the serum. Lots of studies have shown a gender difference in hearing function. And some of them suggested that part of this variation was because of the difference in estrogen levels between the two genders. As for the expression pattern of ERs, there is no gender- or age-related difference to be found. However, the fluorescence intensity of ERα was stronger in female mice than in young male ones. To compare with, ERβ showed no significant difference. Also, the expression of ERs decreased with age. In the old mice, the fluorescence intensities of ERs were significantly decreased in both male and female [9].

Many clinical and basic studies have proved that estradiol plays an important role in auditory physiology, neuronal plasticity, and the metabolic levels of neurotransmitters [18, 19]. ERα might change cochlea and vestibular sensory transduction, and ERβ may have a neuroprotective effect in the inner ear [9]. ERβ protects the auditory system from acoustic trauma in young male and female mice. ERβ in accordance with brain-derived neurotrophic factor (BDNF) promotes neuronal plasticity and protection against trauma in the auditory system [20]. But experimental estrogen-induced hyperprolactinemia leads to hearing loss in the guinea pig. It suggests that otic capsule and hair cell pathology related with estrogen-induced prolonged hyperprolactinemia and conditions such as pregnancy may lead to similar auditory pathology [21]. 17β-estradiol leads to adjustments in the molecular biology of the cochlea and the inferior colliculus of mouse accompanied with behavioral alternations [22]. Estrogen-related receptor gama (ESSR) plays a role in maintenance of hearing in both humans and mice [23].

2.2. Progesterone

Progesterone is secreted principally by the granulosa lutein cells of the corpus luteum, which are formed from granulosa cells after the luteinizing hormone surge. Progesterone is the main hormone of pregnancy, and in pregnancy, after week 8, the placenta replaces the corpus luteum as the main source of progesterone. Several steroids have similar properties and are together classified as the "progestogens." These include 17α-hydroxyprogesterone and pregnenolone as well as progesterone itself.

The two main progesterone receptors are progesterone receptor-A and progesterone receptor-B. And, there are two isoforms of the progesterone receptor encoded by the same gene, but with different start sites for transcription, hence the increased size of progesterone receptor-B compared with progesterone receptor-A. Expression of the progesterone receptor is regulated by estrogens, while progesterone receptors have an important effect, mediated by progesterone receptor-A, in inhibiting the proliferative actions of estrogen. For this reason, progesterone is nearly always given in addition to estrogen therapy, for example, in the oral contraceptive pill and in hormone replacement therapy. The presence of progesterone as a component in hormone replacement therapy leads to poorer hearing in aged women, affecting both the peripheral and central auditory system, and it interferes with the perception of speech in background noise [21].

Nevertheless, there is no direct nuclear effect of progesterone in the inner ear. There is no nuclear progesterone receptor being found in human or rat stria vascularis, organ of Corti or spiral ganglion with immunohistochemistry, or polymerase chain reaction (PCR). But, progesterone receptor-B is being found with Western blot in the cochlea. It probably indicates the staining in the cochlea bone. In this case, the effect of progesterone on hearing is probably not relevant to the action in the inner ear [25].

Progesterone receptors are important for integration of external signals and internal physiological cues in the brain to output an appropriate behavior. In a study using the frog, *Physalaemus pustulosus*, as a model system, progesterone receptor immunoreactivity was found in key brain regions known to modulate the processing of auditory clues [26].

2.3. Androgen

Androgens, which are produced by Leydig cells, like all steroid hormones, are made from cholesterol. A range of androgens is made in the body and, although most of these come from the testes, some are made in the adrenal cortex. The most potent and important of these androgens is testosterone, and by far the highest production of testosterone is in the testes. Testosterone has two main actions: the initiation of spermatogenesis and the development and maintenance of secondary sexual characteristics. In order to achieve the second group of actions, testosterone must be converted to 5α-dihydrotestosterone (DHT). This conversion happens outside the testes, in peripheral tissues. Furthermore, both testosterone and DHT act on the same receptor, the androgen receptor (AR).

In contrast to these well-known effects of estradiol on hearing function, relatively little is known about how androgens might influence hearing or whether androgen receptors (AR) are also expressed in the inner ear of vertebrates. The lack of regenerative ability of adult mammalian cochlea and the irreversible degeneration of cochlear sensory hair cells leads to permanent hearing loss. Whether the androgen receptors (ARs) establish in the inner ear, there are many studies on it, in a transcriptomic analysis of the developing and adult mouse cochlear sensory epithelia, the adult cochlear sensory epithelium overexpressed 2542 transcripts including new transcripts, such as AR, which previously were not reported to be expressed in the adult cochlea [27].

In all major vertebrate animals, androgen receptors have been identified in neural circuits that shape vocalization. Many of those nuclei mentioned above are part of the known vocal and auditory circuit in midshipman. The distribution of androgen receptor mRNA supports that androgens modulate behaviorally defined vocal, auditory, and neuroendocrine circuits in teleost fish and vertebrates in general [28].

Additionally, testosterone in serum increased neural thresholds in females in a frequency-specific way [29]. And hyperandrogenism may be responsible for the elevation of hearing threshold, particularly in the high frequency, in patients with polycystic ovary syndrome [30–32]. On the contrary, hyperandrogenism did not seem to affect otoacoustic emission levels or the medial olivocochlear reflex response in adult female subjects [33].

In audiology, the usage of biomedical interventions and biotherapeutic methods could play an important role in modulating or preventing some kinds of hearing loss. Planar cell polarity is of high importance as it regulates cochlea extension and coordinates orientation of sensory hair cells in the inner ear. If we could use the effect of sex hormone in the inner ear, the establishment of ectopic hair cell-like cell polarity could be built. Testosterone is related to the neuroprotection and regeneration in central nervous system. We could promote an increase in hair cell-like cell polarity in the LER through proliferation and transdifferentiation by using testosterone-3-(O-carboxymethyl) oxime bovine serum albumin and Math1 treatment [34]. In the treatment of immune-mediated sensorineural hearing loss, it was confirmed that testosterone has the preventive and therapeutic effects induced by sensitization using bovine inner ear antigens [35].

3. Physiological variation in sex hormones and effect on inner ear

The levels of sex hormones vary in response to endogenous and exogenous stimuli and many vary in a cyclic fashion. The endocrine changes related to reproductive function (ovarian cycle, pregnancy, and menopause) could in turn affect auditory and balance function. Additionally, there are multiple interactions between the sex hormones involved in these physiological changes and this enhances the possible multidirectional effects on the inner ear.

3.1. Ovarian cycle

In the ovarian cycle, the levels of estrogen and progesterone in the body have a dynamic regulation. Both clinical and basic studies have proved that the changes of auditory and balance system are attributed to estradiol and progesterone. In other words, the fluctuating hearing levels are evident in females during the ovarian cycle. Across the life span, both women and men undergo transitions in reproductive status related in part to changes in sex hormone levels. There is controversy over how hormonal conditions influence cerebral physiology related to evoked potentials and perceptual speech processing in women during ovarian cycle. Hearing thresholds change upon different sex hormone levels during the menstrual cycle [36]. And hearing conduction, measured by auditory brainstem response, is better in postovulatory phase compared with preovulatory phase of menstrual/ovarian cycle [37]. Also, brainstem auditory evoked potentials change in the mid follicular and the mid luteal phases of the ovarian cycle [38]. Moreover, ovarian cycle effects on postural stability but not optokinetic function, and this needs to be considered when conducting studies of postural stability in women [39]. Studies of dichotic listening in women of the reproductive age also show that there is variation in laterality as a function of menstrual cycle phase. The perceptual speech processing of women is highly plastic and operates at varying states of functional asymmetry across days of the menstrual cycle, which are consistent with other works showing menstrual cycle-related changes in lateralized neurocognitive systems in the language domain [40–42].

3.2. Menopause

More organs are found to be influenced by the positive effects of estrogen, and estrogen has been expected to be benefit on auditory system by many investigators. As for the postmenopausal women, many studies suggested that the hearing and balancing problem appeared might be related to their sex hormone levels. Hearing loss in older people usually affects the highest frequencies early on and gradually affects the lower frequencies. Progesterone may have negative effects on the hearing of pre- and postmenopausal women and aging mice. On the contract, estrogen was found in some situation to have a positive influence [25]. The auditory brainstem response thresholds of postmenopausal female are higher than younger men or women [43, 44]. And the lower level of circulating serum estradiol possibly impedes hearing sensitivity in postmenopausal women, which has no relationship with bone mineral densities [45].

Intrinsic estrogen at physiological levels might slow down hearing loss in aging women [46]. At the same time, estrogen therapy may slow down the hearing loss in aging postmenopausal women [47]. Tibolone, a synthetic steroid drug with estrogenic, progestogenic, and weak androgenic actions, is often used in the hormone replacement therapy for menopausal or premenopausal women. And tibolone had no negative effect on hearing function and might decelerate hearing loss in aging postmenopausal women, intrinsic estrogen at physiological levels might slow down hearing loss in aging women [46]. After treatment of healthy menopausal women with tibolone for 6 months, the improvement was more prominent on the right side in audiometry results at low frequency. It may be explained by differences in distribution of ER in the ear. ERs might be more dense in the right ear, so give better response to estrogen therapy [47]. Many studies have showed that estrogen affects hearing function, especially in the postmenopausal women; a recent study gets a result that there may be hearing lateralization in menopausal women, especially significant improvement on right ear can be explained by lower BMD on that side ear bones in turn better response to estrogen therapy due to this, which may be related to ER concentration and the more dense of type ERα and/or ERβ in the right ear [48].

According to the vestibular function, the level of estradiol and progesterone decreases obviously in postmenopausal women with benign paroxysmal positional vertigo, which can cause the inner ear microcirculation disorder, may be a risk factor of BPPV [49].

Although estrogen has been expected to be benefits on auditory system, both clinician and patients need to take into concern that estrogen may have some unwanted side effects, such as increased risk of uterine cancer. Because in the central nervous system, ERβ is highly expressed in neurons and glial cells. And there is little ERβ in the mature uterus, selective ERβ agonists, then they become available [50, 51].

3.3. Pregnancy

Hearing loss appeared in pregnancy is not a commonly reported problem. Some investigators have noticed reversible and physiological sensorineural hearing loss at low frequencies during the period of pregnancy [52, 53]. In some case reports, sudden onset of sensorineural hearing loss during pregnancy has been described [54], and one report concerning a patient who had the hearing loss with each serial pregnancy [55]. But a nationwide population-based study suggested that sudden sensorineural hearing loss (SSNHL) in pregnancy is rare. SSNHL is defined as sudden, idiopathic, usually unilateral deafness developed at most in 72 hours in previously healthy people [56]. It often happens in the third trimester. And SSNHL in pregnancy does not increase the risks of delivery or subsequent stroke [57]. As for the mechanism, there is a hypothesis implied that SSNHL is connected with the changes in cardiovascular system, hematological system, and/or some other systems because of pregnancy. These changes in pregnancy may evoke disorders of cochlea circulation or cochlea fluid homeostasis resulting in SSNHL [57]. Otosclerosis is one of the most common causes of acquired hearing loss and is widely supposed as being related with pregnancy. Another study revealed that resonance frequency of middle ear was found to be low during the third trimester of the pregnancy. And low resonance frequency informs that the acoustic immittance of the middle ear changes during pregnancy [58].

Tinnitus is another auditory symptom in pregnant patients, with proposed theories of pathogenesis, including hyperdynamic circulation, increase in perilymphatic fluid pressure, and hormonal changes. Clinically, it appears that the hearing loss and tinnitus related to pregnancy can spontaneously recover. As for treatment, it depends on the otorhinolaryngologic doctors to decide whether they should administer steroid drugs for acute hearing loss, as it may recover after the delivery [54].

Autophony is a classic complaint of patients suffering from a patulous Eustachian tube (PET). The typical patients with PET have lost a drastic amount of weight, resulting in shrinkage of the peritubal mucous membranes. One third of the patients with PET are either pregnant or taking an estrogen replacement therapy [59]. In order to resolve the symptoms postpartum, management should consist of informative reassurance alone [60].

There is an increase in incidence of Bell's palsy (BP) during pregnancy [61]. One of the reasons could be a brain stem synaptic impairment caused by estrogen, presumably because of ischemic changes [62]. And most of them seem to be concentrated in the third trimester. The most likely explanation about the concentration in the third trimester may be the altered susceptibility to herpes simplex viral reactivation during pregnancy. And the prognosis of pregnant patients may be poorer [63].

3.4. Gender differences in auditory function

Many authors have shown that a gender differences in auditory function and some of them implied that part of this variation was due to the difference in estrogen levels between females and males. There are well-known sex differences in the auditory brainstem response, with women having shorter latencies than men [64]. Hearing loss is more profound in elderly males than females. Many early studies on otoacoustic emissions revealed the existence of sex and ear differences in human beings. Some also revealed that the sex and ear differences in adults are evident in newborns as well. These differences are in the direction of human females having stronger and more numerous spontaneous otoacoustic emissions and stronger click-evoked otoacoustic emissions than do males; also, human right ears have stronger and more numerous spontaneous otoacoustic emissions and stronger click-evoked otoacoustic emissions than do left ears. There is a so-called prenatal-androgen-exposure explanation. Prenatal androgen exposure apparently can alter auditory evoked potentials. The sex difference in otoacoustic emissions in newborns may be that the prenatal androgen exposure in some way weakens the cochlea amplifiers and thereby weakens spontaneous otoacoustic emissions and click-evoked otoacoustic emissions (and perhaps distortion product otoacoustic emissions less markedly) [65].

Sex differences are limited to frequency ranges, which are related to the processing of natural vocalizations and depend on the type of stimulus. In a research using green tree frog, *Hyla cinera*, sex did not change audiogram best frequencies, although sex did make a difference in the sensitivities at those frequencies with males more sensitive in the lower frequency range [29]. The auditory system exhibits differences by sex and by sexual orientation, and the implication is that relevant auditory structures are altered during prenatal development, possibly by exposure to androgens [66].

Gender differences also occur in some pathological situations. In the presence of sex hormone receptors in human middle ear cholesteatoma, stronger expression of progesterone receptor was found in samples from male patients, while stronger expression of estrogen receptor was found in samples from female patients. It suggests that female sex hormones may stimulate proliferation of middle ear cholesteatoma keratinocytes [67]. Estrogen levels between females and males in different ages may influence the function of the auditory systems, and the details of the mechanism should be studied in the future.

4. Sex hormones and auditory and vestibular pathology

Considerable anecdotal evidence and limited information from previous studies suggest that auditory and vestibular functions may be influenced by sex hormones resulting in pathological conditions such as hearing disorders in Turner syndrome, Presbyacusis, Otosclerosis, and Menière's disease.

4.1. Hearing disorders in Turner syndrome

Hearing disorders are obvious in mice and women with Turner syndrome (total or partial loss of one X chromosome) [68]. Approximately one-half of women with TS have a 45,X karyotype, about 20% have 45,X/46,XX mosaicism, and the remainder have structural abnormalities of the X chromosome such as X fragments, isochromosomes, or rings. TS is characterized by bilateral streak gonads, short stature, primary amenorrhea, streak ovaries, and no estrogen production, which often develop an early presbyacusis.

The hearing loss features in patients with Turner Syndrome should be taken into consideration. The common clinical complaints are recurrent otitis media, dysfunction of the Eustachian tube, conductive hearing loss during infancy, and sensorineural hearing loss in the adolescence. The karyotype appears to be important in the hearing loss, with studies demonstrating an increased prevalence in patients with monosomy 45,X or isochromosome 46,i (Xq). It is necessary of morphologic studies of the cochlea to help out in clarifying the etiology of the sensorineural hearing loss [69]. And sensorineural hearing loss is the most common type of hearing loss. It is mostly characterized by a high-frequency loss and/or a mid-frequent dip. It is uncommon for conductive hearing loss in young women with Turner Syndrome. But in a TS cohort, 91% of patients suffered middle ear disease, but the incidence of SNHL was 9%. It is suggested that TS patients should be screened for onset and progression of hearing loss [70]. Consequently, there is a need for hearing rehabilitation in these patients. Questions about hearing must be asked by physicians when treating women with Turner Syndrome to identify those who need hearing rehabilitation, even if they have an audiogram with a normal pure tone average [71].

Both the karyotype and sensorineural dip in hearing could be used to predict the future course of hearing levels for TS patients. And estrogen may have an influence on hearing loss in TS patients [72].

Progressive hearing loss is relatively common in human without a clear molecular basis and medical therapies. A new gene, WBP2, was defined to be involved in the molecular pathway linking hearing impairment to hormonal signaling and provides new therapeutic targets. WBP2 is required for normal glutamatergic synapses in the cochlea and is crucial for hearing [73].WBP2 encodes the protein that acts as a transcriptional coactivator for ERα (ESR1) and progesterone receptor. The loss of Wbp2 expression leads to progressive high-frequency hearing loss in mouse, as well as in two deaf children, each carrying two different variants in the WBP2 gene [73].

4.2. Presbyacusis

Presbyacusis or age-related hearing loss is a complex degenerative disease that affects many people worldwide. Gender does play a role in age-related hearing loss. Longitudinal studies of aging have shown that hearing declines more rapidly in males than females. Elderly people with presbyacusis not only have a loss in sensitivity to sound but also have significant difficulties understanding speech in background noise at supra-threshold, conversational levels. Many researchers have identified sex-specific differences in presbyacusis in humans and animal models [74].

There is growing evidence that interactions between sex hormones and sensory systems are sometimes beneficial, but oftentimes detrimental, such as progesterone with negatively affect hearing in older women, whereas in some cases, estrogen may have positive effects [24]. Data from a large cohort of adults (48–92 years) in the Beaver Dam Epidemiology of Hearing Loss Study show significant age effects in word recognition scores in competing messages for both men and women, but performance is consistently poorer in men than in women at all age groups and hearing loss categories [75].

4.3. Otosclerosis

Otosclerosis is a major cause of acquired hearing loss in adult life affecting exclusively the human temporal bone, which is reported to worsen during periods of intense hormonal activity. Many researchers show a possible link between aggravation of otosclerosis and pregnancy is still debated. Thus, sex hormones were believed to be involved in the progression of the disease. Estrogen deficiency is considered to be a cause of osteoporosis in menopause women, and estrogen substitute therapy has shown beneficial effect in those cases [76].

Otosclerosis becomes manifest between the ages of 20–50 years and is usually bilateral. It affects twice as many females as males [77]. A retrospective study on a sample of 479 women with otosclerosis showed that the risk of subjective hearing deterioration with bilateral otosclerosis increased from 33% after one pregnancy to 63% after six pregnancies [78]. Several reports have suggested that oral contraceptives may increase the risk of hearing loss and in particular otosclerosis, although no clear conclusion has been drawn [79].

Estrogen has an inhibitory effect on bone resorption by directly inhibiting osteoclast activity as well as decreasing auto and paracrine production of cytokines such as interleukin (IL) 1 and IL-6 and tumor necrosis factor, TNF [80]. Researchers investigated the effect of 17β-estradiol on bone remodeling via diastrophic dysplasia sulfate transporter (DTDST) in otosclerosis and in a human osteoblast-like cell line, and they have demonstrated that the response to estrogens in terms of DTDST activity might be related to the expressed receptor type. It is possible that exacerbating effects of estrogens in patients with otosclerosis may be mediated by peculiar profiles of estrogen receptor in otosclerotic cells [81]. However, the regulatory mechanisms of Otosclerosis related to the estrogen receptor profile in the otosclerotic cells need to be further analyzed.

4.4. Menière's disease

Menière's disease is characterized by hearing loss, tinnitus, and vestibular dysfunction. It is thought that endolymph malabsorption is the underlying cause of the swelling of the endolymphatic spaces. Estrogens are known to facilitate the loss of intravascular fluid into the extravascular space, producing edema. Endogenous alterations in concentrations of estrogen and progesterone in the premenstrual syndrome or with the use of exogenous hormones such as oral contraceptives may trigger vertigo in patients with Menière's disease. Many reports show that women with Menière's disease were identified as having premenstrual phase of their monthly cycle or during pregnancy [82]. Genetic factors could contribute, at least partially to it. Many researchers have identified that in some women with Meniere's disease, attacks of vertigo, low frequency hearing loss, aural fullness and tinnitus are exacerbated in the premenstrual phase, when estrogen levels are low with edema in the endolymphatic spaces due to the loss of intravascular fluid into the extravascular space facilitated by estrogens [83–85]. One possible explanation may be estrogen-induced hyperprolactinemia, which was reported to provoke hearing loss and otic capsule dysmorphology in guinea pig [24].

Significant associations have been reported between Menière's disease and genetic polymorphisms. Polymorphisms associated with blood vessel permeability, blood circulation, or inflammation have been reported to be related to the inner ear pathology. AQP5 is known as an exocrine-type water channel with the roles in conveying a high degree of membrane water permeability [86]. Mice lacking AQP5 show lower frequency hearing impairment [87]. Some researchers demonstrated identified AQP5 as an ESα target gene in the mouse uterus using chromatin immunoprecipitation and DNA microarray analyses [88].

5. Summary

Sex hormone-related symptoms of auditory and vestibular systems are common in clinic. Here, we address by recognizing that interactions between sex hormones and sensory systems can be beneficial or detrimental to the peripheral and central auditory and vestibular systems. Knowing how sex steroids can alter hearing ability may give important clues as to how estrogen can preserve hearing in humans. The postmenopausal women have slightly better hearing if administered estrogen replacement therapy, physiological levels of estrogen would seem to have a possible protective effect on hearing function. The association described here shed light to the role of sex hormones and their receptors in the inner ear and behavior and underline the therapeutic potential of specific sex hormone agonists and antagonists.

Acknowledgements

This study was supported by grants from the National Natural Science Foundation of China (NSFC 81420108010, 81370022, 81570920, 81771077 and 81000413), Key Project of Chinese National Programs (2016YFC0905200, 2016YFC0905202), and Zhuo-Xue Plan of Fudan University.

Author details

Zi-Yu He and Dong-Dong Ren*

*Address all correspondence to: dongdongren@fudan.edu.cn

Department of Otology and Skull Base Surgery, Eye, Ear, Nose and Throat Hospital (EENT Hospital), Fudan University, Shanghai, China

References

[1] Nishio N, Teranishi M, Uchida Y, Sugiura S, Ando F, Shimokata H, Sone M, Otake H, Kato K, Yoshida T, Tagaya M, Hibi T, Nakashima T. Polymorphisms in genes encoding aquaporins 4 and 5 and estrogen receptor α in patients with Meniere's desease and sudden sensorineural hearing loss. Life Sciences. Mar 21, 2013;**92**(10):541-546

[2] Stein DG. Brain damage, sex hormones and recovery: A new role for progesterone and estrogen? Trends in Neurosciences. Jul 2001;**24**(7):386-391

[3] Caruso S, Maiolino L, Rugolo S, Intelisano G, Farina M, Cocuzza S, Serra A. Auditory brainstem response in premenopausal women taking oral contraceptives. Human Reproduction. 2003;**18**(1):85-89

[4] Pessina MA, Hoyt RF Jr, Goldstein I, Traish AM. Differential regulation of the expression of estrogen, progesterone, and androgen receptors bysex steroid hormones in the vagina: Immunohistochemical studies. The Journal of Sexual Medicine. Sep 2006;**3**(5):804-814

[5] Stenberg AE, Wang H, Sahlin L, Hultcrantz M. Mapping of estrogen receptors alpha and beta in the inner ear of mouse and rat. Hearing Research. Oct 1999;**136**(1–2):29-34

[6] Forlano PM, Deitcher DL, Bass AH. Distribution of estrogen receptor alpha mRNA in the brain and inner ear of a vocal fish with comparisons to sites of aromatase expression. The Journal of Comparative Neurology. Feb 28, 2005;**483**(1):91-113

[7] Maruska KP, Fernald RD. Steroid receptor expression in the fish inner ear varies sex, social status, and reproductive state. BMC Neuroscience. Apr 30, 2010;**11**:58

[8] Stenberg AE, Wang H, Fish J, Schrott-Fischer A, Sahlin L, Hultcrantz M. Estrogen receptors in the normal adult and developing human inner ear and in Turner's syndrome. Hearing Research. Jul 2001;**157**(1–2):87-92

[9] Motohashi R, Takumida M, Shimizu A, Konomi U, Fujita K, Hirakawa K, Suzuki M, Anniko M. Effects of age and sex on the expression of estrogen receptor alpha and beta in the mouse inner ear. Acta Oto-Laryngologica. Feb 2010;**130**(2):204-214

[10] Simonoska R, Stenberg A, Masironi B, Sahlin L, Hultcrantz M. Estrogen receptors in the inner ear during different stages of pregnancy and development in the rat. Acta Oto-Laryngologica. Nov 2009;**129**(11):1175-1181

[11] Goodson JL, Bass AH. Vocal-acoustic circuitry and descending vocal pathways in teleost fish: Convergence with terrestrial vertebrates reveals conserved traits. The Journal of Comparative Neurology. Jul 1, 2002;**448**(3):298-322

[12] Goodson JL, Bass AH. Forebrain peptides modulate sexually polymorphic vocal circuitry. Nature. Feb 17, 2000;**403**(6771):769-772

[13] Goodson JL, Bass AH. Vasotocin innervation and modulation of vocal-acoustic circuitry in the teleost Porichthys notatus. The Journal of Comparative Neurology. Jul 3, 2000;**422**(3):363-379

[14] Goodson JL, Evans AK, Bass AH. Putative isotocin distributions in sonic fish: Relation to vasotocin and vocal-acoustic circuitry.The Journal of Comparative Neurology. Jul 14, 2003;**462**(1):1-14

[15] Choleris E, Ogawa S, Kavaliers M, Gustafsson JA, Korach KS, Muglia LJ, Pfaff DW. Involvement of estrogen receptor alpha, beta and oxytocin in social discrimination: A detailed behavioral analysis with knockout female mice. Genes, Brain, and Behavior. Oct 2006;**5**(7):528-539

[16] Scordalakes EM, Rissman EF. Aggression and arginine vasopressin immunoreactivity regulation by androgen receptor and estrogen receptor alpha.Genes, Brain, and Behavior. Feb 2004;**3**(1):20-26

[17] Nomura M, McKenna E, Korach KS, Pfaff DW, Ogawa S. Estrogen receptor-beta regulates transcript levels for oxytocin and arginine vasopressin in the hypothalamic paraventricular nucleus of male mice. Brain Research. Molecular Brain Research. Dec 30, 2002;**109**(1–2):84-94

[18] Lee JH, Marcus DC. Estrogen acutely inhibits ion transport by isolated stria vascularis. Hearing Research. Aug 2001;**158**(1–2):123-130

[19] Caruso S, Cianci A, Grasso D, Agnello C, Galvani F, Maiolino L, et al. Auditory brainstem responses in postmenopausal women treated with hormone replacement therapy: A pilot study. Menopause. 2000;**7**:178-183

[20] Meltser I, Tahera Y, Simpson E, Hultcrantz M, Charitidi K, Gustafsson JA, Canlon B. Estrogen receptor β protects against acoustic trauma in mice animal study. Journal of Clinical Investigation. Apr 2008;**118**(4):1563-1570

[21] Horner KC, Cazals Y, Guieu R, Lenoir M, Sauze N.Experimental estrogen-induced hyperprolactinemia results in bone-related hearing loss in the guinea pig.American Journal of Physiology. Endocrinology and Metabolism. 2007 Nov;**293**(5):E1224-E1232 [Epub Aug 21, 2007]

[22] Charitidi K, Meltser I, Canlon B. Estradiol treatment and hormonal fluctuations during the estrous cycle modulate the expression of estrogen receptors in the auditory system and the prepulse inhibition of acoustic startleresponse. Endocrinology. Sep 2012;**153**(9): 4412-4421

[23] Nolan LS, Maier H, Hermans-Borgmeyer I, Girotto G, Ecob R, Pirastu N, Cadge BA, Hübner C, Gasparini P, Strachan DP, Davis A, Dawson SJ. Estrogen-related receptor gamma and hearing function: Evidence of a role in humans and mice. Neurobiology of Aging. Aug 2013;**34**(8):2077.e1-2077.e9

[24] Guimaraes P, Frisina ST, Mapes F, Tadros SF, Frisina DR, Frisina RD. Progestin negatively affects hearing in aged women.Proceedings of the National Academy of Sciences of the United States of America. Sep 19, 2006;**103**(38):14246-14249 [Epub Sep 7, 2006]

[25] Bonnard Å, Sahlin L, Hultcrantz M, Simonoska R. No direct nuclear effect of progesterone in the inner ear: Other possible pathways,Acta Oto-Laryngologica. Dec 2013;**133**(12): 1250-1257

[26] O'Connell LA, Ding JH, Ryan MJ, Hofmann HA. Neural distribution of the nuclear progesterone receptor in the túngara frog, Physalaemus Pustulosus. Journal of Chemical Neuroanatomy. 2011 Apr;**41**(3):137-147

[27] Smeti I, Assou S, Savary E, Masmoudi S, Zine A. Transcriptomic analysis of the developing and adult mouse cochlear sensory epithelia. PLoS One. 2012;**7**(8):e42987

[28] Forlano PM, Marchaterre M, Deitcher DL, Bass AH. Distribution of androgen receptor mRNA expression in vocal, auditory, and neuroendocrine circuits in a teleost fish. The Journal of Comparative Neurology. Feb 15, 2010;**518**(4):493-512

[29] Miranda JA, Wilczynski W. Sex differences and androgen influences on midbrain auditory thresholds in the green treefrog, Hyla Cinerea. Hearing Research. Jun 2009;**252**(1–2):79-88

[30] Oghan F, Coksuer H. Does hyperandrogenism have an affect on hearing loss in patients with polycystic ovary syndrome? Auris, Nasus, Larynx. Aug 2012;**39**(4):365-368

[31] Kucur C, Kucur SK, Gozukara I, Seven A, Yuksel KB, Keskin N, Oghan F. Extended high frequency audiometry in polycystic ovary syndrome. Scientific World Journal. Sep 30, 2013;**2013**:482689

[32] Turan M, Garca MF, Cankaya H. The relationship between hearing thresholds and hyperandrogenism in polycystic ovary syndrome. Medical Science Monitor 2016;**22**:4380-4385

[33] Eren E, Harman E, Arslanoğlu S, Önal K, Katlmiş H. Does hyperandrogenism affect the otoacoustic emissions and medial olivocochlear reflex in female adults? Otology & Neurotology. Jul 2013;**34**(5):784-789

[34] Yang XY, Jin K, Ma R, Yang JM, Luo WW, Han Z, Cong N, Ren DD, Chi FL. Role of the planar cell polarity pathway in regulating ectopic hair cell-like cells induced by Math1 and testosterone treatment. Brain Research. Jul 30, 2015;**1615**:22-30

[35] Yeo SW, Chang KH, Park SN, Suh BD.Effects of testosterone in the treatment of immune-mediated sensorineural hearing loss. European Archives of Oto-Rhino-Laryngology. Jul 2003;**260**(6):316-319 [Epub Jan 28, 2003]

[36] Haggard M, Gaston JB. Changes in auditory perception in the menstrual cycle. British Journal of Audiology. 1978;**12**:105-118

[37] Upadhayay N, Paudel BH, Singh PN, Bhattarai BK, Agrawal K. Pre- and postovulatory auditory brainstem response in normal women. Indian Journal of Otolaryngology and Head & Neck Surgery. Jan 2014;**66**(Suppl 1):133-137

[38] Mann N, Sidhu RS, Babbar R. Brainstemauditory evoked responses in different responses indifferent phases of menstrual cycle. Journal of Clinical and Diagnostic Research. Dec 2012;**6**(10):1640-1643

[39] Darlington CL, Ross A, King J, Smith PF. Menstrual cycle effects on postural stability but not optokinetic function. Neuroscience Letters. Jul 20, 2001;**307**(3):147-150

[40] Cowell PE, Ledger WL, Wadnerkar MB, Skilling FM, Whiteside SP. Hormones and dichotic listening: Evidence from the study of menstrual cycle effects. Brain and Cognition. Jul 2011;**76**(2):256-262

[41] Fernandez G, Weis S, Stoffel-Wagner B, Tendolkar I, Reuber M, Beyenburg S, et al. Menstrual cycle-dependent neural plasticity in the adult human brain is hormone, task, and region specific. Journal of Neuroscience. 2003;**23**(9):3790-3795

[42] Konrad C, Engelien A, Schoning S, Zwitserlood P, Jansen A, Pletziger E, et al. The functional anatomy of semantic retrieval is influenced by gender, menstrual cycle, and sex hormones. Journal of Neural Transmission. 2008;**115**(9):1327-1337

[43] Jerger J, Johnson K. Interactions of age, gender, and sensorineural hearing loss on ABR latency. Ear and Hearing. 1988;**9**:168-176

[44] Wharton JA, Church GT. Influence of menopause on the auditory brainstem response. Audiology. 1990;**29**:196-201

[45] Kim SH, Kang BM, Chae HD, Kim CH. The association between serum estradiol level and hearing sensitivity in postmenopausal women. Obstetrics and Gynecology. May 2002;**99**(5 Pt 1):726-730

[46] Köşüş N, Köşüş A, Turhan NÖ, Kurtaran H. Hearing levels in menopausal women and the effect of tibolone on audiological functions. Journal of Obstetrics and Gynaecology. Apr 2012;**32**(3):294-297

[47] Kilicdag EB, Yavuz H, Bagis T, Tarim E, Erkan AN, Kazanci F. Effects of estrogen therapy on hearing in postmenopausal women. American Journal of Obstetrics and Gynecology. Jan 2004;**190**(1):77-82

[48] Köşüş N, Köşüş A, Turhan NÖ. Discrepancy in improvement of hearing loss between left and right ears after postmenopausal hormone therapy. Medical Hypotheses. Mar 2011; **76**(3):447-449

[49] Wang SF, Zhang L, Li GH, Zhang WW, Wang YP, Geng B. The change of female progesterone level and blood calcium concentration in perimenopausal women with benign paroxysmal positional vertigo. Zhonghua Er Bi Yan Hou Tou Jing Wai Ke Za Zhi. Apr 7, 2017;**52**(4):287-290

[50] Rudziński W, Krejza J. Effects of estrogens on the brain and implications for neuroprotection. Neurologia i Neurochirurgia Polska. Jan–Feb 2002;**36**(1):143-156

[51] Garcia-Segura LM, Azcoitia I, DonCarlos LL. Neuroprotection by estradiol. Progress in Neurobiology. 2001;**63**:29-60

[52] Karan S, Sujata S, Deepak C. Evaluation of audio-rhinological changes during pregnancy. Indian Journal of Otolaryngology and Head & Neck Surgery. 2011;**63**:74-78

[53] Sennaroglu G, Belgin E. Audiological findings in pregnancy. The Journal of Laryngology and Otology. 2011;**115**:617-621

[54] Kenny R, Patil N, Considine N. Sudden (reversible) sensorineural hearing loss in pregnancy. Irish Journal of Medical Science. 2011;**180**(1):79-84

[55] Pawlak-Osinska K, Burduk PK, Kopczynski A. Episodes of repeated sudden deafness following pregnancy. American Journal of Obstetrics and Gynecology. 2009;**200**(4):e7-e9

[56] Kanadys WM, Oleszczuk J. Sudden sensorineural hearing loss during pregnancy. Ginekologia Polska. 2005 Mar;**76**(3):225-227

[57] Hou ZQ, Wang QJ. A new disease: Pregnancy-induced sudden sensorineural hearing loss? Acta Oto-Laryngologica Jul 2011;**131**(7):779-786

[58] Dag EK, Erbek S. Decrease in middle ear resonance frequency during pregnancy. Audiology Research. Apr 20, 2016;**6**(1):147

[59] Reiss M, Reiss G. Patulous eustachian tube – Diagnosis and therapy. Wiener Medizinische Wochenschrift (1946). 2000;**150**(22):454-456

[60] Kumar R, Hayhurst KL, Robson AK. Ear, nose, and throat manifestations during pregnancy. Otolaryngology and Head and Neck Surgery. Aug 2011;**145**(2):188-198

[61] Holland NJ, Weiner GM. Recent developments in Bell's palsy. British Medical Journal. Sep 4, 2004;**329**(7465):553-557

[62] Ben David Y, Tal J, Podoshin L, Fradis M, Sharf M, Pratt H, Faraggi D. Brain stem auditory evoked potentials: Effects of ovarian steroids correlated with increased incidence of Bell's palsy in pregnancy. Otolaryngology and Head and Neck Surgery. Jul 1995;**113**(1):32-35

[63] Vrabec JT, Isaacson B, Van Hook JW. Bell's palsy and pregnancy. Otolaryngology and Head and Neck Surgery. Dec 2007;**137**(6):858-861

[64] Jerger J, Hall J. Effects of age and sex on auditory brainstem response. Archives of Otolaryngology. 1980;**106**:387-391

[65] McFadden D. Masculinization of the mammalian cochlea. Hearing Research. Jun 2009; **252**(1–2):37-48

[66] McFadden D. Sexual orientation and the auditory system. Frontiers in Neuroendocrinology. Apr 2011;**32**(2):201-213

[67] Raynov AM, Choung YH, Moon SK, Park K. Expression of female sex hormone receptors in human middle-ear cholesteatomas. The Journal of Laryngology and Otology. Dec 2005; **119**(12):941-945

[68] Hultcrantz M, Stenberg AE, Fransson A, Canlon B. Characterization of hearing in an X,0 'turner mouse'. Hearing Research. 2000;**143**:182-188

[69] Alves C, Oliveira CS. Hearing loss among patients with Turner's syndrome: Literature review. Brazilian Journal of Otorhinolaryngology. May–Jun 2014;**80**(3):257-263

[70] Parkin M, Walker P. Hearing loss in turner syndrome. International Journal of Pediatric Otorhinolaryngology. Feb 2009;**73**(2):243-247

[71] Bonnard Å, Hederstierna C, Bark R, Hultcrantz M. Audiometric features in young adults with turner syndrome. International Journal of Audiology. 2017 Sep;**56**(9):650-656

[72] Hultcrantz M. Ear and hearing problems in Turner's syndrome. Acta Oto-Laryngologica. Jan 2003;**123**(2):253-257

[73] Buniello A, Ingham NJ, Lewis MA, Huma AC, Martinez-Vega R, Varela-Nieto I, Vizcay-Barrena G, Fleck RA, Houston O, Bardhan T, Johnson SL, White JK, Yuan H, Marcotti W, Steel KP. Wbp2 is required for normal glutamatergic synapses in the cochlea and is crucial for hearing. EMBO Molecular Medicine. Mar 1, 2016;**8**(3):191-207

[74] Willott JF, Bross L. Effects of prolonged exposure to an augmented acoustic environment on the auditory system of middle-aged C57BL/6J mice: Cochlear and central histology and sex differences. The Journal of Comparative Neurology. 2004 May;**472**(3):358-370

[75] Wiley TL, Cruickshanks KJ, Nondahl DM, Tweed TS, Klein R, Klein BK. Aging and word recognition in competing message. Journal of the American Academy of Audiology. 1998; **9**:191-198

[76] Rudic M, Keogh I, Wagner R, Wilkinson E, Kiros N, Ferrary E, Sterkers O, Bozorg Grayeli A, Zarkovic K, Zarkovic N. The pathophysiology of otosclerosis: Review of current research. Hearing Research. 2015 Dec;**330**(Pt A):51-56

[77] Chole RA, McKenna M. Pathophysiology of otosclerosis. Otology & Neurotology. 2001; **22**:249-257

[78] Gristwood RE, Venables WN. Pregnancy and otosclerosis. Clinical Otolaryngology and Allied Sciences. 1983;**8**:205-210

[79] Vessey M, Painter R. Oral contraception and ear disease: Findings in a large cohort study. Contraception. 2001;**63**:61-63

[80] Pacifici R. Estrogen, cytokines, and pathogenesis of postmenopausal osteoporosis. Journal of Bone and Mineral Research. 1996;**11**:1043-1051

[81] Imauchi Y, Laine P, Sterkers O, Ferrary E, Grayeli AB. Effect of 17 betaestradiol ondiastrophic dysplasia sulfate transporter activity in otosclerotic bone cell cultures and SaOS-2 cells. Acta Oto-Laryngologica. 2004;**124**:890-895

[82] Black FO. Maternal susceptibility to nausea and vomiting of pregnancy: Is the vestibular system involved? American Journal of Obstetrics and Gynecology 2002;**186**(5 suppl): S204-S209

[83] Andrews JC, Ator GA, Honrubia V. The exacerbation of symptoms in Meniere's disease during the premenstrual period. Archives of Otolaryngology – Head and Neck Surgery. 1992;**118**:74-78

[84] Morse GG, House JW. Changes in Meniere's disease responses as a function of the menstrual cycle. Nursing Research. 2001;**50**:286-292

[85] Merchant SN, Adams JC, Nadol JB. Pathophysiology of Meniere's syndrome: Are symptoms caused by endolymphatic hydrops? Otology and Neurotology. 2005;**26**:74-81

[86] Kawedia JD, Nieman ML, Boivin GP, Melvin JE, Kikuchi K, Hand AR, Lorenz JN, Menon AG. Interaction between transcellular and paracellular water transport pathways through aquaporin 5 and the tight junction complex. Proceedings of the National Academy of Sciences of the United States of America. 2007;**104**:3621-3626

[87] Merves M, Krane CM, Dou H, Greinwald JH, Menon AG, Choo D. Expression of aquaporin 1 and 5 in the developing mouse inner ear and audiovestibular assessment of an Aqp5 null mutant. Journal of the Association for Research in Otolaryngology. 2003;**4**: 264-275

[88] Kobayashi M, Takahashi E, Miyagawa S, Watanabe H, Iguchi T. Chromatin immunoprecipitation-mediated target identification proved aquaporin 5 is regulated directly by estrogen in the uterus. Genes to Cells. Oct 2006;**11**(10):1133-1143

Permissions

All chapters in this book were first published in SHNPD, by InTech Open; hereby published with permission under the Creative Commons Attribution License or equivalent. Every chapter published in this book has been scrutinized by our experts. Their significance has been extensively debated. The topics covered herein carry significant findings which will fuel the growth of the discipline. They may even be implemented as practical applications or may be referred to as a beginning point for another development.

The contributors of this book come from diverse backgrounds, making this book a truly international effort. This book will bring forth new frontiers with its revolutionizing research information and detailed analysis of the nascent developments around the world.

We would like to thank all the contributing authors for lending their expertise to make the book truly unique. They have played a crucial role in the development of this book. Without their invaluable contributions this book wouldn't have been possible. They have made vital efforts to compile up to date information on the varied aspects of this subject to make this book a valuable addition to the collection of many professionals and students.

This book was conceptualized with the vision of imparting up-to-date information and advanced data in this field. To ensure the same, a matchless editorial board was set up. Every individual on the board went through rigorous rounds of assessment to prove their worth. After which they invested a large part of their time researching and compiling the most relevant data for our readers.

The editorial board has been involved in producing this book since its inception. They have spent rigorous hours researching and exploring the diverse topics which have resulted in the successful publishing of this book. They have passed on their knowledge of decades through this book. To expedite this challenging task, the publisher supported the team at every step. A small team of assistant editors was also appointed to further simplify the editing procedure and attain best results for the readers.

Apart from the editorial board, the designing team has also invested a significant amount of their time in understanding the subject and creating the most relevant covers. They scrutinized every image to scout for the most suitable representation of the subject and create an appropriate cover for the book.

The publishing team has been an ardent support to the editorial, designing and production team. Their endless efforts to recruit the best for this project, has resulted in the accomplishment of this book. They are a veteran in the field of academics and their pool of knowledge is as vast as their experience in printing. Their expertise and guidance has proved useful at every step. Their uncompromising quality standards have made this book an exceptional effort. Their encouragement from time to time has been an inspiration for everyone.

The publisher and the editorial board hope that this book will prove to be a valuable piece of knowledge for researchers, students, practitioners and scholars across the globe.

List of Contributors

Slavi Delchev
Department of Anatomy, Histology and Embryology, Faculty of Medicine, Medical University - Plovdiv, Plovdiv, Bulgaria

Katerina Georgieva
Department of Physiology, Faculty of Medicine, Medical University - Plovdiv, Plovdiv, Bulgaria

Katalin Prokai-Tatrai and Laszlo Prokai
Department of Pharmacology and Neuroscience, University of North Texas Health Science Center, Fort Worth, TX, USA

Tracey A. Quinn
The Ritchie Centre, Monash University, Melbourne, Australia

Stephen R. Robinson and David Walker
School of Health and Biomedical Sciences, RMIT University, Melbourne, Australia

Claire V. Flaherty and Arghavan S. Zangeneh
Department of Neurology, Penn State Hershey Medical Center, Hershey, PA, USA

Marissa A. Harrison
Department of Psychology, Penn State Middletown, Harrisburg, PA, USA

Sanjana Marikunte
Department of Biochemistry and Molecular Biology, Penn State University, PA, USA

Manuela Cristina Russu
"Dr. I. Cantacuzino" Clinic of Obstetrics and Gynecology, "Carol Davila" University of Medicine and Pharmacy, Bucharest, Romania

Alexandra Cristina Antonescu
Intromed Laboratories, Bucharest, Romania

Wafik Said Bahnasy, Yasser A. El-Heneedy and Ehab A. El-Seidy
Department of Neurology, Faculty of Medicine, Tanta University, Tanta, Egypt

Jonathan Martínez Pinto and Ramón Sotomayor-Zárate
Laboratory of Neurochemistry and Neuropharmacology, Center of Neurobiology and Brain plasticity, Institute of Physiology, Faculty of Sciences, Universidad de Valparaíso, Valparaíso, Chile

Rodrigo L. Castillo
Program of Pathophysiology, Institute of Biomedical Sciences, Faculty of Medicine, Universidad de Chile, Santiago, Chile

Tomoya Kataoka
Department of Clinical Pharmaceutics, Graduate School of Medical Sciences, Nagoya City University, Japan

Kazunori Kimura
Department of Clinical Pharmaceutics, Graduate School of Medical Sciences, Nagoya City University, Japan
Department of Hospital Pharmacy, Graduate School of Pharmaceutical Sciences, Nagoya City University, Japan

Manuela Cristina Russu
"Dr. I. Cantacuzino" Clinic of Obstetrics and Gynecology, "Carol Davila" University of Medicine and Pharmacy, Bucharest, Romania

Alexandra Cristina Antonescu
Intromed Laboratories, Bucharest, Romania

Mushap Kuru and Hasan Oral
Department of Obstetrics and Gynecology, Faculty of Veterinary Medicine, Kafkas University, Kars, Turkey

Abdulsamed Kükürt and Metin Öğün
Department of Biochemistry, Faculty of Veterinary Medicine, Kafkas University, Kars, Turkey

Zi-Yu He and Dong-Dong Ren
Department of Otology and Skull Base Surgery, Eye, Ear, Nose and Throat Hospital (EENT Hospital), Fudan University, Shanghai, China

Index

CPSIA information can be obtained
at www.ICGtesting.com
Printed in the USA
LVHW062010100122
708212LV00002B/146

9 781639 873838